Contemporary Pediatric and Adolescent Sports Medicine

Series Editor
Lyle J. Micheli, Boston Children's Hospital
Division of Sports Medicine, BOSTON, MA, USA

This is an appropriate time for a book series focusing on pediatric and adolescent sports medicine. Estimates are that 25 million children regularly engage in organized sports in the United States alone, and due to the increasing intensity of children's and youth sports, there has been a regrettable increase in the incidence of acute sports injuries. Such injuries in young athletes are among the most common reasons medical care is sought. Growing numbers of young athletes with acute injuries are presenting to sports doctors, emergency room physicians, general orthopedists, pediatricians, primary care physicians, athletic trainers, coaches, and parents. High-intensity organized sports and their rigorous training regimens have also precipitated the emergence of a whole type of injury category previously unseen in the growing child: overuse. And yet, despite the explosion in the number of sports-injured young athletes, there is a widespread misunderstanding on how to manage their injuries. This series will fulfill the demand for this knowledge. The titles in the series will encompass four areas: anatomical, sub-specialty, sports-specific, and special populations. The titles in this series will further our knowledge of the management of injuries to the pediatric and adolescent athletes so that we might all better serve our young athletic patients. In particular, we hope that wherever possible we can either prevent injuries or at the very least return these children as quickly and as safely to the athletic fray so that they might better enjoy the thrill and satisfaction of sports participation and grow up to be physically active adults.

Melissa A. Christino • Emily I. Pluhar
Lyle J. Micheli

Editors

Psychological Considerations in the Young Athlete

A Multidisciplinary Approach

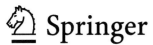 Springer

Editors
Melissa A. Christino
Division of Sports Medicine
Boston Children's Hospital
Boston, MA, USA

Emily I. Pluhar
Division of Sports Medicine and Division of
Adolescent/Young Adult Medicine
Boston Children's Hospital
Boston, MA, USA

Lyle J. Micheli
Division of Sports Medicine
Boston Children's Hospital
Boston, MA, USA

ISSN 2198-266X ISSN 2198-2678 (electronic)
Contemporary Pediatric and Adolescent Sports Medicine
ISBN 978-3-031-25125-2 ISBN 978-3-031-25126-9 (eBook)
https://doi.org/10.1007/978-3-031-25126-9

This Springer imprint is published by the registered company Springer Nature Switzerland AG
The registered company address is: Gewerbestrasse 11, 6330 Cham, Switzerland

For all the young athletes—past, present, and future ...

Preface

Sport participation during the youth and adolescent years provides tremendous opportunities for young people that can positively contribute to their social, emotional, and physical development. Many valuable life lessons, such as teamwork and work ethic, are learned through sports involvement, and many credit their successes in life to a connection with sport. However, despite the myriad of benefits sport participation can offer, there are also many pressures and stressors associated with sport activity in young athletes, and special attention should be paid to psychological considerations in the young athlete.

The world of youth sports continues to grow, with more opportunities for kids to participate in sports, and the ability to specialize in sports or participate in elite teams at younger ages. Sports are supposed to be fun, but for some, the pressure to succeed, get a scholarship, or go to the Olympics can be stifling and lead to burnout. Young athletes can suffer from anxiety, depression, and disordered eating, among other mental health diagnoses, and these conditions can impede sports performance. Injury can also be devastating to youth athletes, who may be abruptly taken out of sport for prolonged periods of time. This can affect one's sense of identity, have significant psychological ramifications, and healthcare providers should be familiar with these issues for the optimal care of young athletes.

The purpose of this text is to provide a broad and multidisciplinary review of psychological aspects of sport participation that are important to consider in young athletes. We will discuss the many psychosocial benefits of sports, describe common mental health and body image issues pediatric athletes may suffer from, explain the psychological effects of injury and surgery on young athletes and the importance of mind-body connection, and we will advocate for safe sport participation and a multidisciplinary approach to the care of young athletes. With the goal of preserving the benefits and fun of sport for young people, the healthcare team, parents, and coaches should strive to provide a nurturing environment that allows athletes achieve their goals, while also supporting their physical and emotional health and overall well-being.

This unique monograph combines the most up-to-date research, as well as perspectives from national experts in the field. To our knowledge, this is the first text to discuss the psychological implications of sport participation in young athletes—a critical topic in today's sport landscape that is often underappreciated and understudied. We hope this collection of chapters provides a valuable resource for our readers, but also stimulates more discussion and research on this very important topic.

Boston, MA, USA   Melissa A. Christino
Boston, MA, USA   Emily I. Pluhar
Boston, MA, USA   Lyle J. Micheli

Contents

Contributors

Kathryn E. Ackerman, MD, MPH Boston Children's Hospital, Boston, MA, USA

Jesse Allen-Dicker, PhD Department of Psychiatry, Lenox Hill Hospital/Northwell Health, New York, NY, USA

Caroline Ames, BA New York, NY, USA

Samantha P. Bento, PhD Department of Psychosocial Oncology & Palliative Care, Dana-Farber Cancer Institute, Boston, MA, USA

Cancer and Blood Disorders Center, Boston Children's Hospital, Boston, MA, USA

Harvard Medical School, Boston, MA, USA

Monique S. Burton, MD Department of Pediatrics, Seattle Children's Hospital, University of Washington, Seattle, WA, USA

Department of Orthopedics and Sports Medicine, Seattle Children's Hospital, University of Washington, Seattle, WA, USA

Melissa A. Christino, MD Division of Sports Medicine, Department of Orthopedic Surgery, Boston Children's Hospital, Boston, MA, USA

Michelle Codner, PsyD Boston Children's Hospital, Boston, MA, USA

Mary M. Daley, MD Division of Sports Medicine, Department of Orthopaedic Surgery, Children's Hospital of Philadelphia, Philadelphia, PA, USA

Pediatrics, Perelman School of Medicine, University of Pennsylvania, Philadelphia, PA, USA

Pierre A. d'Hemecourt, MD, FACSM Division of Sports Medicine, Department of Orthopaedics, Boston Children's Hospital, Boston, MA, USA

The Micheli Center for Sports Injury Prevention, Waltham, MA, USA

Harvard Medical School, Boston, MA, USA

Erika D. Van Dyke, PhD, CMPC Department of Psychology, Springfield College, Springfield, MA, USA

Bianca R. Edison, MD, MS Orthopaedics, Children's Hospital Los Angeles, University Southern California, Los Angeles, CA, USA

Nicole Farnsworth, MS, RD, CSSD, LDN Boston Children's Hospital, Boston, MA, USA

Kelsey L. Griffith, MS Division of Sports Medicine, Boston Children's Hospital, Boston, MA, USA

Shelby Harris, PsyD Department of Neurology, Albert Einstein College of Medicine, Bronx, NY, USA

Department of Psychiatry, Albert Einstein College of Medicine, Bronx, NY, USA

Peter Kadushin, PhD, CMPC Fifth Third Arena, Chicago, IL, USA

Julie McCleery, PhD Research-Practice Partnerships, Center for Leadership in Athletics, University of Washington, Seattle, WA, USA

Kimberly H. McManama O'Brien, PhD Division of Sports Medicine, Department of Orthopedic Surgery, Boston Children's Hospital, Harvard Medical School, Boston, MA, USA

Department of Psychiatry, Boston Children's Hospital, Harvard Medical School, Boston, MA, USA

William P. Meehan III, MD Division of Sports Medicine, Department of Orthopedic Surgery, The Micheli Center for Sports Injury Prevention, Boston Children's Hospital, Boston, MA, USA

Pediatrics and Orthopedics, Harvard Medical School, Boston, MA, USA

Matthew D. Milewski, MD Division of Sports Medicine, Department of Orthopedic Surgery, Boston Children's Hospital, Boston, MA, USA

Michael B. Millis, MD Orthopaedic Surgery, Harvard Medical School, Boston, MA, USA

Child and Adult Hip Program, Boston Children's Hospital, Boston, MA, USA

Aneesh G. Patankar, BS Rutgers Robert Wood Johnson Medical School, New Brunswick, NJ, USA

Emily I. Pluhar, PhD Boston Children's Hospital, Boston, MA, USA

Claudia L. Reardon, MD Department of Psychiatry, University Health Services, University of Wisconsin, Madison, WI, USA

Psychiatry, University of Wisconsin School of Medicine and Public Health, Madison, WI, USA

Laura Reece, MS, RD, CSSD, LDN Boston Children's Hospital, Boston, MA, USA

Katherine Rizzone, MD, MPH Orthopaedics and Pediatrics, University of Rochester Medical Center, Rochester, NY, USA

Miriam Rowan, PsyD Division of Sports Medicine, Department of Orthopedic Surgery, Boston Children's Hospital, Harvard Medical School, Boston, MA, USA

Department of Psychiatry, Boston Children's Hospital, Harvard Medical School, Boston, MA, USA

Samantha R. Sarafin Division of Sports Medicine, Department of Orthopedic Surgery, Boston Children's Hospital, Boston, MA, USA

Jamie Shoop, PhD Minds Matter Concussion Program, Department of Child and Adolescent Psychiatry and Behavioral Sciences, Children's Hospital of Philadelphia, Philadelphia, PA, USA

Christine B. Sieberg, PhD Biobehavioral Pain Innovations Lab, Department of Psychiatry & Behavioral Sciences, Boston Children's Hospital, Boston, MA, USA

Pain & Affective Neuroscience Center, Department of Anesthesiology, Critical Care, & Pain Medicine, Boston Children's Hospital, Boston, MA, USA

Department of Psychiatry, Harvard Medical School, Boston, MA, USA

Andrea Stracciolini, MD, FAAP, FACSM Division of Sports Medicine, Department of Orthopaedics, Boston Children's Hospital, Boston, MA, USA

The Micheli Center for Sports Injury Prevention, Waltham, MA, USA

Harvard Medical School, Boston, MA, USA

Kristin E. Whitney, MD, MA Division of Sports Medicine, Department of Orthopedic Surgery, Boston Children's Hospital, Boston, MA, USA

The Micheli Center for Sports Injury Prevention, Waltham, MA, USA

Harvard Medical School, Boston, MA, USA

Kyra Willoughby Harvard University, Cambridge, MA, USA

Chelsea Butters Wooding, PhD, CMPC Department of Exercise Science, North Park University, Chicago, IL, USA

Chapter 1
Benefits of Sport and Athletic Identity

Bianca R. Edison and Katherine Rizzone

Key Points
- Physical activity and sports participation can benefit individuals and groups under the model of positive human capital attainment, to include physical, emotional, intellectual, financial, social, and individual.
- Specific athlete populations and communities benefit from sport in nuanced ways, and more research is needed to better elucidate these differences.
- Levels of athletic identity have been shown to have both positive and negative effects on athletes' relationship to their sport, physical activity, and mood.
- There is a paucity of research investigating the connection between athlete identity and youth sports; furthermore, athletic identity cannot be studied or exist in isolation from other realms of identity which include age, gender, race, ethnicity, and disability.

Benefits of Sports Participation

Physical activity, a series of different exercises that involve varying parts and muscles of the body, has existed since the beginning of humanity. Organized sports, more structured physical activities that involve teaching a skill with the goal of a

B. R. Edison (✉)
Children's Orthopaedic Center, Children's Hospital Los Angeles, University Southern California, Los Angeles, CA, USA
e-mail: bedison@chla.usc.edu

K. Rizzone
University of Rochester Medical Center, Rochester, NY, USA
e-mail: Katherine_Rizzone@URMC.Rochester.edu

ACTIVE KIDS DO BETTER IN LIFE
WHAT THE RESEARCH SHOWS ON THE COMPOUNDING BENEFITS

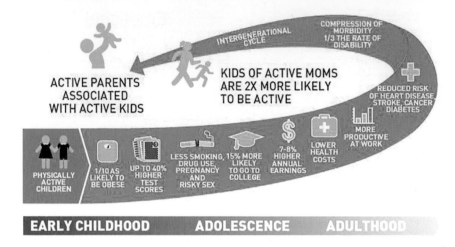

Fig. 1.1 Active kids do better

competition or stated achievement, has also been around for millennia; neolithic rock art from around 10,000 BCE in Egypt showed evidence of swimming and archery [1, 2]. Growing evidence documents that physical movement and sports participation provide physical, mental, social, emotional, cognitive, and academic benefits (Fig. 1.1). Communities that promote policies and develop proper infrastructure to encourage and support participation in sport and recreational activity tend to thrive more [3]. Being physically active is one of the most important actions that people of all ages can take to improve their health [4]. Noncommunicable chronic diseases (NCDs) remain the leading cause of death for individuals worldwide [5], accounting for over 58.8 million deaths worldwide with physical inactivity falling into the top five risk factors for this outcome [6, 7].

Six Realms of Positive Human Capital Attainment

The word, *capital*, can be defined as a supply of useful assets or advantages for a person or society [8]. *Positive capital attainment* describes areas of social organization and networks to bond and bridge individuals with those assets [9]. The report, "Designed to Move," organized by the American College of Sports Medicine, described and organized physical activity and sports participation into six realms of positive capital attainment, into which the benefits of sports participation can be categorized (Fig. 1.2) [10]. These realms include physical, emotional, intellectual,

Human Capital Attainment

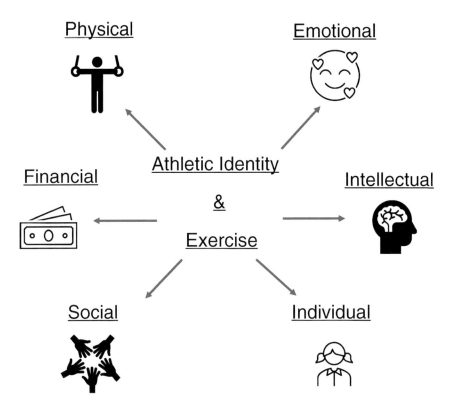

Athletic identity and exercise can affect human capital realms. Capital is defined as a supply of useful assets or advantages. There exist different "capitals" that represent domain-specific human assets. Investment over time can yield future positive dividends.

Fig. 1.2 Human capital attainment

financial, social, and individual capital, and the specifics of these will be described further in the following paragraphs.

Physical Capital

Physical capital is the first realm of positive benefit from sports participation. Physical activity improves one's motor coordination. Lloyd et al. discussed important potential benefits of long-term athletic development as a pathway that could enhance the health, fitness, and performance of all children and adolescents [11].

Other studies have shown that regular physical activity in youth, to include sports participation, results in increased bone density and skeletal muscle power [12, 13]. An essential life skill developed by consistent physical activity is physical literacy, which is defined as "the ability, confidence and desire to be physically active for life" [14, 15]. Building solid physical literacy early on, through purposeful implementation via school learning and community activities, creates a strong launching pad for a lifetime of being physically active [16, 17]. Additionally, several countries associate movement and body cultures with activity [18], and so while activity can be a unifying factor between cultures, it can also affirm individuals' connection to their own community and culture.

While helpful guidelines for weekly activity levels for youth and adolescents [19, 20] exist, unfortunately many youth fall short of those recommendations worldwide [21, 22]. In some countries, schools are cutting amounts of scheduled physical activity like physical education and recess [23–25]. In addition, the COVID-19 pandemic has also led to decreased activity levels for young people [26–28]. Sedentary behavior has a host of negative impacts on health [29, 30]. Future focus needs to continue to increase opportunities and decrease barriers for consistent physical activity for youth. The benefits are well-known, but policy and practice must be focused on improving access and decreasing obstacles.

Exercise is one of the least expensive ways to stay healthy, with studies finding that exercise can prevent chronic diseases as effectively as medication. Cardiorespiratory fitness, to include waist circumference, systolic blood pressure, fasting triglycerides, high-density lipoprotein cholesterol, and insulin, is significantly positively affected by sports participation [31, 32]. Physical activity and sports participation has also been shown to reduce risk and prevalence of other chronic comorbid conditions to include hypertension, stroke, various cancers, coronary heart disease, type 2 diabetes/metabolic syndrome, and overall mortality [33–35]. Recent research reveals that if levels of inactivity are not addressed, our future generations are at significant health risk. Rates of obesity are increasing fastest in countries with low levels of income. According to the research, the estimated rates of overweight and obese children aged 5–19 are up to 65% in the Pacific islands, 39% in the United States, and up to 31% in European countries (Fig. 1.3) [36]. Optimizing strategies to facilitate and increase physical activity in young people should be a focus of schools, governments, and healthcare organizations for both its short- and long-term positive impacts.

Emotional Capital

The second benefit of physical activity participation is described as emotional capital. Mental health is defined as a state of well-being and affective functioning in which individuals realize their own abilities, are resilient to the stresses of life, and have the capacity to make a positive contribution to their community [37].

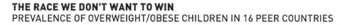

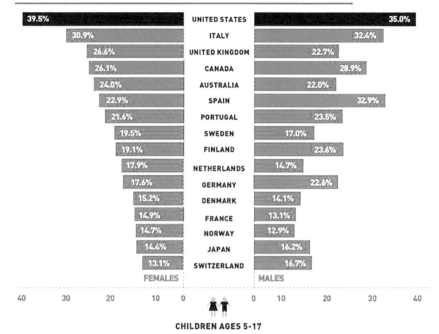

THE RACE WE DON'T WANT TO WIN
PREVALENCE OF OVERWEIGHT/OBESE CHILDREN IN 16 PEER COUNTRIES

Fig. 1.3 Prevelance of overweight/obese children

Participation in sports provides an important social setting with opportunities for promoting mental health and positive youth development [38, 39]. Some prior research has shown an inverse relationship between physical activity participation and depressive symptoms [40–43], and other research has shown that among individuals who experience clinical depression, physical activity leads to statistically significant reductions in score on depression symptom rating scales [44]. The mental and emotional health of youth and young adult athletes has been evaluated with research showing that athletes have lower levels of depression, anxiety, and other mental health-related diagnoses, as compared to their nonathlete student peers during times of non-disruption [45, 46]. In addition, it has been shown that physical activity decreases the risk of substance use like smoking and marijuana in youth [47–49]. While it may not increase abstinence levels for alcohol abusers or smokers, regular physical exercise such as yoga has the potential to improve mood and quality of life for women undergoing detoxification for substance use dependence [47]. Mood enhancement from exercise has the potential to have positive exponential or synergistic effects for both individuals and communities [50].

Intellectual Capital

Another benefit of physical activity participation includes intellectual capital, the attainment of intellectual assets, which includes cognitive-related positive gains. The relationship between physical exercise and cognitive functioning has received much attention in recent years [51, 52]. Particular efforts have focused on evaluating the effects of physical activity and exercise on youth brain development and cognition. The benefits of cognitive functioning that physical exercise can influence creates key elements for children's and adolescents' growth trajectories in their environments [53]. In recent years, several studies have highlighted how sports and physical exercise can improve educational attainment, processing speed, memory, and executive function/mental flexibility [54–58]. Numerous papers have studied the effects of physical activity on cognitive functioning, highlighting the importance of physical fitness [59–65]. Studies show that not only is physical exercise necessary, but it should have specific characteristics that improve study participants' physical condition to include ensuring that a particular activity coincides with the participant's level of development and current skill or ability so as to not interfere with their athletic identity attainment [66, 67]. Research has also shown positive effects of physical activity and sports on brain structure and function. Higher levels of aerobic fitness can promote higher volume in the hippocampus and an increase of white matter microstructure of the corpus callosum [54, 68, 69]. Another group observed a positive relationship between cardiorespiratory function, speed/agility, and the volume of gray matter in frontal, temporal, and subcortical regions of the brain, to include the premotor cortex and hippocampus [70]. Studies have also observed that improvements in physical activity to include aerobic capacity, strength, and body composition can reduce the impact of aging on brain function regression, thus allowing one to maintain cognitive strength and mental skills for longer periods of time and add to quality of life [71–74].

Financial Capital

An additional tier of physical activity and sports participation benefit involves improved financial capital. Athletes face a myriad of experiences in their respective sports, to include physical and mental strengthening, managing adversity by dealing with wins and losses, time management, collaboration, and leadership. Some argue that athletes hold a unique combination of skills that can translate to strengths in the business world, yielding increased financial growth potential. Studies have found adolescent athletes have higher rates of graduation from high school, which positively affect one's professional trajectory and future earning potential [75]. Physical activity participation can potentially contribute to higher income, increased productivity, better performance, and overall job success. Research has shown that those who participate in sports and regular physical activity tend to earn approximately 7–8% more in future income [76]. Furthermore, a collaborative report from EY and ESPNW reported that 94% of women who hold C-suite level positions were formal athletes [77], and 52% played sports at the collegiate level. Global financial success can benefit from increased sports and exercise participation as well because healthier bodies result in decreased absenteeism and less time off/lost productivity time from illness/injury [78]. An example of this is from economic projections and modeling in 2013 which calculated the economic burden associated with physical inactivity from premature morbidity and mortality equated to approximately $53.8 billion [79].

Social Capital

Sports participation offers the opportunity to join a group of diverse individuals to work together toward a common goal, thus leading to stronger social capital as well. Uslaner was one of the first researchers to study sport and social capital. Sport serves as an arena to enable building social capital, as participation widens social contact while building self-confidence and teaches respect for rules [80]. Furthermore, research shows that from sport arises tools related to social inclusion and acceptance, trust, collaboration, civic participation, gender equality, community cohesion, and bridging differences to serve mutually agreed-upon goals [81–83].

Individual Capital

As an athlete participates on a team, they can take opportunities presented to focus on character-related elements of life, one's individual capital. Research has shown that athletes and those participating in regular physical exercise are better able to hone and develop skills to include sportsmanship, time management, commitment to goals, and accountability [84–89]. Specific athlete populations and communities benefit from sport in other nuanced ways, which are important to understand.

Some studies have shown that being a female athlete can be a protective factor for early age sexual intercourse or unintended pregnancy [90, 91]. However, in contrast, recent literature has shown increased rates of teen pregnancy and younger ages of first sexual experience in some athletes [92, 93]. Further research is needed to better understand the risks and benefits of organized sports for young women. Other benefits include school academic achievement and body image. Female athletes are more likely to obtain a high school and college degree than girls who are not involved in sports [94–96]. They also stand to benefit from a more positive body imagery, self-esteem, and lower levels of depression [97–100]. A retrospective study found that girls' high school sports participation affected global self-worth during collegiate years, but mediators included self-perceived physical competence, positive body image, and self-esteem and gender role flexibility [101, 102]. Each sport crafts different subcultures that can influence behaviors, development, and outlook in varying ways. It is important to be mindful of the different cofactors that can impact self-esteem and mental health amidst sports participation.

Individuals with mobility limitation or other disability have even higher levels of inactivity as there are more barriers to activity. Ableism is prevalent and exists in many forms, but individuals with disabilities can potentially experience greater health gains if they are active on a regular basis [103–105]. Unique social, environmental, and financial components must be factored into policy and planning for activity levels to be increased consistently in this population. Each subpopulation of this community (wheelchair users, cerebral palsy, visual and hearing impairment, intellectual disability) must be examined individually to best address the needs of that specific subpopulation [106] and increase inclusiveness.

Youth that identify as lesbian, gay, bisexual, transgender, queer, asexual, and other orientations and identities (LGBTQA+) experience higher rates of violence, homelessness, bullying, self-injurious behavior, and use of substance abuse and other negative aspects of adolescence [107–109]. LGBTQA+ youth, particularly transgender youth, may feel less comfortable participating in activity, even in school [110]. In the adolescent population, Kann's study reported that when compared to heterosexual cisgender high school students, LGBTQA+ high school students had lower median rates of daily participation in moderate to vigorous physical activity for 60 min each day of the week [111]. In a study by Rosario et al., gay and bisexual male high school students differed significantly in rates of moderate to vigorous activity as compared to heterosexual male students; those rates did not differ significantly when comparing among female high school athletes [112]. Other studies report transgender students were less likely to participate in moderate to vigorous aerobic physical activity and muscle strengthening when compared to cisgender students [113]. The multiple benefits of physical activity for this population have been proven [114, 115] and improved inclusiveness should be a priority [110].

During a time of many different touch points of influence during a youth's development, to include family, peers, social media, and news outlets, sports can help young individuals positively shape their trajectory as they grow. It is in this realm that individuals can develop and craft their athletic identity.

Athletic Identity

The psychologist William James proposed the concept of "self" as a primary element of human thoughts, feelings, and actions that can remain fluid [116]. Within psychological research, different theories have been proposed regarding identity that include personal versus social identities as well as singular versus multiple aspects of identity. Early in his career, Erikson argued that one's identity is primarily an unconscious and continually evolving sense of who one is, both as an individual and as a part of a group or society. Furthermore, he argued that an individual's identity cannot exist in a vacuum but is linked to one's culture and environment [117]. Toward the latter stages of his career, Erikson included works that reflected more on identity, particularly in relation to spirituality and the concept of transcendence [118]. Social identity theory views identities of an individual as manifestations of a person's connection with a group or social category. Under identity theory, one's social environment can assign an individual a role, but ultimately, internalization of that role depends on the person accepting that particular role. Members may display preference to that group as identity affirmation, and inclusion is sought [119]. Sports is no exception to this theory of identity.

Britton Brewer was one of the researchers to propose the concept of an athletic identity (AI) and systematically study this area of interest in earnest in the 1990s. Athletic identity refers to the degree of strength and exclusivity to which a person identifies with the athlete role or the degree to which one devotes special attention to sport relative to other engagements or activities in life [120]. Athlete identity can exist to varying degrees for each athlete, ranging as a small part of who someone is to a large encompassing part of his or her life [121]. This component of self-concept can be affected by the experiences, relationships, and involvement in sport activities. Identity can be both psychologically and socially based. Under that premise, a greater athletic identity can influence self-esteem, motivation, and outlook, which can simultaneously be affected by perceptions of athletic competence and performance. Kohn suggested that for some youth, winning would translate to coach's approval, which is also connected to parental acceptance, which in turn affects acceptance of self/self-worth conceptualization [122]. Brewer, Van Raalte, and Linder's prior works suggest that athletic identity arises from a cognitive foundation and exists continually as a social role. Furthermore, they argue that one's athletic identity is tied to both an individual's emotional connection and internalization as well as feedback from social connections, to include teammates, coaches, parents, and spectators [123].

Several instruments have been developed to measure levels of athletic identity. Anderson's Athletic Identity Questionnaire (AIQ) for adolescents has been used out of an interest in evaluating general populations and how the label, "athletic," is assumed, attributed, and maintained [124]. The most commonly used instrument involves the Athletic Identity Measurement Scale (AIMS), which has been validated and applied to elite athletes, recreational athletes, and nonathlete populations. Initially presented as a unidimensional construct involving a ten-item questionnaire, the AIMS tool has been reconceptualized into a seven-item questionnaire that consists of three dimensions: social identity, negative affectivity, and exclusivity (Fig. 1.4) [120]. Social identity involves the extent that an individual connects to and occupies an athlete role. Exclusivity within AIMS describes the level to which an individual's identity and self-work are constructed by the performance within an athletic role. Negative affectivity represents the extent to which one experiences negative sequelae in response to undesirable outcomes within the athletic role [125].

Prior studies have investigated the positive effects athletic identity can have on an individual. Athletic identity has been shown to have a positive effect on one's emotional connection to sport, thereby positively influencing physical activity participation and athletic performance [126]. In addition, emotional health can be improved with physical activity participation and stronger athletic identity [127]. A strong but not exclusive AI level has been associated with improved performance through increased commitment and dedication to one's training and sport goal

Original Athlete Identity Measurement Scale Items

1.	I consider myself an athlete.
2.	I have many goals related to sport.
3.	Most of my friends are athletes.
4.	Sport is the most important part of my life.
5.	I spend more time thinking about sport than anything else.
6.	I need to participate in sport to feel good about myself.
7.	Other people see me mainly as an athlete.
8.	I feel bad about myself when I do poorly in sport.
9.	Sport is the only important thing in my life.
10.	I would be very depressed if I were injured and could not compete in sport.

Reconceptualized Athlete Identity Measurement Scale Items

1.	I consider myself an athlete.
2.	I have many goals related to sport.
3.	Most of my friends are athletes.
4.	Sport is the most important part of my life.
5.	I spend more time thinking about sport than anything else.
8.	I feel bad about myself when I do poorly in sport.
10.	I would be very depressed if I were injured and could not compete in sport.

Factors: Social Identity; Exclusivity: Negative Affectivity

B.W. Brewer, A. E. Cornelius. Norms and factorial invariance of the Athletic Identity Measurement Scale. Academic Athletic Journal 2001, 16: 103–113.

Fig. 1.4 Athlete identity measurement scale

orientation [128]. Higher performance outcomes and sports enjoyment have been found in athletes with stronger athletic identity as compared to those who assume lower athlete roles [129]. When performing well, athletes with stronger AI levels have been found to have more positive athletic experiences and more positive body image and self-confidence [120, 128]. Brewer's research also found that those who adopt more of an athletic role tend to be more physically active than their peers who do not [120, 129]. Strong athletic identity can also foster motivation and self-determination for activities related to one's athletic role from outside approval, encouragement, and goal attainment, thus preventing inactivity and the larger sequelae of burnout and obesity [130, 131].

Conversely, strong athletic identity can be associated with negative outcomes as well. Steinfeldt's work connected higher athletic identity levels with lower tendencies for one to seek help and higher levels of gender role conflict [132]. A strong athletic identity can open an individual's vulnerabilities to mental illness struggles and burnout in the setting of unexpected challenges such as loss, injury/physical illness, and forced retirement [133, 134], especially when athletic identity is a central component to one's overall self-worth. In a systematic review, 34 out of the 35 studies identified found that strong athletic identity negatively correlated with the quality of an athletic career transition [135]. When a strong sense of athletic identity exists at the time of retirement, loss of overall identity is reported, and those individuals tend to take a longer period to adjust to the transition [136, 137], thus opening risk for emotional stress [138].

In a study by Manuel et al., those adolescents in the cohort with higher athletic identity/exclusivity scores were found to have higher Beck Depression Scale scores during their orthopedic injury and depression scores decreasing 6 and 12 weeks after the onset of the injury [139]. Those with an exclusive or very strong athletic identity without other social role connections can face exceptional emotional difficulty adjusting to retirement or the abrupt cessation of sports participation [129, 140]. Lee, Sangwook, and Inwoo found that burnout tended to be a mediator between stress levels and athletic identity in Korean high school athletes; athletic identity had a negative correlation with stress and burnout [141]. Additional studies have found a negative relationship between athletic identity and athlete burnout [108, 131]. Furthermore, individuals with stronger athletic identities may self-impose higher standards of performance and goal attainment. If reality does not align with those standards, one runs the risk of actual-ideal self-discrepancy, which threatens the concept of athletic identity in and of itself and increases risk of burnout [129].

Another negative impact of deep connections to high athletic identity includes performance-enhancing strategies that become detrimental to one's health. As sports become more intense and commercialized, to include youth sports [133], a win at all costs mentality can foster unhealthy hypercompetitive behaviors. Such behaviors include overtraining, playing while injured, using anabolic steroids or other performance-enhancing substances, and displaying disordered eating patterns [121, 142, 143]. Donahue et al. used the dualistic model of passion to examine basketball player aggression, and players were categorized based on their responses as either obsessively passionate (exclusively passionate) or harmoniously passionate (less passionate). They found that obsessively passionate basketball players tended to be more aggressive than those players found as harmoniously passionate, particularly in periods of adversity that may threaten one's concept of athletic identity [144]. In other words, one's love for sport and threat to one's athletic identity can lead to maladaptive social behavior. Visek found contact and collision athletes who maintain high athletic identity as well as identity standards, such as masculine or aggressive, are more likely to exhibit unhealthy behaviors to reaffirm their own identity [145].

Despite these findings, recent research has begun to open the aperture to study the interplay between athletic identity and physical, emotional, and social factors in the youth athlete population. A systematic review conducted in 2019 found ten studies that involved the youth population and included a scale to measure athletic identity with findings supporting a theory that adolescence is a critical time to develop concepts of identity, athletic identity not excluded [119]. Youth tend to adopt a stronger sense of identity as an athlete during their adolescent years as compared to later ages of training and development [146, 147]. This critical time also coincides with research revealing higher rates of burnout/sport dropout in adolescence and among today's youth [148–151]. Strong exclusivity can hamper the development of other elements of one's individual identity or prevent a conglomeration of the interaction of numerous social identity roles. More qualitative and quantitative research regarding athletic identity has recently surfaced, to include levels of athletic identify in youth sports teams, work looking at the personal identification and conceptualization of an athlete, as well as the effects of the COVID-19 pandemic and periods of isolation on athletic identity in athletes [152–154].

Further research in this field is needed to better understand how identity, which can serve as a fluid cognitive structure, aligns with social roles, to include that of athlete in many diverse populations and how that concept can be influenced by or influence factors, such as physical activity or mental health, both individually and within groups. As sports, including youth sports participation, have transformed into a multibillion-dollar industry [155, 156], more research is needed on the intersection of sports participation and social identity, including the effects on a youth development model. Current research and discourse have largely existed in more homogenous populations; however, as with all scientific research, the challenge exists to move more broadly to reflect the multifaceted and diverse population that exists so that scholarship is more inclusive of a larger bandwidth of perspectives. Moreover, athletic identity cannot be studied or exist in isolation from other cultural epistemology to include age, gender, race, ethnicity, and disability. The cultural discourses and life narratives that produce and influence athletic identity cannot be ignored. Schinke argues that "the cultural practices in most sports marginalize female, gay, ageing, racialized bodies that are socially constructed in opposition to white heterosexual masculine standards, taken as normative in defining and giving meaning to sport activities … (leading) to marginalized voices and omitted subject matter" [157, 158]. The power of outside cultural discourses and social normative influences such as media, societal stereotypes, and cultural scripting need to be evaluated regarding how they shape athletes' sense of self and one's interaction with the larger sport milieu.

Conclusion

Sports participation unlocks potential greater physical and emotional health and leads to long-term well-being that cannot be undervalued. Moreover, sports offer an important formative element of identity in youth and young adult athletes that needs further study. Participation in sports offers short- and long-term benefits that reverberate well outside of the arenas of competition. However, if this intrinsic value is suddenly lost because of injury and burnout or for other reasons, that loss is felt deeply by the development of one's mind and body. When athletic identity has high exclusivity levels, it may overshadow the formation of other important and essential traits of individuals. Balancing out the positive and negative impacts of athletic identity is an important equilibrium to foster for providers, parents, coaches, and most importantly, athletes.

Disclosure Statement The authors have nothing to disclose.

References

1. Vörös G. Egyptian temple architecture: 100 years of Hungarian excavations in Egypt, 1907-2007. Cairo: American Univ in Cairo Press; 2007.
2. Crego R. Sports and games of the 18th and 19th centuries. Westport: Greenwood Publishing Group; 2003.
3. Aspen-Institute. Aspen Institute project play. Sport for all play for life: a playbook to get every kid in the game; 2021. https://www.aspenprojectplay.org/sport-for-all-play-for-life. Accessed 27 Jan 2015.
4. Centers for Disease Control and Prevention. US Department of Health and Human Services Physical activity guidelines for Americans. Atlanta, GA: Centers for Disease Control and Prevention (CDC). National Center for Chronic Disease Prevention and Health Promotion; 2008. p. 6–17.
5. Joy EL, et al. Physical activity counselling in sports medicine: a call to action. Br J Sports Med. 2013;47(1):49–53.
6. Forouzanfar MH, et al. Global, regional, and national comparative risk assessment of 79 behavioural, environmental and occupational, and metabolic risks or clusters of risks, 1990–2015: a systematic analysis for the global burden of disease study 2015. Lancet. 2016;388(10053):1659–724.
7. Lee IM, Shiroma EJ, Lobelo F, et al. Lancet physical activity series working group. Effect of physical inactivity on major non-communicable diseases worldwide: an analysis of burden of disease and life expectancy. Lancet. 2012;380:219–29.
8. Merriam-Webster, Inc, editor. Merriam-Webster's dictionary of English usage. Springfield, MA: Merriam-Webster; 1993.
9. Dekker P, Uslaner EM. Social capital and participation in everyday life, vol. 23. London: Routledge; 2001. https://doi.org/10.4324/9780203451571.
10. Designed to Move. https://www.sportsthinktank.com/uploads/designed-to-move-full-report-13.pdf. Accessed 16 Feb 2022.
11. Lloyd RS, et al. Long-term athletic development-part 1: a pathway for all youth. J Strength Cond Res. 2015;29(5):1439–50.
12. Khan KM, et al. Sport and exercise as contributors to the health of nations. Lancet. 2012;380(9836):59–64.
13. Basterfield L, et al. Longitudinal associations between sports participation, body composition and physical activity from childhood to adolescence. J Sci Med Sport. 2015;18(2):178–82.
14. SHAPE America. Physical literacy in the United States: a model, strategic plan and call to action. Society of Health and Physical Educators. https://www.shapeamerica.org/events/physicalliteracy.aspx#:~:text=Physical%20literacy%20is%20the%20ability,development%20of%20the%20whole%20person. Accessed 13 Mar 2022.
15. Spengler JO, Cohen J. Physical literacy: a global environmental scan. The Aspen Institute, Project Play, Robert Wood Johnson Foundation; 2015. https://www.shapeamerica.org/uploads/pdfs/GlobalScan_FINAL.pdf. Accessed 13 Mar 2022.
16. Roetert EP, MacDonald LC. Unpacking the physical literacy concept for K-12 physical education: what should we expect the learner to master? J Sport Health Sci. 2015;4(2):108–12.
17. Bailey R, Hillman C, Arent S, Petitpas A. Physical activity: an underestimated investment in human capital? J Phys Act Health. 2013;10(3):289–308. https://doi.org/10.1123/jpah.10.3.289.
18. Roetert EP, Jefferies SC. Embracing physical literacy. J Phys Educ Recreat Dance. 2014;85(8):38–40.
19. Bevington F, et al. The move your way campaign: encouraging contemplators and families to meet the recommendations from the physical activity guidelines for Americans. J Phys Act Health. 2020;17(4):397–403.
20. U.S. Department of Health and Human Services. Physical activity guidelines for Americans. 2nd ed. Washington, DC: U.S. Department of Health and Human Services; 2018.

21. Ng SW, Popkin BM. Time use and physical activity: a shift away from movement across the globe. Obes Rev. 2012;13(8):659–80.
22. Church TS, et al. Trends over 5 decades in US occupation-related physical activity and their associations with obesity. PLoS One. 2011;6(5):e19657.
23. Marshall J, Hardman K. The state and status of physical education in schools in international context. Eur Phy Educ Rev. 2000;6(3):203–29.
24. Hardman K. An up-date on the status of physical education in schools worldwide: technical report for the World Health Organisation. Book an up-date on the status of physical education in schools worldwide: technical report for the World Health Organisation; 2004.
25. McKenzie TL, Lounsbery MAF. School physical education: the pill not taken. Am J Lifestyle Med. 2009;3(3):219–25.
26. Tulchin-Francis K, et al. The impact of the coronavirus disease 2019 pandemic on physical activity in US children. J Sport Health Sci. 2021;10(3):323–32.
27. Tison GH, et al. Worldwide effect of COVID-19 on physical activity: a descriptive study. Ann Intern Med. 2020;173(9):767–70.
28. Rossi L, Behme N, Breuer C. Physical activity of children and adolescents during the COVID-19 pandemic—a scoping review. Int J Environ Res Public Health. 2021;18(21):11440.
29. Hamilton MT, et al. Too little exercise and too much sitting: inactivity physiology and the need for new recommendations on sedentary behavior. Curr Cardiovasc Risk Rep. 2008;2(4):292–8.
30. Uffelen V, Jannique GZ, et al. Occupational sitting and health risks: a systematic review. Am J Prev Med. 2010;39(4):379–88.
31. Ekelund U, et al. Moderate to vigorous physical activity and sedentary time and cardiometabolic risk factors in children and adolescents. JAMA. 2012;307(7):704–12.
32. Steele RM, Brage S, Corder K, Wareham NJ, Ekelund U. Physical activity, cardiorespiratory fitness, and the metabolic syndrome in youth. J Appl Physiol. 2008;105(1):342–35118369096.
33. Jones-Palm DH, Palm J. Physical activity and its impact on health behaviour among youth. World Health Organization technical paper commissioned from ICSSPE in 2005.
34. Kokkinos P, Sheriff H, Kheirbek R. Physical inactivity and mortality risk. Cardiol Res Pract. 2011;2011:924945.
35. Mitchell T, Church T, Zucker M. Move yourself. Newark, NJ: Wiley; 2008.
36. Martinez JA, et al. Position guidelines and evidence base concerning determinants of childhood obesity with a European perspective. Obes Rev. 2022;23:e13391.
37. World Health Organization. Promoting mental health: concepts, emerging evidence, practice: a report of the World Health Organization, Department of Mental Health and Substance Abuse in collaboration with the Victorian Health Promotion Foundation and the University of Melbourne; 2005. Accessed 1 Mar 2022.
38. Hagell A. The connections between young people's mental health and sport participation: scoping the evidence. London: Association for Young People's Health; 2016.
39. Holt NL, Sehn ZL. Processes associated with positive youth development and participation in competitive youth sport. In: Positive youth development through sport. London: Routledge; 2007. p. 38–47.
40. Mutrie N. The relationship between physical activity and clinically defined depression. Physical activity and psychological well-being; 2000. p. 46–62.
41. O'Neal HA, Dunn AL, Martinsen EW. Depression and exercise. Int J Sport Psychol., 2000;31:110–35.
42. Lawlor DA, Hopker SW. The effectiveness of exercise as an intervention in the management of depression: systematic review and meta-regression analysis of randomised controlled trials. BMJ. 2001;322(7289):763.
43. Teychenne M, Ball K, Salmon J. Associations between physical activity and depressive symptoms in women. Int J Behav Nutr Phys Act. 2008;5(1):1–12.
44. Stathopoulou G, et al. Exercise interventions for mental health: a quantitative and qualitative review. Clin Psychol Sci Pract. 2006;13(2):179.

45. Khubchandani J, et al. The psychometric properties of PHQ-4 depression and anxiety screening scale among college students. Arch Psychiatr Nurs. 2016;30(4):457–62.
46. Connor KM, Davidson JRT. SPRINT: a brief global assessment of post-traumatic stress disorder. Int Clin Psychopharmacol. 2001;16(5):279–84.
47. Wang D, et al. Impact of physical exercise on substance use disorders: a meta-analysis. PLoS One. 2014;9(10):e110728.
48. West AB, et al. A systematic review of physical activity, sedentary behavior, and substance use in adolescents and emerging adults. Transl Behav Med. 2020;10(5):1155–67.
49. Simonton AJ, Young CC, Johnson KE. Physical activity interventions to decrease substance use in youth: a review of the literature. Subst Use Misuse. 2018;53(12):2052–68.
50. Hoffman MD, Hoffman DR. Exercisers achieve greater acute exercise-induced mood enhancement than nonexercisers. Arch Phys Med Rehabil. 2008;89(2):358–63. https://doi.org/10.1016/j.apmr.2007.09.026.
51. Northey JM, et al. Exercise interventions for cognitive function in adults older than 50: a systematic review with meta-analysis. Br J Sports Med. 2018;52(3):154–60.
52. Moran A, Campbell M, Toner J. Exploring the cognitive mechanisms of expertise in sport: progress and prospects. Psychol Sport Exerc. 2019;42:8–15.
53. Gale CR, et al. Cognitive function in childhood and lifetime cognitive change in relation to mental wellbeing in four cohorts of older people. PLoS One. 2012;7(9):e44860.
54. Chaddock L, et al. A neuroimaging investigation of the association between aerobic fitness, hippocampal volume, and memory performance in preadolescent children. Brain Res. 2010;1358:172–83.
55. Scudder MR, et al. The association between aerobic fitness and language processing in children: implications for academic achievement. Brain Cogn. 2014;87:140–52.
56. Donnelly JE, et al. Physical activity, fitness, cognitive function, and academic achievement in children: a systematic review. Med Sci Sports Exerc. 2016;48(6):1197.
57. Li JW, et al. The effect of acute and chronic exercise on cognitive function and academic performance in adolescents: a systematic review. J Sci Med Sport. 2017;20(9):841–8.
58. Xue Y, Yang Y, Huang T. Effects of chronic exercise interventions on executive function among children and adolescents: a systematic review with meta-analysis. Br J Sports Med. 2019;53(22):1397–404.
59. Hillman CH, Castelli DM, Buck SM. Aerobic fitness and neurocognitive function in healthy preadolescent children. Med Sci Sports Exerc. 2005;37(11):1967.
60. Hillman CH, et al. Aerobic fitness and cognitive development: event-related brain potential and task performance indices of executive control in preadolescent children. Dev Psychol. 2009;45(1):114.
61. Hillman CH, et al. The effect of acute treadmill walking on cognitive control and academic achievement in preadolescent children. Neuroscience. 2009;159(3):1044–54.
62. Hillman CH, et al. Effects of the FITKids randomized controlled trial on executive control and brain function. Pediatrics. 2014;134(4):e1063–71.
63. Tomporowski PD, et al. Exercise and children's intelligence, cognition, and academic achievement. Educ Psychol Rev. 2008;20(2):111–31.
64. Lojovich JM. The relationship between aerobic exercise and cognition: is movement medicinal? J Head Trauma Rehabil. 2010;25(3):184–92.
65. Gill SS, Seitz DP. Lifestyles and cognitive health: what older individuals can do to optimize cognitive outcomes. JAMA. 2015;314(8):774–5.
66. Hötting K, Röder B. Beneficial effects of physical exercise on neuroplasticity and cognition. Neurosci Biobehav Rev. 2013;37(9):2243–57.
67. Reigal RE, et al. Relationships between reaction time, selective attention, physical activity, and physical fitness in children. Front Psychol. 2019;10:2278.
68. Chaddock-Heyman L, et al. The effects of physical activity on functional MRI activation associated with cognitive control in children: a randomized controlled intervention. Front Hum Neurosci. 2013;7:72.

69. Chaddock-Heyman L, et al. Physical activity increases white matter microstructure in children. Front Neurosci. 2018;12:950.
70. Esteban-Cornejo I, et al. A whole brain volumetric approach in overweight/obese children: examining the association with different physical fitness components and academic performance. The ActiveBrains project. Neuroimage. 2017;159:346–54.
71. Chang Y-K, et al. The effects of acute exercise on cognitive performance: a meta-analysis. Brain Res. 2012;1453:87–101.
72. Chang Y-K, et al. Effect of resistance-exercise training on cognitive function in healthy older adults: a review. J Aging Phys Act. 2012;20:4.
73. Kerr J, et al. Objectively measured physical activity is related to cognitive function in older adults. J Am Geriatr Soc. 2013;61(11):1927–31.
74. Fernandes J, Arida RM, Gomez-Pinilla F. Physical exercise as an epigenetic modulator of brain plasticity and cognition. Neurosci Biobehav Rev. 2017;80:443–56.
75. Dale D, Corbin CB. Physical activity participation of high school graduates following exposure to conceptual or traditional physical education. Res Q Exerc Sport. 2000;71(1):61–8.
76. Pronk NP, Martinson B, Kessler RC, Beck AL, Simon GE, Wang P. The association between work performance and physical activity, cardiorespiratory fitness, and obesity. J Occup Environ Med. 2004;46(1):19–25.
77. Where Will You Find Your Next Leader? EY © 2015 EYGM limited. https://assets.ey.com/content/dam/ey-sites/ey-com/en_gl/topics/elite-athlete-program/ey-why-female-athletes-make-winning-entrepreneurs.pdf?download. Accessed 3 Mar 2022.
78. Proper KI, Van den Heuvel SG, De Vroome EM, Hildebrandt VH, Van der Beek AJ. Dose-response relation between physical activity and sick leave. Br J Sports Med. 2006;40(2):173–8. https://doi.org/10.1136/bjsm.2005.022327.
79. Ding D, et al. The economic burden of physical inactivity: a global analysis of major non-communicable diseases. Lancet. 2016;388(10051):1311–24.
80. Uslaner EM. Democracy and social capital. In: Warren ME, editor. Democracy and trust, vol. 121; 1999. p. 150.
81. Bailey R. Evaluating the relationship between physical education, sport and social inclusion. Educ Rev. 2005;57(1):71–90.
82. Contribution of Sport to the Millennium Development Goals. United Nations Office on Sport for Development and Peace; 2010. Accessed 26 Feb 2022.
83. Larkin A. Sport and recreation and community building: literature review for the NSW department of the arts, sport and recreation. Sydney: NSW Department of the Arts, sport and Recreation; 2008.
84. Fraser-Thomas J, Côté J, Deakin J. Youth sport programs: an avenue to foster positive youth development. Phys Educ Sport Pedagog. 2005;10(1):19–40.
85. Petitpas AJ, et al. A framework for planning youth sport programs that foster psychosocial development. Sport Psychol. 2005;19:1.
86. President's Council on physical fitness and sports. Washington, DC; 2009.
87. Rosewater A. Learning to play and playing to learn. Team-Up for Youth; 2009.
88. Sheard M, Golby J. Personality hardiness differentiates elite-level sport performers. Int J Sport Exerc Psychol. 2010;8:160–9.
89. Weiss MR. Field of dreams: sport as a context for youth development. Res Q Exerc Sport. 2008;79(4):434–49.
90. Sabo DF, et al. High school athletic participation, sexual behavior and adolescent pregnancy: a regional study. J Adolesc Health. 1999;25(3):207–16.
91. Kulig K, Brener ND, McManus T. Sexual activity and substance use among adolescents by category of physical activity plus team sports participation. Arch Pediatr Adolesc Med. 2003;157(9):905–12.
92. Habel MA, et al. Daily participation in sports and students' sexual activity. Perspect Sex Reprod Health. 2010;42(4):244–50.

93. Taliaferro LA, Rienzo BA, Donovan KA. Relationships between youth sport participation and selected health risk behaviors from 1999 to 2007. J Sch Health. 2010;80(8):399–410.
94. Troutman KP, Dufur MJ. From high school jocks to college grads: assessing the long-term effects of high school sport participation on females' educational attainment. Youth Soc. 2007;38(4):443–62.
95. Lumpkin A, Favor J. Comparing the academic performance of high school athletes and non-athletes in Kansas 2008-2009. J Appl Sport Manag. 2013;4(1):31.
96. Women's Sports Foundation. Teen Sport in America, Part II: Her Participation Matters. April 15, 2021. https://www.womenssportsfoundation.org/articles_and_report/teen-sport-report-ii/. Accessed 18 Mar 2022.
97. Hausenblas HA, Downs DS. Comparison of body image between athletes and nonathletes: a meta-analytic review. J Appl Sport Psychol. 2001;13(3):323–39.
98. Koyuncu M, et al. Body image satisfaction and dissatisfaction, social physique anxiety, self-esteem, and body fat ratio in female exercisers and nonexercisers. Soc Behav Personal Int J. 2010;38(4):561–70.
99. Appaneal RN, et al. Measuring postinjury depression among male and female competitive athletes. J Sport Exerc Psychol. 2009;31(1):60–76.
100. Pluhar E, et al. Team sport athletes may be less likely to suffer anxiety or depression than individual sport athletes. J Sports Sci Med. 2019;18(3):490.
101. Richman EL, Shaffer DR. "If you let me play sports" how might sport participation influence the self-esteem of adolescent females? Psychol Women Q. 2000;24(2):189–99.
102. Daniels E, Leaper C. A longitudinal investigation of sport participation, peer acceptance, and self-esteem among adolescent girls and boys. Sex Roles. 2006;55(11):875–80.
103. Hollis NTD, et al. Physical activity types among US adults with mobility disability, behavioral risk factor surveillance system, 2017. Disabil Health J. 2020;13(3):100888.
104. Waiserberg N, Feder-Bubis P. Enabling physical activity for people living with disabilities. Lancet. 2021;398(10316):2072–3.
105. Carty C, et al. The first global physical activity and sedentary behavior guidelines for people living with disability. J Phys Act Health. 2021;18(1):86–93.
106. Rosenbaum P, Gorter JW. The 'F-words' in childhood disability: I swear this is how we should think! Child Care Health Dev. 2012;38(4):457–63.
107. Taylor J. Mental health in LGBTQ youth: review of research and outcomes. Communique. 2019;48(3):4–6.
108. Gamarel KE, et al. Identity safety and relational health in youth spaces: a needs assessment with LGBTQ youth of color. J LGBT Youth. 2014;11(3):289–315.
109. Rhoades H, et al. Homelessness, mental health and suicidality among LGBTQ youth accessing crisis services. Child Psychiatry Hum Dev. 2018;49(4):643–51.
110. Greenspan SB, Griffith C, Watson RJ. LGBTQ+ youth's experiences and engagement in physical activity: a comprehensive content analysis. Adolesc Res Rev. 2019;4(2):169–85.
111. Kann L, et al. Sexual identity, sex of sexual contacts, and health-related behaviors among students in grades 9–12—United States and selected sites, 2015. Morb Mortal Wkly Rep Surveill Summ. 2016;65(9):1–202.
112. Rosario M, et al. Sexual orientation disparities in cancer-related risk behaviors of tobacco, alcohol, sexual behaviors, and diet and physical activity: pooled youth risk behavior surveys. Am J Public Health. 2014;104(2):245–54.
113. VanKim NA, et al. Weight-related disparities for transgender college students. Health Behav Policy Rev. 2014;1(2):161–71.
114. Kirklewski SJ, Watson RJ, Lauckner C. The moderating effect of physical activity on the relationship between bullying and mental health among sexual and gender minority youth. J Sport Health Sci. Published online 2021. https://doi.org/10.1016/j.jshs.2020.11.013.
115. Clark CM, Kosciw JG. Engaged or excluded: LGBTQ youth's participation in school sports and their relationship to psychological well-being. Psychol Sch. 2022;59(1):95–114.

116. Greenwald AG, Pratkanis AR. The self. In: Wyer Jr RS, Srull TK, editors. Handbook of social cognition, vol. 3. Hillsdale, NJ: Lawrence Erlbaum Associates Publishers; 1984. p. 129–78.
117. Kidwell JS, et al. Adolescent identity exploration: a test of Erikson's theory of transitional crisis. Adolescence. 1995;30(120):785–93.
118. Erikson J. The ninth stage. In: Erikson EH, editor. The life cycle completed. New York: WW. Norton; 1997a. p. 105–15.
119. Edison BR, Christino MA, Rizzone KH. Athletic identity in youth athletes: a systematic review of the literature. Int J Environ Res Public Health. 2021;18(14):7331.
120. Brewer B, Boi P, Petitpas A, Van Raalte J, Mahar M. Dimensions of athletic identity. In: Proceedings of the Annual Meeting of the American Psychological Association, Toronto, ON; 1993. p. 19–22.
121. Coakley J. Sports in society: issues and controversies. Boston, MA: McGraw Hill; 2004.
122. Kohn A. No contest: the case against competition. New York, NY: Houghton Mifflin Harcourt; 1992.
123. Brewer BW, Van Raalte JL, Linder DE. Construct validity of the athletic identity measurement scale. Monterey, CA: Paper presented at the North American Society for the Psychology of Sport and Physical Activity Annual Conference; 1991.
124. Anderson CB, Coleman KJ. Adaptation and validation of the athletic identity questionnaire-adolescent for use with children. J Phys Act Health. 2008;5(4):539–58.
125. Brewer BW, Cornelius AE. Norms and factorial invariance of the athletic identity measurement scale. Acad Athl J. 2001;16:103–13.
126. Babić V, et al. Athletic engagement and athletic identity in top Croatian sprint runners. Coll Antropol. 2015;39(3):521–8.
127. Sanders CE, et al. Moderate involvement in sports is related to lower depression levels among adolescents. Adolescence. 2000;35(140):793.
128. Horton RS, Mack DE. Athletic identity in marathon runners: functional focus or dysfunctional commitment? J Sport Behav. 2000;23:2.
129. Brewer BW, Van Raalte JL, Linder DE. Athletic identity: Hercules' muscles or Achilles' heel? Int J Sport Psychol. 1993;24:237–54.
130. Stets JE, Burke PJ. Identity theory and social identity theory. Soc Psychol Q. 2000:224–37.
131. Martin EM, Horn TS. The role of athletic identity and passion in predicting burnout in adolescent female athletes. Sport Psychol. 2013;27(4):338–48.
132. Steinfeldt JA, et al. Masculinity, moral atmosphere, and moral functioning of high school football players. J Sport Exerc Psychol. 2011;33(2):215–34.
133. Coakley J. Burnout among adolescent athletes: a personal failure or social problem? Sociol Sport J. 1992;9(3):271–85.
134. Gustafsson H, Kenttä G, Hassmén P. Athlete burnout: an integrated model and future research directions. Int Rev Sport Exerc Psychol. 2011;4(1):3–24.
135. Park S, Lavallee D, Tod D. Athletes' career transition out of sport: a systematic review. Int Rev Sport Exerc Psychol. 2013;6(1):22–53.
136. Grove JR, Lavallee D, Gordon S. Coping with retirement from sport: the influence of athletic identity. J Appl Sport Psychol. 1997;9(2):191–203.
137. Houle JLW, Kluck AS. An examination of the relationship between athletic identity and career maturity in student-athletes. J Clin Sport Psychol. 2015;9(1):24–40.
138. Giannone ZA, et al. Athletic identity and psychiatric symptoms following retirement from varsity sports. Int J Soc Psychiatry. 2017;63(7):598–601.
139. Manuel JC, et al. Coping with sports injuries: an examination of the adolescent athlete. J Adolesc Health. 2002;31(5):391–3.
140. Lavallee D, Robinson HK. In pursuit of an identity: a qualitative exploration of retirement from women's artistic gymnastics. Psychol Sport Exerc. 2007;8(1):119–41.
141. Lee K, Kang S, Kim I. Relationships among stress, burnout, athletic identity, and athlete satisfaction in students at Korea's physical education high schools: validating differences between pathways according to ego resilience. Psychol Rep. 2017;120(4):585–608.

142. Coker-Cranney A, et al. How far is too far? Understanding identity and overconformity in collegiate wrestlers. Qual Res Sport Exerc Health. 2018;10(1):92–116.
143. Voelker DK, Gould D, Reel JJ. Prevalence and correlates of disordered eating in female figure skaters. Psychol Sport Exerc. 2014;15(6):696–704.
144. Donahue EG, Rip B, Vallerand RJ. When winning is everything: on passion, identity, and aggression in sport. Psychol Sport Exerc. 2009;10(5):526–34.
145. Visek AJ, et al. Athletic identity and aggressiveness: a cross-cultural analysis of the athletic identity maintenance model. Int J Sport Exerc Psychol. 2010;8(2):99–116.
146. Houle JLW, Brewer BW, Kluck AS. Developmental trends in athletic identity: a two-part retrospective study. J Sport Behav. 2010;33(2):146.
147. Mitchell TO, et al. Exploring athletic identity in elite-level English youth football: a cross-sectional approach. J Sports Sci. 2014;32(13):1294–9.
148. DiFiori JP, Benjamin HJ, Brenner J, et al. Overuse injuries and burnout in youth sports: a position statement from the American medical society for sports medicine. Clin J Sport Med. 2014;24:3–20. Epub 2013/12/25.
149. Kriz PK, MacDonald JP. The youth sports machine: destructive juggernaut or vehicle for success? Curr Sports Med Rep. 2017;16(4):227–9.
150. Wittenberg M. "The role of relatedness in youth athlete burnout." (2018).
151. Gould D. The current youth sport landscape: identifying critical research issues. Kinesiol Rev. 2019;8(3):150–61.
152. Rongen F, et al. Validation of the athletic identity measurement scale in youth academy soccer players. J Athl Dev Exp. 2021;3(3):4.
153. Zanin AC, Preston SL, Adame EA. Athletic identity transformation: a qualitative drawing analysis of implicit constructions of athletes, girls, and the self. Commun Sport. 2021;9(3):395–417.
154. Graupensperger S, et al. Social (un) distancing: teammate interactions, athletic identity, and mental health of student-athletes during the COVID-19 pandemic. J Adolesc Health. 2020;67(5):662–70.
155. Koba M. Spending big on kids' sports? You're not alone, 2014. http://www.cnbc.com/2014/01/13/youth-sports-is-a-7-billion-industryand-growing.html. Accessed 20 Mar 2022.
156. Erdal K. The adulteration of children's sports: waning health and well-being in the age of organized play. Lanham: Rowman & Littlefield; 2018.
157. Schinke, Robert J., and Kerry R. McGannon. Cultural sport psychology and intersecting identities: an introduction in the special section. 2015.
158. Schinke RJ, et al. Cultural sport psychology as a pathway to advances in identity and settlement research to practice. Psychol Sport Exerc. 2019;42:58–65.

Chapter 2
Mental Health Concerns in Athletes

Miriam Rowan, Samantha R. Sarafin, Kyra Willoughby, and Kimberly H. McManama O'Brien

Key Points
- Young athletes experience nearly all the mental health concerns observed in the general population; however, rates of occurrence per mental health disorder may differ from the general population.
- Mental health conditions have significant impacts on athlete health and performance.
- Factors of psychological resilience can reduce vulnerability to mental health concerns.

M. Rowan (✉) · K. H. McManama O'Brien
Division of Sports Medicine, Department of Orthopedic Surgery, Boston Children's Hospital, Harvard Medical School, Boston, MA, USA

Department of Psychiatry, Boston Children's Hospital, Harvard Medical School, Boston, MA, USA
e-mail: miriam.rowan@childrens.harvard.edu; kimberlyh.m.obrien@childrens.harvard.edu

S. R. Sarafin
Division of Sports Medicine, Department of Orthopedic Surgery, Boston Children's Hospital, Boston, MA, USA
e-mail: samantha.sarafin@childrens.harvard.edu

K. Willoughby
Harvard University, Cambridge, MA, USA
e-mail: kyrawilloughby@college.harvard.edu

M. A. Christino et al. (eds.), *Psychological Considerations in the Young Athlete*,
Contemporary Pediatric and Adolescent Sports Medicine,
https://doi.org/10.1007/978-3-031-25126-9_2

Introduction

Athletic pursuits may begin early in childhood or adolescence [1] and continue across the lifespan [2]. Athletes, like all humans, commence their pursuits with various genotypic and phenotypic vulnerabilities to stress [3]. Athletic pursuits include adversity, which in its frequent form include daily hassles and stressors but may also rise to highly concerning traumatic events [2]. Stress responses to such adversities across the athletic lifespan may include mental health challenges [2]. Adversity can facilitate the emergence of new strengths, maturity, and resilience, but it can also prompt mental health conditions and concerns, from anxiety presentations to substance use and beyond [2, 4, 5]. This chapter focuses on common mental health challenges observed in athlete populations. We take the perspective that all athletes experience stress and that emergent mental health concerns exist on a continuum from typical to atypical (the latter defined as those which cause distress/impairment) and we are aware that mental health stigma can be a barrier for athletes in seeking adequate supports [6]. For organizational purposes, attention to our primary clinically trained readership, and a belief that clear identification of an athlete complaint is an important factor in successful treatment outcomes [7], this chapter is loosely organized in parallel with the *Diagnostic and Statistical Manual of Mental Disorders, Fifth Edition (DSM-5)*. We leave out some conditions which have not been readily prevalent in athlete populations (e.g., psychotic symptom disorders). Although these cases have been observed [8] and are no doubt important, they are beyond the scope of this chapter. We begin with providing an overview of mood and anxiety presentations common to athletes. We follow with information on obsessive-compulsive presentations. Next, we define and describe traumatic reactions and PTSD presenting in athletes, followed by a brief section on dissociative presentations. We only lightly touch on eating disorder diagnoses, which given their larger prevalence, existent continuum from disordered eating to clinical eating disorders, and relationship to relative energy deficiency syndrome (RED-S) requires its own chapter. Substance use disorders are covered next. We then discuss neurodevelopmental disorders impacting the athletic experience. Suicide and non-suicidal self-injurious behaviors, which may present across primary DSM-5 presentations, are addressed after neurodevelopmental presentations. In the final section of this chapter, we highlight the unique experiences of minority athletes, including black, indigenous, and people of color (BIPOC); lesbian, gay, bisexual, transgender and queer plus (LGBTQ+); and para-athletes. Woven throughout our primary focus areas are case examples from our direct clinical work as well as guidance on best practices for treatment. Indeed, with proper prevention, identification, and mental health support, athletes can reduce their vulnerability to mental health struggles and be more resilient so as to "bounce back" from all kinds of challenges, including their competitive sport environments, injuries, and beyond.

Mood Conditions and Concerns

Incidences of depressive presentations among athletes have been well documented [9]. The prevalence of depression in athletes ranges from 15.6% to 21%, meaning one in five athletes are affected by this mental health condition [9]. Importantly, most of the sources informing these rates are studies conducted using college athlete samples and have not included young or older-age athletes [9]. The etiology of depressive features in athletes is likely a result of combined biopsychosocial factors. For example, it is suggested that elite athletes may be particularly vulnerable to depression prompted by experiences of athletic failures [10] and injuries [9], while depressive features among athletes have also been linked to biological factors, such as vitamin D deficiencies [11]. Depression in athletes has also been associated with burnout [12]. A case of a young adult female presenting with depression is illustrated in Box 2.1.

Major depressive disorder (MDD) includes major depressive episodes (MDEs) that last at least 2 weeks and are separated by at least 2 months [13]. Symptoms of a MDE include but are not limited to a depressed mood, loss of enjoyment or interest in activities, substantial weight gain or loss, sleeping too much or too little, agitation or a mentally sluggish mental or physical state, fatigue, inability to concentrate, and/or suicidal ideation [13]. In the general population, adolescents (ages of 12–17), accounting for 12% of the US population, suffer from MDD [14]. Among those older than 18 years old, approximately 6% experience MDD [14]. Other studies suggest that 17% of the adult US population suffers from MDD [15]. MDD is also more commonly diagnosed in women versus men [14]. Minorities may be at greater risk. For example, those who self-reported having at least two or more racial identities were most likely to experience a MDE [14].

Persistent depressive disorder (PDD) is distinct in its long-lasting nature, including a persistent depressed mood for at least a period of 2 years [15]. Symptoms non-exhaustively include positive and/or negative changes in appetite and sleep, lethargy, decreased self-esteem, and increased sense of hopelessness, as well as difficulties with concentration and decision-making abilities [15]. Approximately 3% of the US population suffers from PDD [15].

Most studies regarding athletes and mental health do not distinguish between MDD and PDD. However, one study found that at least 34% of elite athletes suffer from depression [16]. A study of NCAA athletes reported that 23.7% report clinical levels of symptoms of depression with moderate to severe cases of depressive symptoms accounting for 6.3% of athletes [17], with female athletes 1.84 times more likely to report clinically relevant depressive symptoms than male athletes [17]. Similarly, other research has found that elite male athletes are 53% less likely to report mild to severe symptoms of depression than female high-performance athletes [18]. Notably, there is conflicting research on whether active or retired collegiate athletes suffer from higher rates of depression [19–21].

Seasonal affective disorder (SAD) is characterized as a pattern of depressive symptoms emerging seasonally with onset of Fall or Winter and receding with the advent of Spring or Summer. The suggested etiological factors of SAD include disruptions of the circadian rhythm, melanopsin signaling pathway altering serotonin reuptake, and hypothalamic-pituitary-adrenal pathway. Lifetime prevalence of SAD in US, Canadian, and UK populations has been estimated at approximately 0.5–2.4%. Interestingly, in a sample of first-year collegiate athletes, although just 5% presented with mild or severe depression, a greater 16.2% reported a history of experiencing SAD [22]. Potential risk factors for the development of SAD include being female, being in early adulthood, having a family history of SAD, or living at a northern latitude with less wintertime light exposure.

Although athletes share many of the same risk factors for depression as the general population, such as sleep deprivation, lack of support system, and significant negative life events, athlete-specific risk factors exist [7]. For example, a higher likelihood of developing depression is suggested for athletes who are concussed [23]. Injury, burnout, and overtraining, as well as playing an individual sport, are suggested contributing factors among athletes [10, 23–25].

Box 2.1

A 21-year-old female college field hockey player reported increased symptoms of depression starting the summer before her junior season. She endorsed having a depressed mood most of the day nearly every day, loss of interest in things she used to enjoy, low energy, difficulty falling asleep, poor appetite, and isolating herself from social activities. She stated that her depressive symptoms got worse after the season ended in late November when she no longer had field hockey to look forward to and keep her busy, and her depressive symptoms have worsened to the point where they are now putting a strain on her relationships with her friends, family, and boyfriend.

Bipolar disorders represent a group of persistent and often serious mood disorders involving manic or hypomanic episodes and sometimes followed by depressive episodes [26], as you will see in a case example in Box 2.2. Symptoms of manic episodes in bipolar presentations include but are not limited to feeling extremely elated, irritable, and on edge; feeling wired; diminished need for sleep; lack of appetite; speaking very fast about many different topics; sensation of racing thoughts; excessive multitasking; feeling extremely gifted, important, or all-powerful; and making risky decisions or engaging in poor decision-making (for instance, spending unreasonable amounts of money or having risky sex) [27]. Bipolar presentations can present as bipolar I disorder, bipolar II disorder, or cyclothymia [26]. Bipolar I disorder, which may include the most acute mania symptoms of these three presentations, is characterized by episodes of mania lasting at least 7 days or by manic symptoms requiring immediate hospitalization [27]. Manic episodes are usually followed by periods of depression lasting for at least 2 weeks [27]. Bipolar presentations can also include mixed periods where an individual presents with co-occurring manic and depressive symptoms [27]. Bipolar II disorder is similarly marked by hypomanic and depressive periods, but the manic symptoms are less severe than those of bipolar I disorder [27].

Approximately 1–2% of the general population suffers from bipolar disorders [26]. Although there is limited research on athlete presentations of bipolar disorder [28], it is relevant that the typical onset of bipolar symptoms is in late adolescence or early adulthood, which corresponds developmentally with athletes' peak in physical abilities and when they are competing at the highest levels of their sports [29]. Bipolar disorders are suggested to be highly heritable at approximately 70% [26]. It appears that bipolar disorders also have genetic risk alleles with other disorders. For instance, schizophrenia is more closely genetically linked to bipolar I disorder than bipolar II disorder [26]. Likewise, bipolar II disorder is closely genetically linked to MDD [26]. A notable risk factor for bipolar disorders is childhood trauma and maltreatment and often specifically presents in a form of bipolar disorder that includes suicidal thoughts and attempts [30]. Indeed, young athletes are not necessarily protected from such risks and circumstances.

> **Box 2.2**
> *A 25-year-old female triathlete reported increased emotion dysregulation and difficulties in her work and athletic team environments over the past few months. She reported experiencing episodes of elevated mood, racing thoughts, and distractibility for weeks at a time that interfered with her training as well as her job at a fitness club. She reported she did not go to sleep at all one night because she was working on video edits for an independent project; however, she was not tired the next day. During these episodes, she has been known to talk incessantly and make statements like "I've always known I've been gifted in life … people always are intimidated by me … I walk in the room and people are looking." She reported she also has periods of severe depression that last weeks at a time where she cannot get out of bed, is tearful most of the day, has low energy and fatigue, and has thoughts of killing herself.*

With regard to the treatment of mood disorders, in general, a combination of psychotropic medication management and psychotherapy is recommended [31]. MDD/MDE are commonly treated with antidepressant medications, such as a selective serotonin reuptake inhibitor (SSRI) [32, 33], such as fluoxetine, whereas bipolar presentations often warrant the introduction of a mood stabilizer [34], such as lithium. Although antidepressants can be helpful in some cases in reducing symptoms of a bipolar depressive episode [34], it is important to note that antidepressants should be prescribed with a high degree of caution including clarifying a unipolar depression diagnosis due to risk of an antidepressant-induced manic episode. The physical and psychological impact of psychotropic medication on the high-performing athletes should also be carefully considered at the outset. Concerns, for example, include medications with side effects of sedation that may be detrimental to athletic training and performance [35]. The suitability and effectiveness of psychotherapy treatments for mood disorders depend somewhat on the maintaining factors of an individual's depression, however may include a cognitive behavioral therapy (CBT) approach, including talk therapy which helps the athlete to identify maintaining problem behaviors and cognitive distortions that they may have about themselves, others, the world, or the future. CBT incorporates behavioral interventions such as behavioral activation [36], including physical exercise, and increases in activities that may bring athletes' experiences of mastery and/or pleasure. We have found that in some cases exercise as treatment for athletes with depression can be less useful as a behavioral intervention simply because their training has already led to maxing out the mental health benefits of exercise, so in these cases, we lean more heavily on opportunities to build in greater experiences of mastery and/or pleasure beyond the athletic realm. That said, in our practice, we sometimes see that when an athlete has an injury that removes her or him from sport and pre-injury exercise plans, it can present with a decreased mood. In such cases, coordination of care with a sports medicine physician is key in determining an exercise plan that supports one's mental health while not exacerbating an injury or thwarting recovery. Complementing CBT interventions, in our practices, we have found that a compassion-focused therapy approach can also be helpful to mitigate depressive symptoms among athletes who experience high degrees of self-criticism and shame [37, 38].

Anxiety Conditions and Concerns

Anxiety conditions can significantly impact one's ability to both function and perform athletically [39]; thus, it is important to know how to recognize these presentations in athlete populations and understand their potential deleterious effects. Anxiety is characterized by heightened emotional responses associated with worry, fear, and apprehension in response to a real or perceived threat [40]. Though the feeling of anxiety is often a normal and productive response to a stressor, anxiety can become a condition or concern when it occurs over an extended period of time; when it causes disruptive mental and/or physical symptoms, impairment, and/or distress; and/or when an individual is unable to control this feeling of anxiety [40]. Though often discussed in combination, anxiety can be further divided into subtypes, such as panic disorder, generalized anxiety disorder (GAD), or social anxiety (social phobia) [40]. Each of these conditions is characterized by more specified symptoms, such as a persistent fear of having a panic attack, or apprehension around an object or setting, among other examples [40]. While many athletes will only identify as having one anxiety concern or condition, there is a known co-occurrence between multiple anxiety disorders presenting themselves in the same patient (e.g., GAD simultaneously occurring with a specific phobia and social anxiety), as well as anxiety presenting itself alongside depression or mood concerns [41]. There are many formalized subtypes of anxiety, and a young athlete can also present with symptoms of anxiety that do not meet criteria for a formal anxiety disorder diagnosis.

The estimated rate of anxiety in the general population is 10.6–12%, making it one of the most common mental health conditions [39, 42, 43]. Though the prevalence and determinants of anxiety among athletes follow trends similar to the general population, with rates of anxiety cited to be around 8.6% among elite athletes, athletes experience additional athlete- and sport-specific determinants of anxiety [25, 39]. Studies have shown that female and younger athletes experience higher levels of anxiety conditions, and other studies have shown that career dissatisfaction, sport injury, adverse life events, sport type, conditions such as attention deficit hyperactivity disorder, and fear of failure may influence anxiety presentations in athletes [39, 44–47].

A specific phobia is an intense and irrational fear triggered by an object or situation whereby the individual as an immediate response of extreme distress and avoidance of the object or situation, despite the fact that the fear reaction is greater than what is proportionate when considering the true danger that is encountered [40]. Among athletes, specific phobias related to sport can impair one's ability to perform at practice or competition. For example, a 15-year-old diver who develops a specific phobia of heights after a recent diving injury may find it difficult to dive during their daily training at the pool, and she may spend much of the day leading up to diving practice worrying about diving off a specific diving board. She may, in fact, refuse to dive altogether. Additionally, phobic reactions can present in the context of other mental health concerns, for example, in some cases of disordered eating or a clinical eating disorder [48] where an athlete has a phobic reaction to food or to the idea or actual weight gain [48].

Social anxiety (SA), defined diagnostically as social anxiety disorder (SAD, a.k.a. social phobia), is characterized by fear and often avoidance of and within social situations and settings prompted by concerns they are being or will be negatively evaluated or scrutinized [40]. Often, individuals with social anxiety experience high levels of distress in situations non-exhaustively including when meeting unfamiliar people, having a conversation, eating or drinking with others, giving a performance, or presenting to a group and/or being in a specific social setting (e.g., a classroom, cafeteria, studio, gym, field, performance venue) [40]. Social anxiety disorder may be performance only in nature [40], whereby an athlete has no anxiety interacting with teammates however during competitions experiences high levels of duress. While some levels of performance anxiety are within normal limits and may even be beneficial for performance [49], many athletes will experience these social- or sport-related performance fears as detrimental to sport participation and performance [50]. For team sport athletes or athletes who are engaging with some sort of sport community, SA might make it difficult or impossible to collaborate, train, compete with, or interact with teammates [50]. Impairments to the social nature of sport can cause not only detriments in sport performance (e.g., a basketball player suffering from SA becomes shaky, feels "frozen," and becomes preoccupied with a worry about being judged by other teammates and spectators that she doesn't communicate to a teammate that she is open for a pass, leading to the team collectively missing a potentially important play), but also for sport and team enjoyment. Interacting with teammates in and outside of practice can have many benefits for performance, health, and happiness, but SA can impact an athlete's ability to engage in this important part of sport [51].

While social anxiety is contained to social and performance domains, a young athlete who has generalized anxiety disorder (GAD) will experience anxiety symptoms prompted by excessive anxiety and worry across several life domains, including about a range of topics, events, or activities [40]. This worry is often paired with physical, emotional, and cognitive symptoms, non-exhaustively including increased muscle aches and soreness, irritability, difficulty sleeping, and impaired concentration [40]. In one study, the overall prevalence of GAD among athletes was 22%, and risk factors for the development of GAD were suggested to include sport injury, attention deficit hyperactivity disorder (ADHD), and fear of failure [44]. In the same study, the construct of mental toughness and one's satisfaction in sport were suggested to be negatively related to GAD [44]. As excessive anxiety can undermine athlete health and performance, among athlete populations, attention should be paid to the potential co-occurrence of GAD with other conditions and stressors. Indeed, a young athlete experiencing acute physical and cognitive symptoms of anxiety while performing on the playing field is unlikely to perform to the best of her or his ability. Similarly, an athlete trying to follow an injury recovery plan may not be able to recover as well or efficiently if they are experiencing abnormal levels of fear, anxiety, or worry.

GAD has been characterized by higher levels of trait anxiety [52] and may be chronic and persistent in their course. But why the ongoing worry? On one hand, planning for potential dangers (a.k.a., prevention), as well as distractions and obstacles (a.k.a., problem solving), can be an important part of effective game strategy and gaining a competitive edge. However, we can't plan for every eventuality and that can be hard to tolerate. Some researchers hypothesize that individuals with GAD tend to engage in chronic, ruminative worry when anticipating (whether accurately or inaccurately) unexpected negative events in the future that they fear would provide an abrupt shift, or contrast, to a negative emotional state [51]. This is called the contrast avoidance hypothesis [53]. The irony for this approach is that for the young athlete, this anticipation of future negative events is likely well intended, but highly ineffective. It serves to increase emotional distress and distract from present-moment training and performance. For illustration, an athlete may fear that they will at some point be injured and then become ineffectively preoccupied with worry about that happening in the future. This approach may lead to present-moment performance decrements and not serve the function of reducing risk of future injury or one's future ability to cope with injury when it occurs.

In contrast to the more chronic course that GAD can take, panic disorder is marked by brief, acute, and often disruptive episodes of distressing physical symptoms and an intense fear reaction to those symptoms [40]. For example, an individual with panic disorder might experience shortness of breath, dizziness, numbness, or elevated heart rate, among other symptoms, and a feeling of loss of control or as if they are dying [40]. For an athlete who experiences panic attacks, there can be significant effects on performance, as you will see in a case example in Box 2.3. Athletes who have had panic attacks often then experience anticipatory worry about a future panic attack occurring at any time, and they consequently bring an element of vigilance to the sport environment, which draws them out of the present moment. This worry, in alignment with the contrast avoidance model, may cause athletes to experience a variety of negative emotions, become unable to train effectively, or feel the need to change their training, recovery, or everyday habits in order to avoid another panic attack [53]. A diagnosis of agoraphobia, where an individual avoids going into public to avoid the chances that one would have a panic attack, may be relevant here also [40].

Box 2.3

A 19-year-old male college baseball pitcher reported a recent onset of events on several occasions where he reported he felt sweaty and shaky, with rapid heart rate, breathlessness, and tightness in his chest. He also reported that in the moment he feared he might be having a heart attack. These episodes appear to have an abrupt onset, reach a peak within 10 min, and then gradually subside. He reported these episodes occurred daily over the past few weeks with no precipitant he could easily identify. Since the onset of these symptoms, he has developed a fear of going to baseball practice because he is afraid he will have one of these episodes while on the mound and will not know what to do. He has consequently started avoiding going to the field for extra pitching sessions and has even started missing some team practices to avoid the possibility of him experiencing a panic attack.

Beyond these common DSM-5 presentations of anxiety, there are anxiety presentations specific to the sport and athlete experience that are described in the literature. Sports-related performance anxiety occurs when an athlete experiences competitive athletic situations as threats, often responding to these threats or fears with worry and anxiety [50]. Sports-related anxiety can occur in the context of a clinical-level anxiety disorder or it can exist independent from this and specific to an athletic setting or situation [50]. Sports-related anxiety is most common among young female athletes, with potential influencing factors being such things as achievement goals, societal pressures, experience, coping skills, difficulty of sport routine, underlying anxiety traits, disordered eating, level of competition, performance setting, and self-confidence [50]. A related concern is competition anxiety, whereby an athlete experiences fear and worry around performing in athletic competition or in other achievement areas, such as music, academics, and business [54–56]. Competition anxiety can lead to decrements in sport performance, enjoyment, and participation [54]. While most athletes will experience some degree of nerves surrounding high-level competition, those experiencing sports-related performance anxiety or competitive anxiety are more likely to prematurely end sport participation and experience greater negative impacts in performance [54].

Despite the large prevalence and number of risk factors for anxiety, treatment for anxiety has not been universalized or historically effective, as different treatments work differently for different individuals, and many individuals often require a combination of treatment modalities [57]. Athletes, as an example, may benefit from a treatment that is tailored to sport-specific stressors, in comparison to other individuals in the general population. The DSM-5 proposes a variety of recommendations to manage or treat anxiety concerns, such as exercise, the use of pharmacological treatments, and psychotherapy, but most often, individuals seeking treatment for anxiety concerns undergo a process of trial-and-error, testing out these recommendations and others [40]. Cognitive behavioral therapy (CBT) is generally a widely accepted, researched, and evidence-based treatment for generalized and social anxiety concerns [58]. CBT enacts methods to change excessive worries associated with anxiety into normal worries through functional analysis, psychoeducation, emotional and behavioral experimentation, and cognitive work [58]. A well-understood maintaining factor in anxiety is avoidance of the feared stimuli, whether an object, situation, or experience [59]. Box 2.4 illustrates this process in a case example of a young athlete demonstrating avoidance of a feared experience and feared outcome. CBT exposure therapy approaches may be more appropriate for specific phobias and panic attacks as they support athletes in blocking avoidant responses to encounter and then habituate to feared stimuli, so they can train and compete to their fullest potential.

Box 2.4

A 14-year-old male soccer player reports fear when in a situation where he must head the soccer ball in practices and games following a recent concussion. This fear has subsequently led him to engage in avoidance behaviors, including skipping practices to not encounter this feared situation. During recent games, whenever the soccer ball is in the air, he has experienced an elevated heart rate, momentary shortness of breath, and feeling light-headed. In his last soccer game, his fear led him to back off the ball which resulted in the ball picked off by the other team. Because he does not engage in heading the ball, he does not get to experience doing so without injury; thus, he continues to fear this situation and avoid it.

Obsessive-Compulsive and Related Presentations

Specific qualities of sport may mask mental health conditions or produce barriers to seeking proper treatment among some young athletes. This can be the case for presentations obsessive-compulsive disorder (OCD) and related presentations in young athletes, where diagnosis and proper clinical care frequently occur later in their development and athletic careers if at all. OCD may include or be associated with unhealthy traits of competitiveness, perfectionism, or secrecy [60–62] that are masked and difficult to differentiate from healthy competitiveness and sports excellence. For example, an athlete may experience body image preoccupation that is both distressing and preoccupying; however, he and those around him may inaccurately believe that this focus is within normal range for someone who uses their body to perform athletically at a high level. He may therefore not identify and seek treatment for what is actually a body dysmorphic disorder (BDD) [60].

Clinicians may encounter the presence of OCD, BDD, and/or compulsive exercise among athletes. Sport activities and athletics, which require high levels of training, focus, and commitment, may increase the vulnerability of developing obsessive-compulsive presentations in higher-risk individuals [63]. OCD is characterized by the presence of obsessions, compulsions, or both [40]. Obsessions are considered recurrent, persistent thoughts, urges, or impulses that often cause anxiety and distress in an individual, as they are typically intrusive and unwanted [40], and the affected individual often makes ineffective efforts to ignore or suppress these obsessions [40]. Compulsions are repetitive behaviors that an individual feels driven to perform as a response to an obsession, and typically, these behaviors or mental acts are an attempt to reduce distress [40]. These mental or behavioral compulsions, which are often irrational and ineffective methods of preventing the feared emotion or event, can often become debilitating [40]. OCD impacts about 2.3% of adults in the general population, and studies show that prevalence may be about 5.3% among college athletes [60, 62]. OCD can co-occur with other mental health concerns, such as depression [64]. The majority of these reported college athletes were undiagnosed and were not receiving care [60]. Clinicians should be aware of the higher prevalence of OCD among athletes, as well as its tendency to be underdiagnosed and untreated.

OCD is often conceptualized through a model of experiential avoidance and a need for control. Experiential avoidance is characterized by an unwillingness to experience or endure uncomfortable internal stimuli (a.k.a., sensory, cognitive, or emotional obsessions), and subsequent behaviors (a.k.a., compulsions) that seek to avoid these uncomfortable stimuli, even if avoidance results in negative consequences for the individual [65]. In many cases, higher experiential avoidance is associated with, and can potentially predict, increased severity of obsessive and/or compulsive symptoms [66]. An athlete's lack of willingness or seeming inability to experience unpleasant internal experiences may result in greater obsessional symptoms when compared to those who are able to approach these unpleasant experiences [66].

Among athlete populations, presentations of obsessive and compulsive behavior might appear as rituals, superstitions, or routines around athletic performance. In one example, an Olympic soccer player has a pregame ritual of placing her shin pads in a repetitive manner from bottom-to-top [67]. When this athlete places the shin pads from top-to-bottom, she does not feel as if she is ready to perform at her best [67]. With this ritual, the athlete is investing time and energy into a regulated behavior that ultimately helps her to minimize anxiety, increase motivation, and feel more in control. Though this ritual does not appear to have any direct function or relationship with the soccer player's athletic performance, the ritual may be acting as a regulatory mechanism, which subsequently helps to improve performance [67].

BDD, another obsessive-compulsive and related disorder in the DSM-5, is defined by an individual's obsession with one or more apparent flaws in his or her physical appearance, whether or not this flaw or these flaws are visible to others [40]. An individual with BDD will often develop repetitive behaviors or compulsions, such as checking one's appearance in a mirror, that simultaneously cause distress or impairment in daily life [40]. Among athlete populations, prevalence of distorted body image, in conjunction with disordered eating and unhealthy dieting, ranges from 12% to 57% [68], and prevalence of specific BDD in the general population ranges from 0.7% to 2.4% [69].

BDD symptoms are observed to be co-occurring alongside disordered eating or clinical eating disorders, as is sometimes seen in ballet dancers [70], as in the example in Box 2.5.

Box 2.5

A 15-year-old female ballet dancer presents with anorexia nervosa, OCD, and BDD. Regarding BDD, she feels clear on a very specific ballerina body ideal that she doesn't feel she has. She reports that when in the locker room changing into clothes for ballet class and during ballet classes, she finds herself checking and re-checking her body and leotard placement on her body in the mirrors. This has become so preoccupying that she often has difficulty attending to the teacher's class instructions. She also finds that despite her efforts to check her body, she never feels satisfied that her body is "okay." She will also suck in her stomach tightly and hold her hands tightly around her waist and measure the distance between her hands on the circumference of her waist to ensure the distance has not gotten wider. She will stare in the mirror as she does this. This behavior has made some of her classmates uncomfortable and some are distancing themselves from her. She reports high levels of distress thinking that she is obese, even though her BMI is on the low end of normal range. When clinicians and parents provide reality-based feedback to help her check her thinking, she reports that she does not believe them and feels they are lying to her.

In a very different athlete group, powerlifters, such as our case example in Box 2.6, and weightlifters have been observed to develop obsessive-compulsive dietary and training schedules for the purposes of maintaining a specific, idealized physique and degree of muscle mass (with or without the assistance of steroids) [71]. Muscle dysmorphia, prompted by an individual's preoccupying beliefs that their muscularity is lacking and related behaviors of body checking and maladaptive efforts to increase muscle mass, has been explored as a form of and/or related to BDD in such athlete populations [72]. Other athletes may present with BDD and simultaneously develop a comorbid substance use disorder in the process of using substances to enhance the self-identified flaws in their appearance.

> **Box 2.6**
> *A 20-year-old female powerlifter reported experiencing muscle dysmorphia, where she believes she is inadequately muscular compared to her competitors, and therefore obsessively checks her appearance in the mirror, compares her appearance to photos of others, or organizes her dietary and training patterns.*

Compulsive exercise is not listed as a DSM-5 disorder or specifically in the OCD category; however, this behavior has been suggested to be co-occurring in the context of several diagnostic presentations and may non-exhaustively function behaviorally as one of the following: obsessive-compulsive, a body or weight manipulation strategy (i.e., in the context of an eating disorder), a non-suicidal self-injurious behavior, or an addiction [73].

Best practice for the treatment of obsessive-compulsive and related disorders includes CBT treatment, which utilizes an Exposure and Response Prevention (ERP) approach [74], as well as psychopharmacology. ERP focuses on having the individual encounter their fear while not acting on urges to engage in the ritual or compulsion typically used to mitigate the emotional distress of the obsession [74].

Trauma- and Stressor-Related Concerns and Relationship to Athletic Injury

An exploration of athlete mental health concerns is not complete without a discussion of acute stress and trauma reactions. Athletes, within and outside of their athletic environments, may encounter a range of experiences from the highly stressful to the life-threatening, and an athlete's reaction to a stressful or traumatic event can vary based on several factors. The DSM-5 organizes trauma- and stressor-related concerns into categories of reactive attachment disorder, disinhibited social engagement disorder, post-traumatic stress disorder (PTSD), acute stress disorder (ASD), adjustment disorders (ADs), and other specified trauma- or stressor-related disorder [40]. Although there will inevitably be cases of athletes with the first two categories, we focus on PTSD, ASD, ADs, and other specified trauma- or stressor-related disorders that we have anecdotally identified as highly relevant to athletes.

An athlete can meet criteria for PTSD in cases where she or her has been directly exposed to, witnessed, or heard about someone close to her or him experiencing at least one event that is life-threatening, involving being seriously injured, or involving sexual violence or she or he has experienced repeated or extreme exposure to aversive details of traumatic events. Symptoms of PTSD include intrusive distressing memories of the event, recurrent distressing dreams about the event, dissociative experiences where the individual feels as if they are reliving the event, psychological distress at and marked physiological reactions to internal and external reminders of the event, as well as avoidance of things associated with the event, onset of negative cognitions and mood, and increased arousal ("hyperarousal") and reactivity to things associated with the event [40]. A diagnosis of PTSD can be given if these symptoms are present for greater than 1 month and can be accompanied by dissociative features, including symptoms of depersonalization and/or derealization [40]. In a systematic review of PTSD in primary care settings, the median point prevalence of PTSD across included studies was found to be 12.5% [75]. In some athlete populations, prevalence of PTSD is cited to range from 13% to 25% [76].

PTSD symptoms can develop for many athletes in the context of injury. This is particularly true for injuries occurring due to high-impact or during a high-stakes moment. Box 2.7 provides an example of PTSD symptoms emerging following a high-impact injury. One small study examining young male and female athletes following anterior cruciate ligament (ACL) rupture found that many had symptoms of PTSD, including avoidance (87.5%), intrusive memories (83/3%), and hyperarousal (75%) with severity of these symptoms being higher for older than younger adolescents, and higher levels of emotional distress were reported by females versus male counterparts [77]. Higher levels of PTSD symptoms have been observed by self-report in athletes within 13 days post-concussion, suggesting a relationship between head injury and PTSD; however, given that these symptoms were measured within a month, these athletes at the time of measurement fell into the category of ASD [78].

Box 2.7
A 16-year-old female ski racer reported increased emotional distress in the months following a ski accident in which she crashed into a tree and broke her leg, requiring her to be taken by med flight to undergo emergency surgery. Since the accident, she has endorsed decreased interest in activities, frequent episodes of overwhelming sadness and anxiety, and difficulty concentrating. She is unable to recall key elements of the trauma and finds herself thinking about the accident often during the day as well as having frequent nightmares, intrusive images, and flashbacks where she is re-experiencing the accident. She has also been engaging in more frequent and severe risky behaviors like driving 60 mph in a 30 mph zone, having the urge to drive off the road into a tree, and drinking alone.

Acute stress disorder (ASD) presents with the same symptoms of intrusion, negative mood, dissociation, avoidance, and/or arousal as seen with PTSD; however, the presentation of these symptoms occur for at least 3 days and within 1 month of the exposure to a traumatic event. Mental health treatment and social support in the ASD phase of an injury response can prevent the later development of PTSD [79].

Symptoms of adjustment disorders (ADs) are particularly common among athletes, as they often are required to make social and emotional adjustments to injury, changes in team and coaches, retirement, and moves across the country. Criteria for ADs include that symptoms occur within 3 months of the stressor and that there is impairment in important areas of functioning and distress is marked and out of greater proportion than the intensity and severity of the stressor [40]. This adjustment-related stress reaction can present with various combinations of disturbance of emotions, disturbance of conduct, depressed mood, and/or anxiety [40].

Other trauma- or stressor-related concerns can also occur among athletes related to the specificities of their sport or performance context. Athletes who report training experiences within an invalidating environment or ongoing abusive coaching experiences across an athlete's training and development can be traumatic in nature and prompt the development of PTSD symptoms [76]. Abusive training environments and coaching practices have been anecdotally documented both in mainstream press [80] and in peer-reviewed literature [81, 82]. Box 2.8 illustrates a case where abuse by a coach led to distressing psychopathology for a young adult skater. Such negative interactions can include shaming, body shaming [83], and online public shaming [84] and have been linked to trauma and dissociative features in non-clinical athlete and dancer populations [85]. The degree of impact can vary depending on the degree of public exposure; the intensity, frequency, or chronicity of the injury; or characteristics of the athlete, among other factors. One 2020 study identified that online public shaming of professional athletes was gendered, with a focus on the objectification of women and the promotion of hyper-masculinity among men [84]. Another stressor that can present for some athletes is that of moral injury [86], whereby the athlete has engaged in behavior aimed at winning that may cross his or her own value system and the value system he or she was raised within [86].

Box 2.8

An 18-year-old female transitioning out of figure skating reported significant levels of anxiety, perfectionism, and emotional distress related to a long history of emotional abuse by her coach. She reported that as a youth, she was frequently called names by her coach such as "elephant" and "fatty" and was told that she would never succeed as a figure skater unless she lost a significant amount of weight. Throughout her skating career, she had a long history of disordered eating including restriction, binge, and purge behaviors. She has always been fixated on achievement as well as approval from her coach and reported she will go to great lengths to meet those expectations. Now that her skating career has ended, these perfectionistic tendencies are resurfacing in her academic and social expectations at her college. She considers anything less than an A to be a failure and anything less than the "top sorority" to be not good enough. She experiences significant emotional distress when she feels she has not met her expectations and responds to these perceived "failures" by further controlling her eating behaviors as well as becoming very rigid in other aspects of her academic and social life.

Athletes have also been examined for perceived stress and traumatic symptoms at the end of their athletic career, and those who experienced an unsupportive career termination endorsed more symptoms of traumatic distress compared to athletes who experienced supportive endings to their career [87]. The nature of combined early-specialization, high athletic identity, and major lifestyle change that characterizes retirement for some athletes can sometimes present as a persistent complex bereavement disorder, which is a condition noted for further study in the DSM-5 [87].

Several treatments for PTSD exist, although treatment is not one-size-fits-all. Within the CBT tradition, the dominant treatments involve exposure to counter avoidance of the feared stimuli associated with a past trauma and emotional and cognitive processing of that trauma. A predominant treatment for PTSD among children and adolescents is Trauma-Focused CBT (TF-CBT) [88]. An adult adaptation of this model is Cognitive Processing Therapy (CPT) [89]. Another well-researched CBT-based trauma treatment is Prolonged Exposure (ED). Eye Movement Rapid Desensitization (EMDR) also has an evidence base for reducing PTSD symptoms [90]. It is important to carefully assess that an individual meets full criterion for a PTSD diagnosis before embarking on any of these treatments.

Dissociative Experiences in Athletic Pursuits

Many researchers and theorists consider dissociative features on a continuum ranging from a momentary lapse in attention to a depersonalization/derealization disorder. We will focus our discussion of dissociative experiences on two presentations most common to athlete populations: depersonalization and derealization. Both involve experiences that lie outside of reality and characterized by "detachment" that are not better explained by the effects of a substance or a physical condition. Depersonalization involves detachment from oneself with a feeling of being outside of and an observer of oneself, including one's emotions, sensations, thoughts, and behaviors [40]. Athletes can present reporting an experience of feeling physically or emotionally "numb." Derealization involves more of a feeling of perceptual distortion occurring outside of themselves in their environment [40]. For example, an athlete reporting they felt during a game a sense of their surrounding being distorted or unreal in some way, as if in a "fog" or "wobbly," that cannot be explained by a physical condition.

Dissociative processes can be particularly problematic, and sometimes dangerous, in the context of athletic training and performance. In more recent media following the 2020 Olympic Games, the general population has been exposed to the phenomenon of the "twisties" among high-level athletes, which may be a result of depersonalization, derealization, or both following psychic trauma or PTSD [91]. With sports disciplines that require large amounts of coordination skills, self- and body-awareness, and emotional processing, "twisties"—or a sense of a detachment from oneself or one's surroundings, like that of depersonalization and derealization—can be extremely dangerous, as an athlete may not be able to effectively execute their coordination skills when they detach from themself or their surroundings [91]. For example, a 14-year-old gymnast who is predisposed to depersonalization and derealization following a traumatic event may be at increased risk of injury or failure during athletic performance when he is trying to vault into the air. In general, when an athlete becomes detached from their emotions or from their environment during a training session or competition, they become more vulnerable to physical and psychological harm.

Another feature of dissociation is dissociation from emotional experiencing. This occurs when an individual consciously or unconsciously disconnects from a strongly valanced emotional experience or affective state as a coping or emotion regulation strategy. Some researchers have identified a common factor of experiential avoidance underlying the development of different mental and behavioral concerns and illnesses [92], including anxiety, as we outlined earlier, as well as addictive behaviors [93]. Interventions created for this teach patients to stay connected with their emotions and their surroundings while being exposed to greater and greater intensity of aversive experiences as a way of building tolerance.

Dissociative processes are not all maladaptive. In the context of traumatic experiences, some individuals adaptively and involuntarily disconnect from the trauma experience, and this can have some protective results [94]. One's ability to "turn off" certain perceptions and experiences to hyper-focus on other in the moment tasks may be an important part of athletic mental performance. For example, dissociative strategies have been observed in runners, and significantly so for less experienced runners, to cope when engaging in more challenging runs [95], although these authors did not suggest the degree to which such processes are helpful versus problematic.

Treatments for maladaptive dissociative responses would focus on identifying with emotions and sensory information in the body, employing anti-dissociation skills, and connecting with and exposing oneself to emotional experiences while avoiding engaging in urges to avoid or escape that experience, so as to learn and practice new ways of emotional experience [94].

Feeding and Eating Conditions

We are clear that the prevalence of eating disorders (EDs) in athletes is higher than in that of the general population [96]. In our clinics, eating disorders are a frequently occurring concern which often sadly co-occurs with injury. Given the high incidence of EDs in athletes, complicating body image issues, influences of sport culture and the sporting environment, and overlap with RED-S symptoms, ED conditions as they relate to the young athlete require their own chapter. We aim to simply introduce DSM-5 clinical ED presentations occurring in athlete populations here. These include avoidant/restrictive food intake disorder (ARFID), anorexia nervosa (AN), bulimia nervosa (BN), and binge-eating disorder (BED).

Avoidant/restrictive food intake disorder (ARFID) is included here to attend to the fact that a young athlete can have highly avoidant ("picky") or restrictive eating due to sensory aversions to food, fear of aversive consequences to eating (e.g., fear of nausea after eating), or disinterest in food, without having a drive for thinness in their clinical picture, which can lead to poor nutritional intake and low-energy availability status and compromise their health and performance, including development of RED-S symptoms. Although there are no rates available for ARFID prevalence among young athletes, one specific 12-year-old youth athlete case presented to our clinic following her bone stress injury and physical workup revealed nutritional deficiencies, including scurvy, and recognition that she was falling off her normal growth curve. She denied any desire to be at low weight and rather had a limited range of foods, mostly plain pasta, that she would eat. She was flagged for ARFID. In these cases, given specialized CBT for ARFID (CBT-AR) [97] treatment is indicated, we recommend a referral to a specialist in this approach. Prevalence rates for ARFID are not fully established and are wide in range [98]. There has been only one study of prevalence rates in a community school-based sample in Switzerland that noted a point prevalence of 3.2% [99].

Anorexia nervosa (AN) includes a criteria of significantly low weight, extreme fear of weight gain or change in body shape, and body image disturbance often accompanied by poor insight into the seriousness of consequences of low body weight [40]. We often see cases of anorexia athletica [100], which is common among athletes participating in lean and aesthetic sports.

Bulimia nervosa (BN) is identified by a repeated pattern of binge-eating episodes that involve consuming a large amount of food in a brief window of time, followed by efforts of compensate (a.k.a. "purge" via engagement in vomiting, laxative abuse, overexercise, extended restriction of food, or diuretics, among other strategies) for the binge-eating episode in an attempt to avoid weight gain [40]. The athlete in this case often has some problems with a self-esteem highly dependent on body image and the binge-purge cycle must occur at a minimum for at least one time per week for at least 3 months to meet criteria [40].

Binge-eating disorder (BED)'s core criteria is the same as the binge eating episode seen in BN, however individuals with BED to not engage in compensatory behavior following a binge [40]. Binges occur at least weekly for at least 3 months, and it is common for individuals to feel out of control, ashamed, and/or disgusted by their binge eating, as is also common in BN [40]. Anecdotally, we have seen binge-eating episodes in athletes when they are winding down from an evening performance and games.

For an in-depth study of eating disorders and body image issues presenting in athletes, and their relationship to RED-S, including prevalence rates and treatments, please refer to Chap. 3.

Neurodevelopmental Conditions

Neurodevelopmental conditions, such as autism spectrum disorder (ASD) and learning disorders (LDs), can significantly impact the health and performance of athletes—interestingly, in both positive and negative ways [101]. Though many of the symptoms that characterize these different conditions can impair one's ability to perform athletically and should therefore be treated in order to maximize the athlete's potential, sport has also been found to be extremely beneficial tool for some individuals seeking behavioral, psychosocial, or physical improvement of symptoms in conditions like ASD and attention deficit hyperactivity disorder (ADHD) [102]. Typically developing at a young age, neurodevelopmental conditions are defined by deficits that produce impairments of functioning [40]. ASD, ADHD, intellectual disability (ID), communication disorders, neurodevelopmental motor disorders, and specific LDs all fall under the classification of neurodevelopmental conditions [103]. Neurodevelopmental conditions have a high rate of comorbidity with other disorders and conditions, and many can also be associated with related genetic disorders or environmental factors [103].

Though these conditions most often affect one's ability to develop, learn, participate in social life, and conduct cognitive functions, the effects of these conditions also bleed into one's ability to perform on the playing field, court, and rink [104]. Despite the pervasiveness of neurodevelopmental conditions and their prevalence among athlete populations, there exists limited evidence on the presence and impact of these conditions on athletes, likely due to the unfortunately common assumption that mental disorders and concerns are less common among athletes compared to the general population [105]. Most literature focuses on children and young athletes, because though these conditions do typically arise in early development, there is a common misconception that individuals and athletes are not impacted by these conditions later in life [104]. By examining each of the individual neurodevelopmental conditions and understanding their impact both for the life of the individual and for their sport-specific experience, it is clear this is not the case.

Attention deficit hyperactivity disorder (ADHD) is a neurodevelopmental disorder characterized by behavioral concerns with hyperactivity, impulsivity, and/or inattention, causing impairment or negative effects in one's daily life [40]. Like many other neurodevelopmental conditions, ADHD exists on a spectrum, with individuals experiencing different degrees of symptoms and behaviors. Individuals with ADHD are also at increased risk of comorbid psychological concerns, such as anxiety disorders, depression, and other learning and neurodevelopmental conditions [105]. Though ADHD incidence is cited between 3% and 10% among American children, evidence suggests that the percentage is higher among athletes, as sport participation is often used as a coping mechanism for symptoms of ADHD, both emotionally and physically [105]. For example, an athlete who often experiences feelings of hyperactivity may find it helpful to run during soccer practice, or another athlete who struggles with impulsivity may be able to make efficient decisions on the playing field.

However, because ADHD may often have negative impacts on an athlete's ability to function socially, athletically, academically, and in their daily life, there have been an increasing number of articles pointing toward both psychosocial interventions and medications tailored toward the athlete [104]. Because the invasive symptoms of ADHD can be treated by both stimulant and nonstimulant medications, it is crucial to consider an athlete's level of participation in sport and the medications allowed by the athlete's sports league or organization guidelines [105]. Doing so will allow the athlete to maximize treatment of their symptoms, avoid banned substances, and capitalize on relative symptomatology that might be advantageous during athletic play (e.g., timing the administration of medication intake for athlete participating in a competition where spontaneity and impulsive movements are helpful for their sport) [105]. Substance and stimulant abuse concerns should be factored into treatments for ADHD in athletes, but if the measures are taken to understand the athlete's case, medical history, symptomatology, and effects of ADHD fully, treatments can be prescribed safely on an individual basis in order to aid both the athlete's health and their sport performance. However, psychosocial and behavioral treatments and interventions should not be undervalued for athletes in comparison to pharmacological treatments [104].

Autism spectrum disorder (ASD) is a developmental condition that often poses challenges to social, behavioral, and communicative functioning [40]. Like ADHD, ASD exists on a spectrum, and affected individuals experience a wide variety and degree of symptoms [40]. For example, many individuals with ASD struggle with communication, social, and behavioral skills and may have trouble understanding others' feelings or interactions, adapting to changes in routine, and maintaining eye contact, among many other varying symptoms [106]. Approximately 1 in 59 children is diagnosed with ASD, and the prevalence among athlete-specific populations is unknown [107]. Often, athletic participation can help to improve psychological, cognitive, or behavioral functioning in athletes with ASD, though it may also be difficult for athletes with ASD to participate or excel in sport due to difficulty communicating with coaches and teammates or other symptoms that may translate to the playing field [108]. Therefore, as necessary, accommodations, modifications, and treatment should be sought out for athletes with ASD to support them in their athletic and daily endeavors.

Learning disorders (LDs) are developmental conditions characterized by difficulty with information processing and learning, which often prevents individuals from effectively learning and using skills and information [40]. Though there are many different types of LDs, the DSM-5 estimates the prevalence of deficits in reading to be about 4–9% in the general population, and 3–7% in mathematics [40]. When thinking about LDs, one might imagine symptoms of difficulty learning a topic in a classroom or being unable to learn how to write or do math. However, LDs may also pose struggles on the athletic field if athletes find it difficult or are unable to learn and absorb skills and information necessary for the sport. Many athletes with LDs may not participate in sport or might face negative repercussions in their self-esteem or confidence on the playing field if they are not properly supported [109]. Despite these direct implications of LDs on sport performance, it continues to be an understudied intersection in sports medicine, and one that should be further explored to properly encourage these athletes toward participation and success.

For athletes with neurodevelopmental conditions, concussions are of a higher concern, as these athletes are at a higher risk of developing concussions and taking longer to recover from concussions [110]. Though minimal literature exists examining the relationship between neurodevelopmental conditions and athletic performance more generally, there is a growing body of literature seeking to understand the relationship between concussion incidence and neurodevelopmental conditions. In one study, it was found that individuals with neurodevelopmental conditions, irrespective of sex, were at increased risk of one or multiple concussions, and when accounting for concussion history, male athletes with ADHD and LDs were at greater risk [110]. In another study, athletes with ADHD and with LDs were found to report greater numbers of concussions [111]. Because concussions and many neurodevelopmental conditions, such as ADHD, involve memory, attention, and concentration, these conditions are known to impact both risk of and recovery from concussions [105]. As concussions significantly impair not only an athlete's ability to perform athletically but also their ability to perform cognitively, it is important to view these neurodevelopmental conditions as risk factors for concussions, in addition to the understanding of concussions as a stand-alone issue impacting athletes [110]. Box 2.9 provides a case example from our clinic of a young adult who experienced successive concussions that impacted her ability to engage in activities of daily living.

Box 2.9
A 20-year-old runner with history of three concussions over the past 2 years reported persistent symptoms of headache, balance issues, strained eyes, poor concentration, anxiety, depressed mood, and tearfulness. She stated that before the concussions, she was training for a half marathon and was very active and happy but does report always having been a slightly anxious person. She described that since her most recent concussion, her mood has been significantly anxious and depressed and that it has been hard for her to get up in the morning or "put effort into anything." She reported she has been isolating herself because of this, which has seemed to worsen her mood.

Substance-Related Concerns

Substance use in athletes can serve many functions, from relaxation to social connection to emotional avoidance to (perceived) performance enhancement. While one athlete may use one substance to connect socially with teammates outside of practice, another athlete may be using a substance to perform better during their next game, or to improve their symptoms from a co-occurring condition or concern, such as depression. Among elite athletes, the main recreational motivations for using substances include socialization, recreational pleasure, self-treatment strategies, and increases in alertness, energy, or self-confidence [112–114]. There is also a high performance-enhancing motivation, as some substances will increase strength, power, and endurance, support better focus or recovery, or improve specific sport skills and traits, such as aggression for a combat sport [112, 114].

Substance use can involve the use of illegal or banned substances as well as legal substances and is generally characterized by social, recreational, or episodic engagement with substances on occasion, without serious or harmful problems [115]. However, there is a difference between substance use and substance misuse, as well as the characterization of a substance use disorder or concern. Substance misuse is defined as the use of substances, but in a way in which they are not supposed to be used or in a manner that could be dangerous to the individual or others [116]. Misuse of substances does not necessarily characterize a disorder. Substance use disorders or concerns are problematic patterns of using one or multiple substances, resulting in daily life impairment or distress [117]. When substance use develops into a substance use disorder, there tends to be significant impacts on one's health, social relationships, work, school, and/or athletic performance.

If substance use exists on a continuum from recreational use, to misuse, to the development of substance use disorders, one might understand substance use on a scale of both prevalence (occasional or social vs. heavy or harmful) and symptomatology (no harmful symptoms due to experimentation with recreational substances vs. hazardous or dangerous symptoms associated with risky use of substances) [112]. For athletes, common longitudinal factors associated with substance use and misuse are cited to include "(1) sport context and culture (e.g., normative beliefs about heavy peer drinking or illicit drug use); (2) situational temptation (e.g., availability of alcohol or other drugs); (3) permissive attitudes among athletes, coaches and parents; (4) sensation-seeking personality; and (5) male sex" [75, [81–83]. Cross-sectional factors are cited to include "(1) current use of performance enhancing substances or tobacco; (2) identification as lesbian, gay, bisexual or transgender; (3) party lifestyle or drinking game participation; (4) overestimating peer use; (5) achievement orientation; (6) lower use of protective measures (e.g., avoiding serious intoxication, using a designated driver); (7) leadership position; (8) fraternity/sorority membership; (9) problem gambling; and (10) injury" [75].

Among athlete populations, rates of substance abuse and substance abuse disorders differ by sport and substance type, but are largely similar to the general population, if not lower in prevalence [112]. Substance use disorders may be more common in retired athletes as opposed to active athletes [112]. In one literature review, it was found that US collegiate athletes engaged in lower annual use of many substances, including alcohol, cigarettes, marijuana, amphetamines, AAS, cocaine, ecstasy, and lysergic acid diethylamide, than nonathletes, but some athletes in certain sports use and misuse some substances (such as alcohol, cannabis, nicotine, and prescribed stimulants/opioid pain medications) at increased rates [112]. Exner and colleagues' [118] narrative review of psychotropic substance use among elite athletes found that this group's predominant use was of alcohol, stimulants, (prescription) opioids, nicotine, and cannabis [118]. In both the general population and in elite athletes, alcohol, caffeine, nicotine, cannabis, and stimulants are the most frequently used and misused [112]. However, because elite athletes experience the unique pressure to perform at high levels compared to those in the general population who are not competing athletically, there may be a greater pressure to use, and subsequently misuse, performance-enhancing substances such as anabolic androgenic agents and stimulants. Still, there is a variation in both prevalence and impact depending on the specific type of substance and its usage.

Alcohol use, and binge drinking more specifically, is an identified concern among athlete populations, such as in our case example in Box 2.10. Alcohol use prior to competition or training may reduce anxiety or boost self-confidence, but it also might increase the prevalence of dehydration, insomnia, injury, accidents, hangovers, lateness, reduced metabolic recovery/glycogen resynthesis, and impaired psychomotor skills and thermoregulation [75]. In the long term, alcohol use can also contribute to slower recovery times, weight gain, higher injury rates, and academic underperformance that could contribute to athletic eligibility among specific populations of student-athletes [75]. Though athletes often perceive they may benefit from the use of alcohol if they struggle to feel comfortable and confident while interacting with their teammates, they also put themselves at risk when they are running down the field with impaired thermoregulation of their body temperature or are generally at greater risk of injury. Overall, alcohol negatively impacts performance, particularly aerobic performance, but continues to be widespread among athlete populations [119].

Box 2.10
A 17-year-old female hockey player reported anxiety and depressive symptoms in the context of hockey including not connecting with other girls on team, having issues with the coach, and experiencing stress about college recruitment. She recently revealed that she has been drinking five to six beers every night for over a year to help her fall asleep. She reported she frequently drinks alone to "take the edge off" and distract herself when she is having negative thoughts and emotions.

Among both elite athletes and nonathletes, cannabis containing primarily tetra-hydrocannabinol (THC) is the most widely used substance, though elite athletes do tend to use cannabis less in comparison [112, 120]. In 2018, self-reported use of cannabis among US collegiate athletes was about 25%, and prevalence of synthetic cannabis use has also increased [120]. Cannabis can produce positive effects such as reduced anxiety, in addition to improved sleep and reduced pain, but it can also inhibit an athlete's ability to react quickly, properly maintain a lower heart rate and blood pressure, remain motivated to compete, and maintain coordination of their body [112]. For many athletes, the improved reaction time, memory, energy, and concentration that often come with stimulant use can sound appealing, but in larger doses, stimulants can often produce side effects such as anxiety and insomnia that make it difficult to perform at one's best [112].

The literature and discourse regarding nicotine use among athletes is mixed and controversial. The World Anti-Doping Agency (WADA) does not currently prohibit nicotine use in sport. Nicotine has been observed to enhance anaerobic performance in nicotine-naive individuals [121, 122]. Nicotine products range from cigarettes, e-cigarettes, snus, chewing tobacco, and gum, among others. Use is observed to be widespread among "team/strength" sports, including ice hockey, bobsleigh, wrestling, gymnastics, skiing, rugby, and America football, with Mündel's 2017 review noting that 25–50% of such athletes used nicotine in competition [123]. Electronic nicotine delivery systems (ENDS), also known as vaping or e-cigarettes, have gained increased use among athletes and have concerning potential consequences to health and athletic performance. In 2019, it was estimated by the NCAA that only 8% of athletes used ENDS products [112]. One study found that youth athletes in the sports of softball, baseball, and wrestling were at higher risk of ENDS use and that sport participation did not protect athletes from using ENDS [124]. Consequences of ENDS use to the cardiovascular [125] and pulmonary [126] systems have been noted, including risk concern for serious to lethal pulmonary injury [127]. Decrements to athletic recovery processes, including sleep and recovery from injury, have also been hypothesized [128].

Though stimulants are often used to treat athletes with ADHD and/or related conditions, one review argues for a number of considerations prior to the administration of stimulants to athletes, including the likelihood of performance enhancement following stimulant use, the potential dangerous side effects of stimulant use, policies and regulations of sports organizations and governing bodies, poor inter-rater reliability of ADHD diagnosis in relation to therapeutic use, and the psychiatric treatment of diagnosed mental illness [129]. Given the potential dangerous side effects, stimulants are not generally recommended for athletes [129], but there is still a high prevalence of stimulant use given the common side effects of increased concentration, alertness, safety, competitiveness, and aggression [130]. These perceived benefits of stimulant use do not override the potential dangers, which can often include headaches, anxiety, difficulty sleeping, heatstroke, cardiac arrest, increased temperature, increased heart rate, increased blood pressure, constricted blood vessels, dizziness, and confusion, in addition to many other symptoms [131]. In a study of college-level athletes, prevalence of stimulant use was 3% of athletes over 1 year [114, 132].

Athletes have also fallen victim to the "Opioid Epidemic." A recent systematic review of opioid use in athletes found that use is highly prevalent among athletes, and, notably, studies found similar prevalence of opioid use among high school athletes as compared to professional athletes [133]. In a 2021 survey of collegiate student-athletes, 9% of student-athletes reported use of narcotic pain medication with a prescription, and 2% of student-athletes reported using narcotic pain medication without a prescription in the past year—making narcotic pain medication one of the most prevalent drugs used specifically to prepare for athletic practice among student-athletes [134]. Athletes may be especially vulnerable to misuse of opioids, as they are often prescribed narcotics for the treatment of severe athletic injuries or pain [134]. Though opioids may temporarily relieve pain and improve energy, motivation, and mood, they are also likely to produce substance use disorder overdose, abnormal pain sensitivity, low testosterone and reduced energy, drive, and additional symptoms [119]. Many opioids and other narcotics are banned from use while in sport [114].

Anabolic androgenic agents (AAS), or performance-enhancing substances, are among the most frequently used performance-enhancing substances and continue to be one of the most common doping methods among athletes [119]. In one study, the use of anabolic agents was cited to be between 31% and 37.1% among Italian athletes, with an average consumption of 18.4% [130]. For many individuals, performance-enhancing substances and AASs can produce effects that improve their ability to perform athletically, such as the development of increased muscle mass, strength, power, endurance, muscle recovery, and explosiveness, in addition to other effects [119]. One study reveals that the development of a steroid use disorder is often a result of three main factors, including "(1) a strong desire to maintain a certain physique; (2) suppression of the hypothalamic-pituitary-gonadal axis, causing testosterone production to shut down; and (3) attempts to reverse common side effects of use (i.e., loss of libido, impaired erectile function, decreased energy and depression)" [75, 95]. However, though athletes may feel that AAS can improve athletic performance, AAS can also lead to long-lasting and extremely damaging side effects, such as kidney damage [120].

In general, substance use disorders produce significant effects on athletic performance, and often, athletic eligibility. In a study of student-athletes representing the National Association of Intercollegiate Athletics (NAIA), alcohol, drug, and tobacco use and misuse were found to have long-lasting biopsychosocial impacts on athletes [134]. These biopsychosocial impacts often vary by substance type. For example, alcohol use can cause dehydration, damage to the athlete's central nervous system, and greater likelihood of engaging in risky or dangerous behaviors that may impact both performance and athletic eligibility [134]. Both alcohol and cannabis may result in lower levels of concentration and attention during athletic competition, which could subsequently produce both decreased performance and an increased risk of injury [134]. Stimulants and AAS may produce negative cardiovascular side effects [134]. Anabolic steroids can lead to kidney damage and increased aggression [130]. The misuse of substances often leads to physical side effects that may make it extremely difficult to perform at one's best.

Many substances can also lead to several detrimental consequences that manifest psychologically in sport. Stimulants specifically may produce large increases in anxiety, loss of concentration, irritability, and perceptual misjudgments [131]. Therefore, while substance use can cause an athlete to experience elevated heart rate or temperature while they are trying to athletically perform, they also may experience anxiety that inhibits their ability to showcase their skills or interact with their teammates, or they may misjudge their movements. Additionally, many substances can lead to sleeping difficulties, which may impact one's psychological and mental health in the long term [131, 135].

In treating substance use disorders and concerns, there are a number of reliable screening instruments and effective treatment interventions, though there is room for these interventions to be expanded toward the specific athlete population [113, 136]. Medical practitioners should identify those athletes at risk and attempt to eliminate risk factors [137]. Treatment may include these preventative measures, in addition to education, motivational interviewing, and pharmacologic interventions

[114]. For example, if a practitioner learns of an athlete's substance use through recognizing the signs and symptoms of drug abuse, the practitioner may attempt to inform the athlete of the dangerous side effects of substance use for both health and athletic performance and then refer the athlete to a mental health professional for treatment [114]. While treating substance use and misuse among athletes, practitioners should also screen for polysubstance use, as many athletes who display concerns with one substance may have other unaddressed concerns or conditions [138].

Suicide and Non-suicidal Self-Injurious Behavior

Recent suicides of high-profile athletes such as Aaron Hernandez, Junior Seau, Madison Holleran, and Katie Meyer have demonstrated that elite athletes are not immune to suicide and, in fact, may have unique risk factors for suicide that are specific to their identity as an athlete [139]. In a study of active and recently retired elite athletes, prevalence of suicidal ideation was 15.6% [140]. The overall suicide rate of US collegiate athletes is estimated to be 1 out of 100,000 per year [139–142]. Still, there is a debate regarding whether athletic participation increases or decreases risk for suicide [139]. It is posited that high-level athletes experience a level of pressure that can contribute to emotional disturbance that may be a risk factor for suicide, but that the social support in physical activity offered by athletics can buffer against suicide [140].

In one study of collegiate student-athletes, difficulty in romantic or other social relationships was identified as a potential marker of risk for suicidal behavior and/ or ideation [143]. In addition, traumatic brain injury and end-of-career concerns have been identified as relevant factors that may be more commonly implicated as contributors to athlete vs. nonathlete suicide [139]. Despite sport-specific contributors to suicide prevalence, athletics and sport participation have also been cited to lower prevalence of suicidal ideation and attempts, particularly among youth [144]. One study found the suicide rate in NCAA athletes to be lower than that of the general and collegiate population of similar age [139]. Among NCAA athletes, males were found to have a significantly higher rate of suicide compared with females, with football athletes at greatest risk [139].

In addition to suicidal behavior, athletes may also engage in non-suicidal self-injury (NSSI)—another serious concern that practitioners should preventatively look for and treat. NSSI, including cutting, burning, scratching, and head banging, among others, can have a variety of different functions, with difficulties regulating emotions in intrapersonal functioning being a predominant function [145]. Athletes with abuse experiences have been documented to also engage in other forms of NSSI, including disordered eating, substance abuse, sexual risk behaviors, or abuse of prescription painkillers reportedly in efforts to independently cope with deeply distressing emotional experiences [146].

Among athletes, as well as the general population, suicide and suicidal ideation are large concerns for which practitioners should consistently screen. Practitioners should understand the signs and symptoms of these concerns in order to effectively administer prevention and treatment mechanisms in predisposed or presently affected athletes. Screening for other psychiatric illnesses and concerns may help to identify individuals at risk, but it is also crucial to create environments in which disclosure and treatment of mental health concerns is safe and acceptable, and trusted individuals frequently inquire about athlete well-being [139].

Suicide is extremely devastating, and it, along with suicidal ideation, attempts, and NSSI, has significant impacts on both the affected athlete and their surrounding communities [139]. It is important that athletes, though often represented as models of peak health, wellness, and athletic performance, are simultaneously viewed as individuals who are not immune to mental health concerns and conditions, and who should be looked after, treated, and supported in a similar manner to the general population.

Minority Experiences

Overall, youth who endure trauma are more likely to have mental health disorders and struggle academically in school [147]. Those who experience trauma are also less likely to have accessible mental healthcare services or treatment options [147]. Underrepresented minority youth are more likely to experience adversity, live in poverty, and have worse health outcomes than white youth [148]. Research suggests that because underrepresented minority youth are more likely to experience adverse childhood experiences (ACEs), they are more likely to have worse long-term mental and physical health [148]. This trend of worse mental health outcomes extends past childhood into college for racial minorities [149]. In one study examining access to mental health resources for underrepresented minority athletes (African American, Latinos, and Asian American), they estimated about 78% of underrepresented minority athletes needed access to mental health resources, while only 11% of those in need of mental health services received care in the past year [149]. Likewise, research has shown that while underrepresented minority adolescents are far more likely to suffer from mental illness, they are also less likely to actually use mental healthcare services than nonminority counterparts [150]. Moreover, collegiate minority athletes report higher levels of stress [149].

In general, those who identify as LGBTQ+ report higher levels of depression than heterosexual peers, particularly during adolescence to early adulthood [151]. Sexual minority adolescents were also more likely to report being cyberbullied, lower family satisfaction, and unsatisfactory medical care [151]. Research has found a significant relationship between internalized homophobia of sexual minority individuals and depression [152]. Box 2.11 discusses emergent symptoms experienced by an adolescent athlete in distress around how their fully expressed gender minority identity could potentially negatively impact their family support and athletic career.

For LGBTQ+ athletes, there is substantial overlap with the experiences of the general LGBT population as athletes can also face stereotyping, harassment, and discrimination during their athletic careers [153]. Even during youth athletics, LGBT athletes are more likely to view sports as an unsafe and unwelcoming environment and thus may be unable to benefit from the physical and psychological health that sports provide [153]. By the time they reach college, LGBT athletes fear being "outed" to their community and of experiencing peer rejection, and are also concerned they may not receive institutional support [153]. Research suggests that athletic trainers and sports medicine physicians may be the key to improving health outcomes for LGBT athletes in college as they are able to address unique LBGT health risks, provide affirming gender and sexual identity care, and promote inclusivity in athletic communities [153].

Adults with physical disabilities are more likely to suffer from mental health conditions than those without disabilities [154]. One study has found that ableist microaggression against people with disabilities significantly contributes to poor mental health outcomes in individuals with physical disabilities [155]. Those with more visible and noticeable disabilities are more likely to experience ableist microaggressions [155]. Like LGBTQ athletes, para-athletes are also more likely to suffer from mental health issues—even among high-level para-athletes who can be part of the Paralympics [156]. Researchers have proposed that elite athletes with disabilities suffer from poorer mental health in comparison to nondisabled peers [156]. It has been posited that the high rate of mental illness in disabled athletes is because of harmful stereotypes about those with disabilities [156].

Box 2.11

A 16-year-old rower reported emotional distress related to thoughts about coming out to family and coaches as transgender. They reported they have already come out to some friends at school and have been supported, but they are worried about potential rejection from family and about how coming out would affect their future in rowing. Having been assigned female at birth, they are unsure about whether to medically transition before or after college rowing because they want to row at the highest level possible but know that if they medically transition, they will be unable to compete on a women's collegiate team. This pervasive anxiety and distress can often reach a peak and lead them to feel out of control and overwhelmed. Six months ago, they began self-harming by cutting as a way to relieve intense emotions and regain some control, and now they report feeling "addicted" to the behavior as a primary way of decreasing intense distress in the short term.

Psychological Resilience

Athletes frequently encounter stressors and adversity, both in their athletic pursuits and in their daily life [2]. While adversity can often facilitate the emergence of positive traits, it can prompt mental health conditions and concerns, such as those described throughout this chapter, that significantly impact athlete health and performance [2, 4, 5]. In the process of considering how athletes may better encounter adversity to mitigate vulnerability to mental health concerns, one might turn to the concept of psychological resilience. Psychological resilience is defined as "the process of adapting well in the face of adversity, trauma, tragedy, threats, or significant sources of stress," or more simply, a dynamic process of adapting to stress [157, 158]. With greater psychological resilience, an athlete will be better equipped to "bounce back" from adversity or stress, and may be better able to cope with mental health concerns, or not develop mental health issues at all [158]. Generally, psychological resilience can reduce vulnerability to mental health concerns, as well as improve athletic performance [158]. Regardless of mental health status, psychological resilience may act as a powerful skill for reducing athletic burnout, coping with sport injury, and enhancing personal growth [158–161].

Some factors that can enhance psychological resilience, and therefore support athletes who are particularly vulnerable to mental health concerns, include positive adaptation to adversity, stress coping ability, and supportive athletic environments [158], though there is a need for more rigorous research on how psychological resilience can be used as a tool for addressing mental health concerns and bolstering positive coping among athletes. While learning about the mental health conditions described in this chapter, it is important to reflect on how psychological resilience may be harnessed to improve the overall well-being and athletic performance of these affected athletes.

Conclusion

As is evident in this chapter, various mental health concerns and challenges can present in young athletes. We take an overarching perspective that all athletes experience stress, that emergent mental health concerns exist on a continuum from typical to atypical, and that mental health stigma can be a barrier for athletes in seeking adequate support [6]. We have sought to underline crucial considerations for the identification and treatment of athletes to better support their psychological and physiological well-being, in addition to their athletic performance. Through loosely organizing this chapter around the DSM-5 and outlining specific conditions as they relate to athletic performance, this chapter has showcased a range of mental health challenges, in addition to those not outlined in this chapter, that impact athlete populations just as they do nonathlete populations. Through a variety of case examples from our clinic, we have illustrated some common signs and symptoms of these challenges among athletes to provide guidance for future practitioners working closely with athlete populations. Finally, through an introduction to the concept of psychological resilience, we have established the relationship between these mental health concerns, psychological resilience, experiences of adversity, and specific vulnerabilities among young athletes.

References

1. Hyde E, Omura J, Fulton J, Lee S, Piercy K, Carlson S. Disparities in youth sports participation in the U.S., 2017–2018. Am J Prev Med. 2020;59(5):e207–10.
2. Malm C, Jakobsson J, Isaksson A. Physical activity and sports—real health benefits: a review with insight into the public health of Sweden. Sports. 2019;7(5):127.
3. Smoller JW. The genetics of stress-related disorders: PTSD, depression, and anxiety disorders. Neuropsychopharmacology. 2016;41(1):297–319.
4. Miller-Graff LE. The multidimensional taxonomy of individual resilience: trauma violence abuse, vol. 23; 2020. p. 660. https://journals.sagepub.com/doi/10.1177/1524838020967329. Accessed 14 Mar 2022.
5. Seery MD, Holman EA, Silver RC. Whatever does not kill us: cumulative lifetime adversity, vulnerability, and resilience. J Pers Soc Psychol. 2010;99(6):1025.
6. Bauman NJ. The stigma of mental health in athletes: are mental toughness and mental health seen as contradictory in elite sport? Br J Sports Med. 2016;50(3):135–6.
7. Purcell R, Gwyther K, Rice SM. Mental health in elite athletes: increased awareness requires an early intervention framework to respond to athlete needs. Sports Med Open. 2019;5(1):1–8.
8. Oforeh K, Nkemjika S, Olayinka O, Azim S. Role of suboptimal psychiatric evaluation in the development of first episode psychosis in an athlete: a case report. Sports Psychiatry J Sports Exerc Psychiatry. 2022;1:70. https://psycnet.apa.org/fulltext/2022-33811-001.pdf. Accessed 14 Mar 2022.
9. Wolanin A, Gross M, Hong E. Depression in athletes: prevalence and risk factors. Curr Sports Med Rep. 2015;14(1):56–60.
10. Hammond T, Gialloreto C, Kubas H, Hap Davis H IV. The prevalence of failure-based depression among elite athletes. Clin J Sport Med. 2013;23(4):273. https://pubmed.ncbi.nlm.nih.gov/23528842/. Accessed 14 Mar 2022.
11. Schaad KA, Bukhari AS, Brooks DI, Kocher JD, Barringer ND. The relationship between vitamin D status and depression in a tactical athlete population. J Int Soc Sports Nutr. 2019;16:40. https://www.ncbi.nlm.nih.gov/pmc/articles/PMC6734287/. Accessed 14 Mar 2022.
12. Francisco CD, Arce C, Vílchez MP, Vales Á. Antecedents and consequences of burnout in athletes: perceived stress and depression. Int J Clin Health Psychol. 2016;16(3):239.
13. Saltiel PF, Silvershein DI. Major depressive disorder: mechanism-based prescribing for personalized medicine. Neuropsychiatr Dis Treat. 2015;11:875.
14. Center for Behavioral Health Statistics and Quality. 2020 National Survey on drug use and health: methodological summary and definitions; 2021. https://www.samhsa.gov/data/sites/default/files/reports/rpt35330/2020NSDUHMethodSummDefs092421/2020NSDUHMethodsSummDefs092421.htm. Accessed 15 Mar 2022.
15. Patel RK, Rose GM. Persistent depressive disorder. StatPearls. Treasure Island, FL: StatPearls Publishing; 2021. https://www.ncbi.nlm.nih.gov/books/NBK541052/. Accessed 14 Mar 2022.
16. Gouttebarge V, Castaldelli-Maia JM, Gorczynski P, Hainline B, Hitchcock ME, Kerkhoffs GM, et al. Occurrence of mental health symptoms and disorders in current and former elite athletes: a systematic review and meta-analysis. Br J Sports Med. 2019;53(11):700–6.
17. Wolanin A, Hong E, Marks D, Panchoo K, Gross M. Prevalence of clinically elevated depressive symptoms in college athletes and differences by gender and sport. Br J Sports Med. 2016;50(3):167–71.
18. Gorczynski PF, Coyle M, Gibson K. Depressive symptoms in high-performance athletes and non-athletes: a comparative meta-analysis. Br J Sports Med. 2017;51(18):1348–54.
19. Weigand S, Cohen J, Merenstein D. Susceptibility for depression in current and retired student athletes. Sports Health. 2013;5(3):263.

20. Armstrong S, Oomen-Early J. Social connectedness, self-esteem, and depression symptomatology among collegiate athletes versus nonathletes. J Am Coll Heal. 2010;57:521. https://www.tandfonline.com/doi/abs/10.3200/JACH.57.5.521-526. Accessed 14 Mar 2022.
21. Kontos A, Covassin T, Elbin R, Parker T. Depression and neurocognitive performance after concussion among male and female high school and collegiate athletes. Arch Phys Med Rehabil. 2012;93(10):1751–6.
22. Covassin T, Bretzin A, Japinga A, Teachnor-Hauk D, Nogle S. Exploring the relationship between depression and seasonal affective disorder in incoming first year collegiate student-athletes. Athl Train Sports Health Care. 2018;11(3):124–30.
23. Rice SM, Parker AG, Rosenbaum S, Bailey A, Mawren D, Purcell R. Sport-related concussion and mental health outcomes in elite athletes: a systematic review. Sports Med Auckl Nz. 2018;48(2):447.
24. Frank R, Beckmann J, Nixdorf I. Depressionen im Hochleistungssport: Prävalenzen und psychologische Einflüsse. Dtsch Z Für Sportmed. 2013;2013(11):1. http://www.zeitschrift-sportmedizin.de/artikel-online/archiv-2013/heft-11/depressionen-im-hochleistungssport-praevalenzen-und-psychologische-einfluesse/. Accessed 14 Mar 2022.
25. Schaal K, Tafflet M, Nassif H, Thibault V, Pichard C, Alcotte M, et al. Psychological balance in high level athletes: gender-based differences and sport-specific patterns. PLoS One. 2011;6(5):e19007.
26. McIntyre RS, Berk M, Brietzke E, Goldstein B, López-Jaramilo C, Kessing LV, et al. Bipolar disorders. Lancet. 2020;396(10265):1841–56.
27. National Institute of Mental Health (NIMH). Bipolar disorder. Bethesda, MD: National Institute of Mental Health (NIMH); 2020. https://www.nimh.nih.gov/health/topics/bipolar-disorder. Accessed 14 Mar 2022.
28. Currie A, Gorczynski P, Rice SM, Purcell R, McAllister-Williams RH, Hitchcock ME, et al. Bipolar and psychotic disorders in elite athletes: a narrative review. Br J Sports Med. 2019;53(12):746–53.
29. Daley M, Reardon C. Bipolar disorder and athletes: a narrative review. Curr Sports Med Rep. 2021;20(12):638–44.
30. Aas M, Henry C, Andreassen OA, Bellivier F, Melle I, Etain B. The role of childhood trauma in bipolar disorders. Int J Bipolar Disord. 2016;4(1):1–10.
31. Treatment for Adolescents With Depression Study (TADS) Team. Fluoxetine, cognitive-behavioral therapy, and their combination for adolescents with depression: treatment for adolescents with depression study (TADS) randomized controlled trial. JAMA. 2004;292(7):807.
32. Clevenger SS, Malhotra D, Dang J, Vanle B, IsHak WW. The role of selective serotonin reuptake inhibitors in preventing relapse of major depressive disorder. Ther Adv Psychopharmacol. 2018;8(1):49.
33. Stahl SM, Morrissette DA, Faedda G, Fava M, Goldberg JF, Keck PE, et al. Guidelines for the recognition and management of mixed depression. CNS Spectr. 2017;22(2):203–19.
34. Sidor MM, MacQueen GM. Antidepressants for the acute treatment of bipolar depression: a systematic review and meta-analysis. J Clin Psychiatry. 2010;71(2):953.
35. Reardon CL, Creado S. Psychiatric medication preferences of sports psychiatrists. Phys Sportsmed. 2016;44:397. https://www.tandfonline.com/doi/abs/10.1080/00913847.2016.1216719. Accessed 15 Mar 2022.
36. Sturmey P. Behavioral activation is an evidence-based treatment for depression. Behav Modif. 2009;33:818. https://journals.sagepub.com/doi/10.1177/0145445509350094?url_ver=Z39.88-2003&rfr_id=ori%3Arid%3Acrossref.org&rfr_dat=cr_pub++0pubmed. Accessed 14 Mar 2022.
37. Leaviss J, Uttley L. Psychotherapeutic benefits of compassion-focused therapy: an early systematic review. Psychol Med. 2015;45(5):927.

38. Mosewich AD, Kowalski KC, Sabiston CM, Sedgwick WA, Tracy JL. Self-compassion: a potential resource for young women athletes. J Sport Exerc Psychol. 2011;33(1):103–23.

39. Rice SM, Gwyther K, Santesteban-Echarri O, Baron D, Gorczynski P, Gouttebarge V, et al. Determinants of anxiety in elite athletes: a systematic review and meta-analysis. Br J Sports Med. 2019;53(11):722.

40. American Psychiatric Association. Diagnostic and statistical manual of mental disorders: DSM-5. 5th ed. Washington, DC: American Psychiatric Association; 2013. 947 p.

41. Tiller JWG. Depression and anxiety. Med J Aust. 2013;199:S28–31.

42. Somers JM, Goldner EM, Waraich P, Hsu L. Prevalence and incidence studies of anxiety disorders: a systematic review of the literature. Can J Psychiatr. 2006;51:100. https://journals.sagepub.com/doi/10.1177/070674370605100206?url_ver=Z39.88-2003&rfr_id=ori%3Arid%3Acrossref.org&rfr_dat=cr_pub++0pubmed. Accessed 14 Mar 2022.

43. Wittchen H-U, Jacobi F. Size and burden of mental disorders in Europe—a critical review and appraisal of 27 studies. Eur Neuropsychopharmacol. 2005;15(4):357–76.

44. Li C, Fan R, Sun J, Li G. Risk and protective factors of generalized anxiety disorder of elite collegiate athletes: a cross-sectional study. Front Public Health. 2021;9:607800. https://www.ncbi.nlm.nih.gov/pmc/articles/PMC7902705/. Accessed 14 Mar 2022.

45. Reardon CL, Hainline B, Aron CM, Baron D, Baum AL, Bindra A, et al. Mental health in elite athletes: International Olympic Committee consensus statement (2019). Br J Sports Med. 2019;53(11):667–99.

46. Hussey JE, Donohue B, Barchard KA, Allen DN. Family contributions to sport performance and their utility in predicting appropriate referrals to mental health optimization programmes. Eur J Sport Sci. 2019;19:972. https://www.tandfonline.com/doi/abs/10.1080/17461391.2019.1574906. Accessed 14 Mar 2022.

47. Kilic Ö, Aoki H, Haagensen R, Jensen C, Johnson U, Kerkhoffs GMMJ, et al. Symptoms of common mental disorders and related stressors in Danish professional football and handball. Eur J Sport Sci. 2017;17:1328. https://www.tandfonline.com/doi/abs/10.1080/17461391.2017.1381768. Accessed 14 Mar 2022.

48. Mairs R, Nicholls D. Assessment and treatment of eating disorders in children and adolescents. Arch Dis Child. 2016;101(12):1168–75.

49. Nurfatehah Mat Salleh F, et al. Determination of psychological correlates of peak performance in developmental archers. J Phys Educ Sport. 2020;20:344. https://www.iat.uni-leipzig.de/datenbanken/iks/nwls/Record/4059460. Accessed 21 Mar 2022.

50. Patel D, Omar H, Terry M. Sport-related performance anxiety in young female athletes. J Pediatr Adolesc Gynecol. 2010;23(6):325–35.

51. Eime RM, Young JA, Harvey JT, Charity MJ, Payne WR. A systematic review of the psychological and social benefits of participation in sport for children and adolescents: informing development of a conceptual model of health through sport. Int J Behav Nutr Phys Act. 2013;10:98.

52. Mohammadzadeh J-K. The comparison of personality traits, trait â state anxiety and existential anxiety among patients with generalized anxiety disorder and normal people. J Clin Psychol. 2016;8(1):83–92.

53. Newman MG, Llera SJ. A novel theory of experiential avoidance in generalized anxiety disorder: a review and synthesis of research supporting a contrast avoidance model of worry. Clin Psychol Rev. 2011;31(3):371.

54. Grossbard J, Smith R, Smoll F, Cumming S. Competitive anxiety in young athletes: differentiating somatic anxiety, worry, and concentration disruption. Anxiety Stress Coping. 2009;22(2):153. https://pubmed.ncbi.nlm.nih.gov/18937102/. Accessed 14 Mar 2022.

55. Gould D, Greenleaf C, Krane V. Arousal-anxiety and sport behavior. In: Horn TS, editor. Advances in sport psychology. Champaign, IL: Human Kinetics; 2002. p. 207–36. https://psycnet.apa.org/record/2002-17365-007. Accessed 14 Mar 2022.

56. Smith R, Smoll F. Youth sports as a behavior setting for psychosocial interventions. In: Van Raalte JL, Brewer BW, editors. Exploring sport and exercise psychology. Washington,

DC: American Psychological Association; 2002. p. 341–71. https://psycnet.apa.org/doiLanding?doi=10.1037%2F10465-017. Accessed 14 Mar 2022.

57. Locke AB, Kirst N, Shultz CG. Diagnosis and management of generalized anxiety disorder and panic disorder in adults. Am Fam Physician. 2015;91(9):617–24.

58. Borza L. Cognitive-behavioral therapy for generalized anxiety. Dialogues Clin Neurosci. 2017;19(2):203.

59. Aupperle RL, Paulus MP. Neural systems underlying approach and avoidance in anxiety disorders. Dialogues Clin Neurosci. 2010;12(4):517.

60. Cromer L, Kaier E, Davis J, Stunk K, Stewart SE. OCD in college athletes. Am J Psychiatry. 2017;174:595. https://ajp.psychiatryonline.org/doi/abs/10.1176/appi.ajp.2017.16101124. Accessed 14 Mar 2022.

61. Reardon CL, Factor RM. Sport psychiatry. Sports Med. 2010;40(11):961–80.

62. Ruscio AM, Stein DJ, Chiu WT, Kessler RC. The epidemiology of obsessive-compulsive disorder in the national comorbidity survey replication. Mol Psychiatry. 2010;15(1):53.

63. Marazziti D, Parra E, Amadori S, Arone A, Palermo S, Massa L, et al. Obsessive-compulsive and depressive symptoms in professional tennis players. Clin Neuropsychiatry. 2021;18(6):304.

64. Browning ME, Kirk NPV, Krompinger JW. Examining depression symptoms within OCD: the role of experiential avoidance. Behav Cogn Psychother. 2022;50:367.

65. Hayes SC, Strosahl K, Wilson KG, Bissett RT, Pistorello J, Toarmino D, et al. Measuring experiential avoidance: a preliminary test of a working model. Psychol Rec. 2004;54(4):553–78.

66. Blakey SM, Jacoby RJ, Reuman L, Abramowitz JS. The Relative Contributions of experiential avoidance and distress tolerance to OC symptoms. Behav Cogn Psychother. 2016;44(4):460–71.

67. Hobson NM, Bonk D, Inzlicht M. Rituals decrease the neural response to performance failure. PeerJ. 2017;5:e3363. https://www.ncbi.nlm.nih.gov/pmc/articles/PMC5452956/. Accessed 16 Mar 2022.

68. Montenegro S. Disordered eating in athletes. Athl Ther Today. 2006;11(1):60. https://www.researchgate.net/publication/237706553_Disordered_Eating_in_Athletes. Accessed 15 Mar 2022.

69. Bjornsson AS, Didie ER, Phillips KA. Body dysmorphic disorder. Dialogues Clin Neurosci. 2010;12(2):221.

70. Nascimento AL, Luna JV, Fontenelle L. Body dysmorphic disorder and eating disorders in elite professional female ballet dancers. Am Acad Clin Psychiatr. 2012;24(3):191–4.

71. MacPheil D, Oberle C. Seeing shred: differences in muscle dysmorphia, orthorexia nervosa, depression, and obsessive-compulsive tendencies among groups of weightlifting athletes. Perform Enhanc Health. 2022;10(1):100213.

72. Tod D, Edwards C, Cranswick I. Muscle dysmorphia: current insights. Psychol Res Behav Manag. 2016;9:179.

73. Lichtenstein MB, Hinze CJ, Emborg B, Thomsen F, Hemmingsen SD. Compulsive exercise: links, risks and challenges faced. Psychol Res Behav Manag. 2017;10:85.

74. Fineberg NA, Hollander E, Pallanti S, Walitza S, Grünblatt E, Dell'Osso BM, et al. Clinical advances in obsessive-compulsive disorder: a position statement by the International College of Obsessive-Compulsive Spectrum Disorders. Int Clin Psychopharmacol. 2020;35(4):173.

75. Spottswood M, Davydow DS, Huang H. The prevalence of posttraumatic stress disorder in primary care: a systematic review. Harv Rev Psychiatry. 2017;25(4):159.

76. Aron CM, Harvey S, Hainline B, Hitchcock ME, Reardon CL. Post-traumatic stress disorder (PTSD) and other trauma-related mental disorders in elite athletes: a narrative review. Br J Sports Med. 2019;53(12):779–84.

77. Padaki AS, Noticewala MS, Levine WN, Ahmad CS, Popkin MK, Popkin CA. Prevalence of posttraumatic stress disorder symptoms among young athletes after anterior cruciate ligament rupture. Orthop J Sports Med. 2018;6(7):2325967118787159. https://www.ncbi.nlm.nih.gov/pmc/articles/PMC6083780/. Accessed 21 Mar 2022.

78. Brassil HE, Salvatore AP. The frequency of post-traumatic stress disorder symptoms in athletes with and without sports related concussion. Clin Transl Med. 2018;7:25. https://www.ncbi.nlm.nih.gov/pmc/articles/PMC6056355/. Accessed 14 Mar 2022.

79. Bryant RA, Mastrodomenico J, Felmingham KL, Hopwood S, Kenny L, Kandris E, Cahill C, Creamer M. Treatment of acute stress disorder: a randomized controlled trial. Arch Gen Psychiatry. 2008;65(6):659. https://pubmed.ncbi.nlm.nih.gov/18519824/. Accessed 15 Mar 2022.

80. Gervis M, Dunn N. The emotional abuse of elite child athletes by their coaches. Child Abuse Rev. 2004;13(3):215–23.

81. Sabato TM, Walch TJ, Caine DJ. The elite young athlete: strategies to ensure physical and emotional health. Open Access J Sports Med. 2016;7:99.

82. Lopez Y, Dohrn S, Posig M. The effect of abusive leadership by coaches on Division I student-athletes' performance: the moderating role of core self-evaluations. Sport Manag Rev. 2020;23(1):130–41.

83. McMahon J, McGannon KR, Palmer C. Body shaming and associated practices as abuse: athlete entourage as perpetrators of abuse. Sport Educ Soc. 2021;27:578. https://www.tandfonline.com/doi/abs/10.1080/13573322.2021.1890571. Accessed 14 Mar 2022.

84. MacPherson E, Kerr G. Online public shaming of professional athletes: gender matters. Psychol Sport Exerc. 2020;51:101782.

85. Thomson P, Jaque SV. Exposing shame in dancers and athletes: shame, trauma, and dissociation in a nonclinical population. J Trauma Dissociat. 2013;14:439. https://www.tandfonline.com/doi/abs/10.1080/15299732.2012.757714. Accessed 14 Mar 2022.

86. Griffin BJ, Purcell N, Burkman K, Litz BT, Bryan CJ, Schmitz M, et al. Moral injury: an integrative review. J Trauma Stress. 2019;32(3):350–62.

87. Wippert P-M, Wippert J. Perceived stress and prevalence of traumatic stress symptoms following athletic career termination. J Clin Sport Psychol. 2008;2(1):1–16.

88. de Arellano MAR, Lyman DR, Jobe-Shields L, George P, Dougherty RH, Daniels AS, et al. Trauma-focused cognitive behavioral therapy: assessing the evidence. Psychiatr Serv. 2014;65(5):591.

89. Ito M, Horikoshi M, Resick PA, Katayanagi A, Miyamae M, Takagishi Y, et al. Study protocol for a randomised controlled trial of cognitive processing therapy for post-traumatic stress disorder among Japanese patients: the Safety, Power, Intimacy, Esteem, Trust (SPINET) study. BMJ Open. 2017;7(6):e014292. https://www.ncbi.nlm.nih.gov/pmc/articles/PMC5734443/. Accessed 15 Mar 2022.

90. Shapiro F. The role of eye movement desensitization and reprocessing (EMDR) therapy in medicine: addressing the psychological and physical symptoms stemming from adverse life experiences. Perm J. 2014;18(1):71.

91. Casiglia E, Tikhonoff V. "Twisties" and Olympic games: a role for hypnosis in top-level athletes who have lost the sense of the self in aerial space? Psychology. 2021;12(9):1379–83.

92. Berghoff CR, Tull MT, DiLillo D, Messman-Moore T, Gratz KL. The role of experiential avoidance in the relation between anxiety disorder diagnoses and future physical health symptoms in a community sample of young adult women. J Contextual Behav Sci. 2017;6(1):29.

93. García-Oliva C, Piqueras JA. Experiential avoidance and technological addictions in adolescents. J Behav Addict. 2016;5(2):293.

94. Lanius RA. Trauma-related dissociation and altered states of consciousness: a call for clinical, treatment, and neuroscience research. Eur J Psychotraumatol. 2015;6:27905. https://www.ncbi.nlm.nih.gov/pmc/articles/PMC4439425/. Accessed 15 Mar 2022.

95. McDonald D, Kirkby RJ. Use of dissociation strategies when running becomes difficult: levels of ability and gender differences. Eur J High Abil. 2011;6:73. https://www.tandfonline.com/doi/abs/10.1080/0937445950060108. Accessed 15 Mar 2022.

96. Sundgot-Borgen J, Torstveit MK. Prevalence of eating disorders in elite athletes is higher than in the general population. Clin J Sport Med. 2004;14(1):25. https://journals.lww.com/cjs-

portsmed/Fulltext/2004/01000/Prevalence_of_Eating_Disorders_in_Elite_Athletes.5.aspx. Accessed 21 Mar 2022.
97. Thomas JJ, Becker KR, Kuhnle MC, Jo JH, Harshman SG, Wons OB, et al. Cognitive-behavioral therapy for avoidant/restrictive food intake disorder (CBT-AR): feasibility, acceptability, and proof-of-concept for children and adolescents. Int J Eat Disord. 2020;53(10):1636.
98. Norris ML, Spettigue WJ, Katzman DK. Update on eating disorders: current perspectives on avoidant/restrictive food intake disorder in children and youth. Neuropsychiatr Dis Treat. 2016;12:213.
99. Kurz S, van Dyck Z, Dremmel D, Munsch S, Hilbert A. Early-onset restrictive eating disturbances in primary school boys and girls. Eur Child Adolesc Psychiatry. 2015;24(7):779.
100. Sudi K, et al. Anorexia athletica. Nutrition. 2004;20(7–8):657–61.
101. Ludyga S, Puhse U, Gerber M, Kamijo K. How children with neurodevelopmental disorders can benefit from the neurocognitive effects of exercise. Neurosci Biobehav Rev. 2021;127:514–9.
102. Montalva-Valenzuela F, Andrades-Ramírez O, Castillo-Paredes A. Effects of physical activity, exercise and sport on executive function in young people with attention deficit hyperactivity disorder: a systematic review. Eur J Investig Health Psychol Educ. 2022;12(1):61–76.
103. Morris-Rosendahl DJ, Crocq M-A. Neurodevelopmental disorders—the history and future of a diagnostic concept. Dialogues Clin Neurosci. 2020;22(1):65.
104. Putukian M, Kreher J, Coppel D, Glazer J, McKeag D, White R. Attention deficit hyperactivity disorder and the athlete: an american medical society for sports medicine position statement. Clin J Sport Med. 2011;21(5):392–400.
105. Stewman CG, Liebman C, Fink L, Sandella B. Attention deficit hyperactivity disorder: unique considerations in athletes. Sports Health. 2018;10(1):40.
106. Lai M-C, Lombardo MV, Baron-Cohen S. Autism. Lancet. 2014;383(9920):896–910.
107. Baio J, Wiggins L, Christensen DL, Maenner MJ, Daniels J, Warren Z, et al. Prevalence of autism spectrum disorder among children aged 8 years — autism and developmental disabilities monitoring network, 11 sites, United States, 2014. MMWR Surveill Summ. 2018;67(6):1.
108. Yu CCW, Wong SWL, Lo FSF, So RCH, Chan DFY. Study protocol: a randomized controlled trial study on the effect of a game-based exercise training program on promoting physical fitness and mental health in children with autism spectrum disorder. BMC Psychiatry. 2018;18(1):1–10.
109. Contributor NT. Encouraging physical activity in people with learning disabilities. Nurs Times. 2018;114:18. https://www.nursingtimes.net/roles/learning-disability-nurses/encouraging-physical-activity-in-people-with-learning-disabilities-16-07-2018/. Accessed 14 Mar 2022.
110. Gunn BS, McAllister TW, McCrea MA, Broglio SP, Moore RD. Neurodevelopmental disorders and risk of concussion: findings from the National Collegiate Athletic Association Department of Defense Grand Alliance Concussion Assessment, Research, and Education (NCAA-DOD CARE) Consortium (2014–2017). J Neurotrauma. 2022;39:379. https://www.liebertpub.com/doi/abs/10.1089/neu.2020.7446. Accessed 14 Mar 2022.
111. Nelson LD, Guskiewicz KM, Marshall SW, Hammeke T, Barr W, Randolph C, McCrea MA. Multiple self-reported concussions are more prevalent in athletes with ADHD and learning disability. Clin J Sport Med. 2016;26(2):120. https://pubmed.ncbi.nlm.nih.gov/25915144/. Accessed 14 Mar 2022.
112. McDuff D, Stull T, Castaldelli-Maia JM, Hitchcock ME, Hainline B, Reardon CL. Recreational and ergogenic substance use and substance use disorders in elite athletes: a narrative review. Br J Sports Med. 2019;53(12):754–60.
113. McDuff DR, Baron D. Substance use in athletics: a sports psychiatry perspective. Clin Sports Med. 2005;24(4):885–97.
114. Reardon CL, Creado S. Drug abuse in athletes. Subst Abus Rehabil. 2014;5:95.

115. Durrant R, Thakker J. Substance use & abuse: cultural and historical perspectives. Thousand Oaks, CA: Sage; 2022. https://sk.sagepub.com/books/substance-use-and-abuse.
116. Health (UK) NCC for M. Drug misuse. London: British Psychological Society; 2008. https://www.ncbi.nlm.nih.gov/books/NBK53227/. Accessed 14 Mar 2022.
117. Hasin DS, O'Brien CP, Auriacombe M, Borges G, Bucholz K, Budney A, et al. DSM-5 Criteria for substance use disorders: recommendations and rationale. Am J Psychiatry. 2013;170(8):834.
118. Exner J, Bitar R, Berg X, Pichler E-M, Herdener M, Seifritz E, et al. Use of psychotropic substances among elite athletes – a narrative review. Swiss Med Wkly. 2021;151(7):w20412. https://smw.ch/article/doi/smw.2021.20412. Accessed 14 Mar 2022.
119. Stull T, Morse E, McDuff D. Substance use and its impact on athlete health and performance. Psychiatr Clin North Am. 2021;44(3):405–17.
120. National Collegiate Athletic Association. National study on substance abuse habits of college student-athletes. Indianapolis, IN: NCAA; 2018. http://www.ncaa.org/sites/default/files/2018RES_Substance_Use_Final_Report_FINAL_20180611.pdf.
121. Mündel T, Olfert IM. Nicotine and exercise performance: another tool in the arsenal or curse for anti-doping? Eur J Appl Physiol. 2018;118(4):679.
122. Johnston R, Crowe M, Doma K. Effect of nicotine on repeated bouts of anaerobic exercise in nicotine naïve individuals. Eur J Appl Physiol. 2018;118(4):681–9.
123. Mündel T. Nicotine: sporting friend or foe? A review of athlete use, performance consequences and other considerations. Sports Med Auckl Nz. 2017;47(12):2497.
124. Veliz P, McCabe SE, McCabe VV, Boyd CJ. Adolescent sports participation, E-cigarette use and cigarette smoking. Am J Prev Med. 2017;53(5):e175.
125. Olfert IM, DeVallance E, Hoskinson H, Branyan KW, Clayton S, Pitzer CR, et al. Chronic exposure to electronic cigarettes results in impaired cardiovascular function in mice. J Appl Physiol. 2018;124(3):573.
126. Chun LF, Moazed F, Calfee CS, Matthay MA, Gotts JE. Pulmonary toxicity of e-cigarettes. Am J Physiol-Lung Cell Mol Physiol. 2017;313:L193. https://journals.physiology.org/doi/abs/10.1152/ajplung.00071.2017. Accessed 15 Mar 2022.
127. Christiani DC. Vaping-induced acute lung injury. N Engl J Med. 2019;382:960. https://www.nejm.org/doi/full/10.1056/nejme1912032. Accessed 15 Mar 2022.
128. Young S, Henderson C, Couperus K. The effects of electronic nicotine delivery systems on athletes. Curr Sports Med Rep. 2020;19(4):146–50.
129. Reardon CL, Factor RM. Considerations in the use of stimulants in sport. Sports Med. 2016;46(5):611–7.
130. Mazzeo F, Raiola G. An investigation of drugs abuse in sport performance. J Hum Sport Exerc. 2018;13:S309. https://www.researchgate.net/publication/326442276_An_investigation_of_drugs_abuse_in_sport_performance. Accessed 16 Mar 2022.
131. Avois L, Robinson N, Saudan C, Baume N, Mangin P, Saugy M. Central nervous system stimulants and sport practice. Br J Sports Med. 2006;40(Suppl 1):i16–20.
132. Johnston L, O'Malley P, Bachman J, Schulenberg J. Monitoring the future national survey results on drug use, 1975-2009 - Volume II: College students & adults ages 19-50, vol. 2. Bethesda, MD: National Institute on Drug Abuse; 2010. p. 283.
133. Ekhtiari S, Yusuf I, AlMakadma Y, MacDonald A, Leroux T, Khan M. Opioid use in athletes: a systematic review. Sports Health. 2020;12(6):534.
134. Moore M, Abbe A. The National Association of Intercollegiate Athletics substance use and abuse survey. J Issues Intercoll Athl. 2021. http://csri-jiia.org/wp-content/uploads/2021/02/RA_2021_05.pdf.
135. Hosker D, Elkins RM, Potter M. Promoting mental health and wellness in youth through physical activity, nutrition, and sleep. Child Adolesc Psychiatr Clin N Am. 2019;28(2):171–93.
136. Leshner AI. Science-based views of drug addiction and its treatment. JAMA. 1999;282(14):1314.
137. Nelson LF, Weitzman ER, Levy S. Prevention of substance use disorders. Med Clin North Am. 2022;106(1):153–68.

138. Orsini MM, Milroy J, Wyrick D, Sanders L. Polysubstance use among first-year NCAA college student-athletes. J Child Adolesc Subst Abuse. 2018;27:1–7.
139. Rao AL. Athletic suicide - separating fact from fiction and navigating the challenging road ahead. Curr Sports Med Rep. 2018;17(3):83–4.
140. Timpka T, Spreco A, Dahlstrom O, Jacobsson J, Kowalski J, Bargoria V, et al. Suicidal thoughts (ideation) among elite athletics (track and field) athletes: associations with sports participation, psychological resourcefulness and having been a victim of sexual and/or physical abuse. Br J Sports Med. 2021;55(4):198–205.
141. Rao AL, Asif IM, Drezner JA, Toresdahl BG, Harmon KG. Suicide in National Collegiate Athletic Association (NCAA) athletes: a 9-year analysis of the NCAA resolutions database. Sports Health. 2015;7(5):452.
142. Maron B, Haas T, Murphy C, Ahluwalia A, Rutten-Ramos S. Incidence and causes of sudden death in U.S. college athletes. J Am Coll Cardiol. 2014;63(16):1636–43.
143. Anchuri K, Davoren AK, Shanahan A, Torres M, Wilcox H. Nonsuicidal self-injury, suicidal ideation, and suicide attempt among collegiate athletes: findings from the National College Health Assessment. J Am Coll Heal. 2019;68:815. https://www.tandfonline.com/doi/abs/10.1080/07448481.2019.1616743. Accessed 16 Mar 2022.
144. Taliaferro LA, Eisenberg ME, Johnson KE, Nelson TF, Neumark-Sztainer D. Sport participation during adolescence and suicide ideation and attempts. Int J Adolesc Med Health. 2011;23(1):3. https://www.degruyter.com/document/doi/10.1515/ijamh.2011.002/html. Accessed 16 Mar 2022.
145. Taylor P, Jomar K, Dhingra K, Forrester R, Shahmalak U, Dickson J. A meta-analysis of the prevalence of different functions of non-suicidal self-injury. J Affect Disord. 2018;227:759–69.
146. McMahon J, McGannon KR. 'I hurt myself because it sometimes helps': former athletes' embodied emotion responses to abuse using self-injury. Sport Educ Soc. 2019;26(2):161–74.
147. Larson S, Chapman S, Spetz J, Brindis CD. Chronic childhood trauma, mental health, academic achievement, and school-based health center mental health services. J Sch Health. 2017;87(9):675–86.
148. Liu S, Kia-Keating M, Nylund-Gibson K. Patterns of adversity and pathways to health among White, Black, and Latinx youth. Child Abuse Negl. 2018;86:89–99.
149. Ballesteros J, Tran AGTT. Under the face mask: racial-ethnic minority student-athletes and mental health use. J Am Coll Heal. 2018;68:169. https://www.tandfonline.com/doi/abs/10.1080/07448481.2018.1536663. Accessed 15 Mar 2022.
150. Lu W, Todhunter-Reid A, Mitsdarffer ML, Muñoz-Laboy M, Yoon AS, Xu L. Barriers and facilitators for mental health service use among racial/ethnic minority adolescents: a systematic review of literature. Front Public Health. 2021;9:641605. https://www.frontiersin.org/articles/10.3389/fpubh.2021.641605/full. Accessed 15 Mar 2022.
151. Luk JW, Gilman SE, Haynie DL, Simons-Morton BG. Sexual orientation and depressive symptoms in adolescents. Pediatrics. 2018;141(5):e20173309. https://publications.aap.org/pediatrics/article/141/5/e20173309/37851/Sexual-Orientation-and-Depressive-Symptoms-in. Accessed 15 Mar 2022.
152. Yolaç E, Meriç M. Internalized homophobia and depression levels in LGBT individuals. Perspect Psychiatr Care. 2021;57(1):304–10.
153. DeFoor MT, Stepleman LM, Mann PC. Improving wellness for LGB collegiate student-athletes through sports medicine: a narrative review. Sports Med Open. 2018;4(1):1–10.
154. Tough H, Siegrist J, Fekete C. Social relationships, mental health and wellbeing in physical disability: a systematic review. BMC Public Health. 2017;17(1):1–18.
155. Kattari SK. Ableist microaggressions and the mental health of disabled adults. Community Ment Health J. 2020;56(6):1170–9.
156. Swartz L, Hunt X, Bantjes J, Hainline B, Reardon CL. Mental health symptoms and disorders in Paralympic athletes: a narrative review. Br J Sports Med. 2019;53(12):737–40.

157. Palmiter D, Alvord M, Dorlen R, Comas-Diaz L. Building your resilience; 2020. https:// www.apa.org, https://www.apa.org/topics/resilience. Accessed 17 Mar 2022.
158. O'Brien KHM, Rowan M, Willoughby K, Griffith K, Christino MA. Psychological resilience in young female athletes. Int J Environ Res Public Health. 2021;18(16):8668. https://www. ncbi.nlm.nih.gov/pmc/articles/PMC8392459/. Accessed 17 Mar 2022.
159. Tamminen KA, et al. Exploring adversity and the potential for growth among elite female athletes. Psychol Sport Exerc. 2013;14(1):28–36.
160. Lu F, Lee WP, Chang Y-K, Chou C-C, Hsu Y-W, Lin J-H, et al. Interaction of athletes' resilience and coaches' social support on the stress-burnout relationship: a conjunctive moderation perspective. Psychol Sport Exerc. 2016;22:202–9.
161. Day MC, Wadey R. Researching growth following adversity in sport and exercise: methodological implications and future recommendations. Qual Res Sport Exerc. Health. 2017;9:1. https://www.tandfonline.com/doi/abs/10.1080/2159676X.2017.1328460. Accessed 17 Mar 2022.

Chapter 3
Eating Disorders and Relative Energy Deficiency in Sport (RED-S)

Laura Reece, Nicole Farnsworth, Kristin E. Whitney, and Kathryn E. Ackerman

Key Points
- Youth athletes are at risk for developing low energy availability (EA), whether through high training demands, inadequate nutritional status, or a combination of both.
- The causes of relative energy deficiency in sport (RED-S) can be unintentional, misconceived, or uncontrollable; determination of the potential cause(s) will assist providers in implementing appropriate treatment measures.
- Disordered eating (DE) and eating disorders (EDs) are prevalent in the youth athlete population, especially in those sports emphasizing weight, physique, or thinness.
- Treatment of DE/EDs in adolescent athletes should include a multidisciplinary team.

L. Reece (✉) · N. Farnsworth · K. E. Ackerman
Boston Children's Hospital, Boston, MA, USA
e-mail: Laura.Reece@childrens.harvard.edu; Nicole.Farnsworth@childrens.harvard.edu;
Kathryn.Ackerman@childrens.harvard.edu

K. E. Whitney
Division of Sports Medicine, Department of Orthopedic Surgery, Boston Children's Hospital, Boston, MA, USA

The Micheli Center for Sports Injury Prevention, Waltham, MA, USA

Harvard Medical School, Boston, MA, USA
e-mail: Kristin.Whitney@childrens.harvard.edu

© The Author(s), under exclusive license to Springer Nature Switzerland AG 2023
M. A. Christino et al. (eds.), *Psychological Considerations in the Young Athlete*, Contemporary Pediatric and Adolescent Sports Medicine, https://doi.org/10.1007/978-3-031-25126-9_3

Introduction

Sports and exercise participation provide an environment in which athletes can challenge themselves both physically and mentally. Individuals can train their bodies to perform at an optimal level to achieve their goals in their athletic endeavors. At times, athletes may find themselves inadequately fueled for their body's basal needs and training demands, which can negatively impact health and performance outcomes. This inadequacy can stem from many causes, may be intentional or unintentional, and can be further amplified in the youth athlete with increased energy needs of growth and development. This chapter will discuss the definitions of low energy availability (EA), relative energy deficiency in sport (RED-S), disordered eating (DE) and eating disorders (EDs), the epidemiology of these in the young athlete population, consequences of RED-S and DE/EDs, risk factors/warning signs, screening tools available, intervention and treatment approaches, and possible preventive measures.

Low Energy Availability and Relative Energy Deficiency in Sport

EA is defined as dietary energy intake (EI) minus exercise energy expenditure (EEE) normalized to fat-free mass (FFM): $EA = (EI - EEE)/FFM$ [1]. Athletes with low EA are more likely to be classified as having increased risk of hormonal dysfunction, poor bone health, metabolic dysfunction, hematological impacts, psychological disorders, cardiovascular risks, and gastrointestinal dysfunction than athletes with adequate EA. Performance variables that have been associated with low EA include decreased training response, decreased endurance performance, impaired judgment, decreased coordination, decreased concentration, increased irritability, and depression [2–5].

As EA diminishes, energy is diverted away from the reproductive axis to more vital bodily systems, such as cell maintenance and immune function. The bodies of energy-restricted athletes develop energy-conserving mechanisms [6]. In fact, female athletes with functional hypothalamic amenorrhea (FHA) have been shown to have lower resting energy expenditure (REE) and triiodothyronine (T3) than their eumenorrheic athletic counterparts [7, 8]. Male athletes also exhibit physiological changes as a result of lowering EA, including decreased testosterone levels and low bone mineral density [9]. Studies in adult female exercisers have suggested that an EA of at least 30 kcal/kg of FFM per day is necessary to maintain proper functioning of the hypothalamic-pituitary-ovarian axis and at least 45 kcal/kg of FFM per day to maintain proper bone metabolism [10]. In male athlete studies, the cutoff for low EA is not as well established, as it has been postulated that male athletes have a differing critical threshold [11, 12]. These numbers may vary from individual to individual and no ideal set point has been established in the growing, adolescent athlete.

Female athletes are at risk for the "Female Athlete Triad" (Triad), a term referring to the interrelationship among energy availability, menstrual function, and bone mineral density (BMD). According to the 2007 Triad position stand of the American College of Sports Medicine (ACSM), an athlete may be at different points along

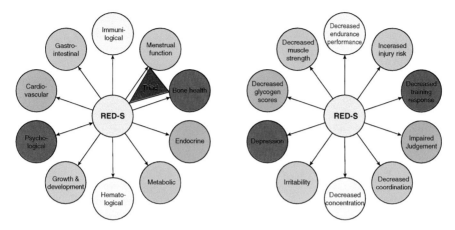

Fig. 3.1 Health and performance consequences of relative energy deficiency in sport (RED-S) [14, 18]

three spectra from optimal health to significant disease [6]. At one end of the spectra, an athlete has optimal energy availability, eumenorrhea, and optimal bone health. Further along the spectra, an athlete may have reduced EA with or without DE, subclinical menstrual disorders (e.g., oligomenorrhea, luteal deficiency, anovulation), and/or low BMD. At the pathologic end of the spectra are the combination of low EA with or without an ED, functional hypothalamic amenorrhea (FHA; absence of menses caused by suppression of the hypothalamic-pituitary-ovarian axis without a known anatomic or organic disease cause), and osteoporosis [6]. The Male Athlete Triad has been more recently introduced to describe a similar relationship among energy availability, testosterone levels, and BMD [13].

Appropriate EA is paramount for overall health and performance, and in 2014 the International Olympic Committee (IOC) expanded the concept of Triad by introducing the term "RED-S" (relative energy deficiency in sport) [14]. RED-S can apply to both men and women and refers to impaired physiological function caused by relative energy deficiency involving menstrual function, metabolic rate, bone health, immunity, protein synthesis, and cardiovascular health. In addition to the known reproductive and bone health consequences, inadequate caloric intake and maladaptive eating behaviors can lead to impaired growth, decreased stamina, muscle strength, coordination, concentration, and speed, in addition to higher risk of muscle strains, ligamentous sprains, and fractures [5, 14–18] (Fig. 3.1).

Disordered Eating vs. Eating Disorder

Oftentimes, the personality traits and behaviors that contribute to an athlete's success in sport are similar to those thought to correlate with the development of an ED, including perfectionism, discipline, and sacrifice for distinction, among others [19]. The focus and drive that an athlete puts into maximizing performance can contribute to the development of a hyperfocus on the physical form and an obsession with achieving what they or others believe to be an "ideal body" for her/his sport. Athletes with DE/EDs often have a preoccupation with food that correlates with experiencing isolation, a sense of being misunderstood, difficulty with interpersonal relationships, and depression [20, 21]. More serious consequences of EDs such as AN include electrolyte abnormalities, cardiac arrhythmias, severe bradycardia, hypotension, and even death [22].

The terms ED/DE are often used interchangeably; however, it is important to differentiate the two and understand recent changes in feeding and ED terminology. DE is typically used to describe individuals who have restrictive eating habits and/ or purging behaviors, but do not meet diagnostic criteria for a clinical ED. Individuals with DE often cycle through periods of severe food restricting, dieting, and/or overexercising and run the risk of developing a clinical ED. In the most recent version of the American Psychiatric Association's *Diagnostic and Statistical Manual of Mental Disorders* (DSM-5), an ED is diagnosed as anorexia nervosa (AN), bulimia nervosa (BN), avoidant/restrictive food intake disorder (ARFID), pica, rumination disorder, binge eating disorder (BED), other specified feeding or ED (OSFED), or unspecified feeding or ED (UFED) [23]. Some diagnoses include a dimensional component, which allows for specification of illness severity. AN is characterized by a distorted body image and restriction of EI that leads to severe weight loss with a pathological fear of gaining weight, and an undue influence of weight and shape on the individual's self-worth. While low body mass index (BMI) and amenorrhea are often associated with AN, a BMI cutoff and menstrual irregularity are no longer required to fit the diagnosis of AN as it had been in past editions of the DSM [24]. BN is characterized by frequent episodes of binge eating followed by inappropriate behaviors such as self-induced vomiting or exercising excessively to avoid weight gain. Such compensatory behaviors occur at least once a week to meet BN diagnostic criteria [23].

ARFID is a feeding or eating disturbance that leads to persistent failure to meet appropriate nutritional and/or energy needs with one or more of the following: (a) significant weight loss (or failure to gain weight in a child), (b) significant nutritional deficiency, (c) dependence on enteral feeding or oral nutritional supplements, and/or (d) significant interference with psychological functioning. In ARFID, however, there is no evidence of a disturbance in the way one's body weight or shape is experienced [23]. Other ED diagnoses that, like ARFID, do not involve disturbance in one's body image include pica, the compulsive eating of nonnutritive substances, and rumination disorder, repeated regurgitation of food not associated with other EDs.

One of the most notable changes in DSM-5 compared to DSM-IV and its text revision (DSM-IV-TR) [24] is the inclusion of BED. BED involves recurring episodes of eating significantly more food in a much shorter amount of time than most people would eat under similar circumstances, with such episodes marked by feelings of lack of control. Those with BED may eat too quickly, even when not hungry; may have feelings of guilt, embarrassment, or disgust; and typically have such binges at least once a week for at least 3 months [23].

Other DSM-5 feeding and ED diagnoses include OSFED and UFED. OSFED involves feeding or eating behaviors that cause clinically significant distress and impairment in areas of functioning, but do not meet the full criteria for any of the other feeding and EDs. Some diagnoses are given caveats, such as "atypical AN," which may include an individual who meets all diagnostic criteria of AN, but despite significant weight loss, still has a weight within or above the normal range. UFED involves behaviors that cause clinically significant distress/functional impairment but do not meet full clinical criteria for any of the other named feeding or EDs. This may be because of a lack of information at the time of the patient presentation [23].

Orthorexia nervosa, while not a term listed in the DSM-5, was first coined by Bratman in 1997 and is an unofficial term to describe excessively "healthy eating" [25]. It typically stems from a desire for one to achieve optimal health and wellness through diet, but often shares symptoms with AN [25, 26].

Certain types of DE may now fall into the DSM-5 categories of OSFED, ARFID, or UFED. While the semantics may seem cumbersome, the terminology updates help include broader categories of DE. Recognizing that these diagnoses exist and should be treated is imperative, as they are associated with medical and performance consequences [2, 18, 27].

Prevalence of Low EA, DE, and EDs

Recent studies looking at low EA found prevalence ranging from 22% to 58% in various team sports and performing artist athletes [28–33]. Matt et al. assessed energy availability and nutrient intake in 72 (60 female, 12 male) high school cross-country runners and found that 30% of males and 60% of females were below 30 kcal/kg FFM/day and considered to have low EA.

Adolescent elite athletes have a higher prevalence of ED than nonathlete controls [34]. Adolescence, a vulnerable period of rapid growth, hormonal fluctuations, personality development, and increased social pressures, is the most common time of ED onset in the general population [35]. Adolescent athletes have the added pressures of increased training volume and intensity, coach expectations, and trying to improve performance and achieve an "ideal sports physique" to adapt to a world of adult athletics. Thus, it is not surprising that in one study, most adult female athletes who met criteria for an ED reported that they started dieting and developing their EDs during puberty/adolescence [36]. Other studies utilizing ED questionnaires found that 18.2–35.4% of high school female athletes had DE, with higher rates in aesthetic sport athletes [37, 38]. When more aesthetic sport athletes were included, DE rates were higher [38].

Male athletes are susceptible to athletic performance pressures in addition to sociocultural influences including body shape pressure and gender role expectations [39–41]. Research on DE/EDs in males has been historically minimal [42]. In the United States, research looking at adolescent boys attempting to change their body weight or shape found 30% of adolescent boys have tried to gain weight compared to 6.5% of girls [43]. In another study, 22% of adolescent males engaged in disordered eating behaviors aimed at defining musculature [44].

The reported prevalence of DE and EDs has ranged from 6% to 60% among female athletes and 0–85.5% for male athletes [45–47]. This wide range can be attributed to varied athlete populations, the inaccuracy of different screening tools, and the DE/ED definitions utilized [48]. In particular, athletes participating in leanness sports, in which a lean frame or specific body weight may be considered important to either traditional expectations of sport-specific aesthetics or weight-based classification criteria systems (e.g., gymnastics, ballet, figure skating, cheerleading, synchronized swimming, wrestling, and lightweight rowing), have been extensively studied and were found to have higher rates of DE and EDs than those participating in non-leanness sports and nonathletes [49, 50]. In a study of the entire population of Norwegian elite athletes in 1 year, the prevalence of EDs among female athletes was 42% in aesthetic sports, 24% in endurance sports, 17% in technical sports, and 16% in ball game sports [51]. In male athletes, the prevalence of EDs was 22% in antigravitational sports, 9% in endurance sports, and 2% in ball sports [51]. Additionally, in a study of elite, recreational, and noncompetitive female athletes ages 17–30 years, those from leanness-focused sports, reported more DE symptomatology regardless of participation level [50].

Screening for Low EA and DE/EDs

Screening for DE/EDs, Triad, and RED-S can be challenging as the symptomatology may sometimes be subtle. There are a few assessment tools that exist to identify athletes with DE, EDs, Triad, and/or RED-S [10, 52, 53]. There are also screening tools that exist for nonathlete populations, which can be applied to athletes to help diagnose DE behaviors or a clinical ED [54–59]. However, many of these questionnaires depend upon self-disclosure, which is often very challenging for individuals with eating pathology. Such individuals frequently feel a great deal of shame, embarrassment, denial, or even a protective nature around their maladaptive eating behaviors. In an athlete population, there are the additional fears of other negative consequences including ineligibility to play and/or potential loss of scholarship or position on a team.

To identify athletes at risk for DE/ED and their related health consequences, it may be helpful to leverage preexisting forums where athletes are required to have medical clearance screenings, such as the pre-participation physical evaluation (PPE) setting [60]. This is required by many high schools, colleges, universities, and athletic clubs to clear an athlete for participation in her respective sport, thus presenting an optimal time to screen athletes for eating concerns. The Female Athlete Triad Coalition (FATC) now recommends the screening questions listed in Table 3.1 [10]. From what we know about the prevalence of DE/ED among athletes, the physician should always have signs of the Triad on his/her radar when assessing female athletes. If a female athlete presents with oligo-/amenorrhea and/or frequent injuries, such as bone stress injuries, the physician should be sure to screen the athlete for the other Triad components [6, 61]. Although the PPE can be quite beneficial, a survey of 347 National Collegiate Athletic Association (NCAA) Division 1 universities found that of the responding 257 universities, all required PPEs for incoming athletes, however only 32% required annual follow-up, and only 9% included all of the FATC-recommended questions as part of their screening processes. In fact, 44%

Table 3.1 Female Athlete Triad Coalition pre-participation examination screening questions [10]

1. Have you ever had a menstrual period?
2. How old were you when you had your first menstrual period?
3. When was your most recent menstrual period?
4. How many periods have you had in the past 12 months?
5. Are you presently taking any female hormones (estrogen, progesterone, birth control pills)?
6. Do you worry about your weight?
7. Are you trying to or has anyone recommended that you gain or lose weight?
8. Are you on a special diet or do you avoid certain types of foods or food groups?
9. Have you ever had an eating disorder?
10. Have you ever had a stress fracture?
11. Have you ever been told you have low bone density (osteopenia or osteoporosis?)

of the responding schools' screening forms had just four Triad-related questions or fewer [62]. In a separate study of 239 NCAA athletes in 16 sports, the electronic PPE did not adequately detect athletes with increased risk for Triad or DE behaviors, suggesting that the PPE may benefit from a validated screening tool designed to better detect athletes with low EA [63].

In conjunction with the RED-S diagnostic criteria, the IOC developed the RED-S Clinical Assessment Tool (RED-S CAT) to assist in the screening of athletes for RED-S. It is an integrative model that utilizes red, yellow, and green lights as indicators of the severity of RED-S and is an aid to determine an athlete's return to play [53] (Fig. 3.2).

The Low Energy Availability in Females Questionnaire (LEAF-Q) was developed to detect persistent low EA and Triad conditions, with or without DE/ED, and was published in 2014 in a validation study. The LEAF-Q is intended for use as a complement to other DE/ED screening tools as it is not meant to discriminate between normal and pathological eating patterns [52].

As mentioned above, there are many questionnaires that have been validated in nonathletes, to screen for subclinical DE as well as ED behaviors and patterns. These include the Eating Attitudes Test (EAT-26) [56], the Eating Disorder Examination Questionnaire (EDE-Q) [58], the Eating Disorder Inventory (EDI) [54], and the Three-Factor Eating Questionnaire (TFEQ) [64]. The EDE-Q, EDI, and TFEQ have been used to screen for subclinical DE in athletes and recreational exercisers, and scores demonstrating high drive for thinness (DT) or high dietary restraint (DR) correlated with increased risk for Triad [65–69]. The Eating Disorder Examination interview performed by a licensed mental health professional remains the gold standard for successful diagnosis of EDs [70]. However, there is no consensus on which screening tool is most efficient and effective in a sports medicine clinic, PPE, or training room environment.

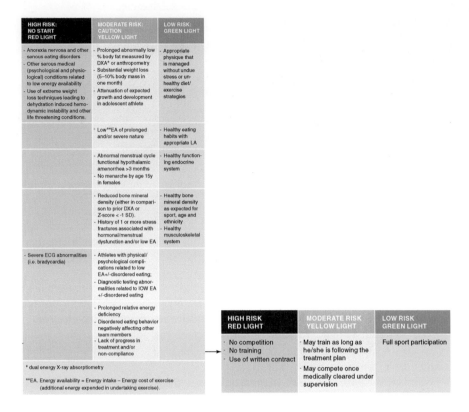

Fig. 3.2 RED-S Clinical Assessment Tool (RED-S CAT) [53]

A promising athlete-specific ED screen is the Brief Eating Disorder in Athletes Questionnaire (BEDA-Q) [71]. Results from prior studies of athletes using various traditional nonathlete validated ED questionnaires found that elite athletes were underreporting and nonathletes were overreporting symptoms associated with ED, resulting in a high percentage of athletes classified as false negative when comparing results from a clinical interview to diagnose ED [71]. Thus, in developing the BEDA-Q, researchers screened elite adolescent athletes with various ED questionnaire components followed by the Eating Disorder Examination interview. Based on results, they then extracted items with good predictive abilities for an ED diagnosis from the EDI-Body dissatisfaction, EDI-Drive for thinness, and EDI-Perfectionism subscales to develop the nine-question BEDA-Q (Table 3.2). This new tool demonstrated excellent ability to distinguish between elite adolescent female athletes with and without EDs, but needs to be tested in larger, more diverse athlete populations [71].

Table 3.2 Brief Eating Disorder in Athletes Questionnaire (BEDA-Q) (Based on [71])	1. I feel extremely guilty after overeating
	O always O usually O often O sometimes O rarely O never
	2. I am preoccupied with the desire to be thinner
	O always O usually O often O sometimes O rarely O never
	3. I think that my stomach is too big
	O always O usually O often O sometimes O rarely O never
	4. I feel satisfied with the shape of my body
	O always O usually O often O sometimes O rarely O never
	5. My parents have expected excellence of me
	O always O usually O often O sometimes O rarely O never
	6. As a child, I tried very hard to avoid disappointing my parents and teachers
	O always O usually O often O sometimes O rarely O never
	7. Are you trying to lose weight now?
	O Yes O No
	8. Have you tried to lose weight?
	O Yes O No
	9. If yes, how many times have you tried to lose weight?
	O 1–2 O 3–5 O >5 times

Education

The key to appropriate treatment and prevention of RED-S and DE/ED in athletes continues to be education of athletes and those around them. Several clinical studies have assessed the knowledge of athletes, physicians, physical therapists, high school nurses, and coaches on all three components of the Triad. They have reported that less than 50% of such respondents were able to identify all three components of the Triad [45–48]. Studies assessing knowledge of RED-S have shown low understanding of RED-S concepts in athletes [72]. In another study of 931 physicians from a variety of specialties at three large academic hospitals, only 37% had heard of Triad [73]. Additionally, evidence suggests that coaches lack the knowledge to recognize the signs and symptoms of DE/EDs and do not feel well-equipped to confront athletes when they suspect eating pathology [74–76]. Due to complications that exist around self-disclosure by athletes, educating coaches and certified athletic trainers (ATCs) about the Triad and DE/EDs can increase awareness and enable early identification and intervention [2]. In fact, coaches' encouragement to seek help has been cited by athletes with EDs as a significant reason for their seeking out support services for their EDs [76–78].

Signs and symptoms of DE/EDs may include weight loss, ritualistic eating, isolating behavior, excessive concern with body image, mood changes, fatigue, frequent illness and injury, decreased exercise performance, and prolonged recovery time after injury. Under-fueled athletes may notice lightheadedness, difficulty concentrating, excessive fatigue, bowel changes, generalized weakness, as well as oligo- or amenorrhea. As mentioned previously, a variety of musculoskeletal, cardiovascular, gastrointestinal, renal, and neuropsychiatric symptoms may also present as a consequence of low EA or RED-S [6, 18, 79].

Intervention

If athletic team personnel have strong suspicion that an athlete is struggling with low EA, an ED, or DE, a conversation with the athlete should be the next step. Creating a rapport in a comfortable environment is important for establishing trust between coaching staff and the athlete. According to NCAA recommendations, those with influence in the sport environment can play an important role in recommending and encouraging appropriate treatment, and they themselves should be trained by healthcare professionals with experience and expertise in EDs and athletes [80]. The ATC or team physician is sometimes in a better position than the coach to have this initial discussion with the athlete. It is important to approach the athlete in a nonjudgmental, non-accusatory way in a private setting. This will help to minimize any further embarrassment or shame for the athlete. Concern for the athlete's health should be the primary focus of the discussion rather than targeting specific behaviors. Targeting specific behaviors may lead to resistance and denial in response to a feeling of being accused. The secondary focus is the intervention recommendations, which begin with a physical examination to assess medical status and stability to determine a treatment approach. The athlete needs to feel supported by the coach and athletic staff, as fear of loss of scholarship or position on the team may cause the athlete to resist getting the help that she needs to recover.

Treatment

If an athlete has been diagnosed or suspected of low EA, determining the cause for this inadequate energy status will help in determining the appropriate treatment. Young athletes can fall into low EA status unintentionally due to lack of knowledge regarding energy needs, commitment to demanding training and competition schedules, gastrointestinal dysfunction or malabsorption, and decreased appetite due to exercise, mental health status, or medications [81]. Addressing low EA in these instances may involve psychoeducation, dietary modifications, and/or referral to specialists for medical management [82]. Low EA can be reversed fairly quickly in athletes with a prompt diagnosis and full engagement in recommendations on the part of the athlete [14, 18, 81].

If the cause of low EA is due to DE/ED, an interdisciplinary, biopsychosocial approach is optimal to treat and prevent further complications. The treatment team often involves a primary care and/or sports medicine physician, a sports dietitian, and a mental health professional. Broadening the team to provide more support can be quite helpful and may include family members, coaches, ATCs, exercise physiologists, and/or other medical professionals. The initial goal of treatment is to increase EA and often body weight to achieve normal physiologic function. This is typically done with both diet and exercise modification [10, 83–85].

The physician should conduct initial as well as subsequent physical examinations to get a better understanding of the patient's health status and gauge the safety of athletic participation throughout treatment. If a significant ED and/or low weight is appreciated at the initial visit, specific labs should be obtained. Additional studies based on the suspicion of other aspects of RED-S may also need to be included initially, with follow-up studies based upon results (Table 3.3).

Once a patient's baseline health is assessed and it is determined if an ED is present, a proper treatment plan can be created. Caloric needs for an individual struggling with DE/ED vary greatly depending on such factors as activity level, BMI, body fat percentage, type of DE/ED, and the presence of electrolyte abnormalities. The pace of the caloric increases are at the discretion of the dietitian and physician, often based on the patient's ability to meet caloric goals set between sessions and

Table 3.3 Initial lab and other testing recommended for athletes presenting with low EA/DE/ED. Modified from Nazem TG and Ackerman KE. The female athlete triad. Sports Health. 2012;4(4):302–11 [61]

Component of triad	Diagnostic testing
Low energy availability/DE/ED	• Complete blood count with differential, comprehensive metabolic panel, phosphorus, magnesium
	• Urinalysis with specific gravity if water loading suspected
	• ECG if low weight, bradycardia, or other physical findings warrant testing
	• Triiodothyronine (T3)
Menstrual dysfunction	• Urine human chorionic gonadotropin (hCG), follicle-stimulating hormone (FSH), thyroid-stimulating hormone (TSH) and free thyroxine (free T4), prolactin, ± estradiol
	If hyperandrogenism is suspected:
	• Luteinizing hormone (LH) to assess LH/FSH ratio, total testosterone, sex hormone binding globulin, dehydroepiandrosterone sulfate (DHEA-S), 8am 17-hydroxyprogesterone
	To confirm estrogen status:
	• Progesterone challenge (e.g., medroxyprogesterone 10 mg daily for 10 days followed by observation for withdrawal bleed)
Male hypogonadism	• Serum testosterone, prolactin, FSH, and LH [86]
Low bone mineral density, multiple bone stress injuries or fractures	• Dual-energy X-ray absorptiometry (DXA) with metabolic bone work-up to follow as needed
	(DXA of an adolescent should include the total body and spine and Z-scores of the total body less head and spine should be reported. Body composition will be included in the whole body scan, which may aid in determining energy needs)

the weight goals determined by the treatment team. The Society for Adolescent Health and Medicine recommends a two-step process to determine treatment goal weight. The first step is to determine the degree of malnutrition as compared to the reference population based on median BMI, BMI z-score, and rate of weight loss. The second step is to review the adolescent's growth charts for height, weight, and BMI trajectories while also considering the pubertal stage of development. It is recommended to re-evaluate goal weights every 3–6 months in the adolescent population [17]. Based on the severity of the condition and patient's clinical progress, close follow-up may be very useful in management, and the frequency and duration of follow-up appointments are at the discretion of the physician and other team members [87]. The team will also work with the athlete to determine the role of sport in their identity, self-esteem, and teammate relationships. This information can help the treatment team better understand the athlete and improve a tailored treatment approach. Individual treatment can vary greatly based on needs. It may include hospitalization; residential, day, and/or intensive individual outpatient treatment; family therapy; and/or group therapy. Communication between treatment team members as well as with the athlete, the family, and the "sport family" (i.e., athletic coaches, ATCs, PTs) can help to ensure that all involved are aware of the treatment plan, as well as what will be required medically before the athlete is able to return to play. Trust is of the utmost importance to help engage the athlete in the recommended treatment plan.

Medical treatment for any comorbidity or injury associated with the DE/ED/low EA should also be included. For example, serum 25-hydroxy vitamin D levels <30 ng/mL are associated with increased incidence of bone stress injury [88]. Vitamin D intake of 600–800 IU daily is recommended by the US Department of Agriculture dietary guidelines [89], but higher intake may be required in order to reach goal serum 25-hydroxy vitamin D levels of over 30 ng/mL [90, 91]. If an athlete's menstrual cycle does not return to normal after a trial of nutritional, psychological, and/or activity modification interventions, transdermal estradiol (E2) therapy with cyclic oral progestin can be considered [92]. Transdermal E2 has been shown to increase BMD and improve bone microarchitecture in oligo-amenorrheic athletes [93, 94].

The registered dietitian (RD) plays an essential role on this interdisciplinary treatment team. RDs are responsible for providing the affected individual with medical nutrition therapy (MNT) to nourish the body, normalize the metabolism, and repair any nutritional deficiencies consequential of the ED [95]. An RD can also utilize tactics such as motivational interviewing to engage the patient in treatment and enhance her motivation. Depending on which ED the individual is suffering with, the treatment approach may differ. However, there is a common thread of reducing stigma around certain foods, creating a varied diet, and providing the body with the appropriate balance of macro- and micronutrients to help the individual remain in a positive energy balance [95, 96]. For an athlete, an RD who is a certified specialist in sports dietetics (CSSD) can be particularly helpful, as they can help the athlete meet increased energy needs as well as teach proper pre-, during-, and post-activity fueling [97, 98]. Determining energy needs for an adolescent athlete with an

ED or DE can present some challenges. Most formulas for estimating number of calories utilized through sports activity have been developed for the adult athletic population and not validated for use in adolescents [98–102]. Determining energy needs in adolescent athletes includes evaluating physical activity levels (PAL) and resting energy expenditure (REE). Given the limitations, PAL can be used as a starting point and adjusted based on the dietitian's discretion and pending further information from clinical interview of intensity and duration of activities [103]. If available, REE can be determined via indirect calorimetry, although this is not always practical. Predictive equations such as Harris Benedict [102], Mifflin St. Jeor [99], Cunningham [100], or Schofield [101] can help to estimate resting energy expenditure (REE). In an adolescent, it is important to consider not only calories for activity level but also calories required for growth and development. A dietitian should be sure to re-evaluate caloric estimates as an adolescent athlete progresses through treatment to ensure she continues to stay in a positive energy balance with increases in lean body mass, fat mass, and height, as well as increases in activity level.

Psychotherapy is an essential component of the treatment of athletes struggling with EDs. Cognitive behavioral therapy (CBT) is the most effective treatment for individuals struggling with BN and is the first line of defense for individuals struggling with BED [104]. CBT is a form of psychotherapy used with BN and BED that focuses on identifying and restructuring irrational thoughts in order to change maladaptive behaviors and negative feelings. CBT also teaches individuals about identifying situations, as well as cognitive distortions, that might trigger symptom use. It is most successful in those motivated to change, as it requires outside homework involving self-monitoring and practicing techniques learned in sessions. Studies in adolescents are limited [105]. Dialectical behavior therapy (DBT) is a very structured mindfulness-based third-wave CBT treatment that focuses on clearly identifying chains of events, including emotional experiences and, in some cases, emotional avoidance prompting problem ED behaviors. The treatment includes the use of mental and behavioral skills to enhance a patient's capacity for mindfulness, emotional regulation, distress tolerance, and interpersonal effectiveness. DBT has been shown to be effective in decreasing BED and purging in certain populations [105]. In addition to DBT, another mindfulness-based third-wave CBT treatment for eating disorders is acceptance and commitment therapy (ACT), which has been shown to be particularly effective in reducing body image problems in the treatment of AN [106].

Family-based therapy (FBT) is an increasingly adopted treatment approach in adolescents struggling with EDs and has been found most effective in adolescents struggling with AN [107]. Formerly known as "Maudsley family therapy," FBT is recommended as first-line therapy by the Society for Adolescent Health and Medicine for treatment of AN in adolescents [17]. FBT is primarily an outpatient-based intensive treatment program, usually of 6–12 months of duration, that requires the parents manage the refeeding/weight restoration of the affected adolescent. An FBT team is comprised of a physician and an FBT therapist and may include a dietitian, whose role is often intended for occasional guidance but not meal planning [108]. In many cases, the dietitian will even meet with the parents of the athlete alone to help empower them in the refeeding process. A study by Couturier et al. found that FBT was superior to individual therapy at follow-up for adolescents struggling with AN and BN [109], and Lock et al. found FBT to have a lower remission rate at 1 year follow-up compared to adolescents with AN treated with individual therapy [110]. However, it is important to note that FBT may not be appropriate for all adolescents, particularly older adolescents or those with families who are not close by or cannot commit to the intensive meal monitoring. In such instances, individual therapy may be the more appropriate intervention. A newer form of CBT known as enhanced CBT (CBT-E) has been examined for use in adolescents as an alternative to FBT and was found to be well-accepted and effective at 6- and 12-month follow-ups for this population [111, 112].

The ED treatments recommended above may be effective in and applicable to the athlete population, but more research in athletes is needed. It is important that those working with an affected athlete have clinical ED and sports-related expertise. Members of the interdisciplinary team should be individuals who understand the value of sport in the athlete's life [80]. An individual with influence in the sport environment is often ideal to spearhead this initiative. This may help alleviate some of the shame and resistance that can be associated with participating in psychotherapy and help athletes to be more open to seeking treatment and remaining consistent with it [80].

Return to Play

When the time comes to consider the athlete's readiness to return to play, the RED-S CAT can be utilized to assist in this process. The model is designed to integrate a clinical assessment as well as return to play guidelines into a functional model that is easy to understand for all those involved [53]. The model may be customized for the individual athlete to meet her needs, and then the written contract can be used to ensure consistency of messages from all members of the treatment team. It can also be shown to parents, coaches, and athletes to manage expectations [53]. Both the RED-S CAT and the Triad Coalition's Return to Play models are expert attempts to quantify medical risk and offer guidelines for safe return to play for those with DE/EDs [10, 53]. They are both works in progress, as they are currently being studied to determine their clinical utility and effectiveness, and will likely have future iterations for improvement.

Depending on the diagnosis and severity of illness, an athlete may be asked to completely refrain from activity until they are more medically stable and able to participate. Once the athlete does begin reintegrating into sport, it is helpful to set guidelines around the frequency as well as duration of activity so that there is no confusion about or manipulation of the amount of activity that is occurring. Several studies have shown that there is a psychological and possibly medical benefit to allowing a medically stable sport participant to continue to do some form of monitored exercise during treatment [113–115]. Helping an athlete learn how to use exercise in a healthy way during treatment may prevent confusion later as they to integrate back into sports and a society rife with media messages about body image, diet, and fitness. It is also beneficial to have an athlete work with a dietitian while reincorporating sport to understand associated increased fueling needs.

Prevention

Structuring specific initiatives within the athletic community to help support and encourage proper fueling and positive body image may be helpful in preventing the development of RED-S, DE, and EDs. Some organizations have worked on establishing preventive guidelines for athletes. The NCAA's Sport Science Institute is a new resource that has been established with the focus of health and safety in collegiate athletes. Its website has a list of resources aimed at the prevention of EDs in the athletic community [80]. The National Eating Disorders Association (NEDA) has developed a "toolkit" focused on educating coaches and ATCs on how to recognize EDs, as well as how to prevent them and create a supportive and healthy environment for their athletes [116]. Peer-led ED prevention programs for college athletes are also being tested and have thus far shown promising results in decreasing ED behaviors and motivating athletes to seek help when needed [117–119].

Summary

Because of the high prevalence and significant consequences, those working with youth athletes should have an understanding of the signs of symptoms of low EA and an index of suspicion for DE/EDs. Terminology for DE/EDs has changed over time, particularly with recent definitions presented in the DSM-5, but it is most important that low EA and maladaptive eating behaviors are recognized and treated, regardless of their labels. Early detection and treatment leads to improved outcomes, and clinic visits and PPEs are good opportunities to screen for DE/EDs. An athlete's DE/ED treatment team should typically include a physician, dietitian, and mental health specialist, all of whom have familiarity with DE/EDs and sport. Treatment is often enhanced by including members of the athlete's "sport family" and other individuals important in their life. Treatment models may vary and can be modified on a case-by-case basis, but a contract to delineate goals and return to play criteria is consistently helpful in keeping the team and athlete aware of the plan and in managing expectations. Finally, decreasing the stigma around mental health issues in sport and enhancing education about such topics is vital to combatting the prevalence of DE/ED in our student-athlete communities. More research is needed on how best to reach athletes, coaches, ATCs, and others with this message.

References

1. Ihle R, Loucks AB. Dose-response relationships between energy availability and bone turnover in young exercising women. J Bone Miner Res. 2004;19:1231–40.
2. Ackerman KE, Holtzman B, Cooper KM, Flynn EF, Bruinvels G, Tenforde AS, Popp KL, Simpkin AJ, Parziale AL. Low energy availability surrogates correlate with health and performance consequences of Relative Energy Deficiency in Sport. Br J Sports Med. 2019;53:628–33.
3. Keay N, Francis G, Hind K. Low energy availability assessed by a sport-specific questionnaire and clinical interview indicative of bone health, endocrine profile and cycling performance in competitive male cyclists. BMJ Open Sport Exerc Med. 2018;4:e000424.
4. Degoutte F, Jouanel P, Bègue RJ, Colombier M, Lac G, Pequignot JM, Filaire E. Food restriction, performance, biochemical, psychological, and endocrine changes in judo athletes. Int J Sports Med. 2006;27:9–18.
5. Vanheest JL, Rodgers CD, Mahoney CE, De Souza MJ. Ovarian suppression impairs sport performance in junior elite female swimmers. Med Sci Sports Exerc. 2014;46:156–66.
6. Nattiv A, Loucks AB, Manore MM, Sanborn CF, Sundgot-Borgen J, Warren MP, American College of Sports Medicine. American College of Sports Medicine position stand. The female athlete triad. Med Sci Sports Exerc. 2007;39:1867–82.
7. Souza MJD, Lee DK, VanHeest JL, Scheid JL, West SL, Williams NI. Severity of energy-related menstrual disturbances increases in proportion to indices of energy conservation in exercising women. Fertil Steril. 2007;88:971–5.
8. O'Donnell E, Harvey PJ, De Souza MJ. Relationships between vascular resistance and energy deficiency, nutritional status and oxidative stress in oestrogen deficient physically active women. Clin Endocrinol (Oxf). 2009;70:294. https://doi.org/10.1111/j.1365-2265.2008.03332.x.
9. Hooper DR, Kraemer WJ, Saenz C, Schill KE, Focht BC, Volek JS, Maresh CM. The presence of symptoms of testosterone deficiency in the exercise-hypogonadal male condition and the role of nutrition. Eur J Appl Physiol. 2017;117:1349–57.
10. De Souza MJ, Nattiv A, Joy E, et al. 2014 Female Athlete Triad Coalition Consensus Statement on Treatment and Return to Play of the Female Athlete Triad: 1st International Conference held in San Francisco, California, May 2012 and 2nd International Conference held in Indianapolis, Indiana, 2013. Br J Sports Med. 2014;48:289.
11. Fagerberg P. Negative consequences of low energy availability in natural male bodybuilding: a review. Int J Sport Nutr Exerc Metab. 2018;28:385–402.
12. Loucks AB, Kiens B, Wright HH. Energy availability in athletes. J Sports Sci. 2011;29:S7–S15.
13. Nattiv A, De Souza MJ, Koltun KJ, Misra M, Kussman A, Williams NI, Barrack MT, Kraus E, Joy E, Fredericson M. The male athlete triad—a consensus statement from the female and male athlete triad coalition. Part 1: Definition and scientific basis. Clin J Sport Med. 2021;31:335–48.
14. Mountjoy M. The IOC consensus statement: beyond the Female Athlete Triad—Relative Energy Deficiency in Sport (RED-S). Br J Sports Med. 2014;48:491.
15. El Ghoch M, Soave F, Calugi S, Dalle Grave R. Eating disorders, physical fitness and sport performance: a systematic review. Nutrients. 2013;5:5140–60.
16. Fogelholm M. Effects of bodyweight reduction on sports performance. Sports Med. 1994;18:249–67.
17. Society for Adolescent Health and Medicine, Golden NH, Katzman DK, Sawyer SM, Ornstein RM, Rome ES, Garber AK, Kohn M, Kreipe RE. Position Paper of the Society for Adolescent Health and Medicine: medical management of restrictive eating disorders in adolescents and young adults. J Adolesc Health. 2015;56:121–5.
18. Mountjoy M, Sundgot-Borgen JK, Burke LM, et al. IOC consensus statement on relative energy deficiency in sport (RED-S): 2018 update. Br J Sports Med. 2018;52:687–97.

19. Thompson RA, Sherman RT. Eating disorders in sport. New York, NY: Routledge; 2010.
20. Shanmugam V, Jowett S, Meyer C. Eating psychopathology as a risk factor for depressive symptoms in a sample of British athletes. J Sports Sci. 2014;32:1587–95.
21. Shanmugam V, Jowett S, Meyer C. Interpersonal difficulties as a risk factor for athletes' eating psychopathology. Scand J Med Sci Sports. 2014;24:469–76.
22. Yager J, Andersen AE. Clinical practice. Anorexia Nervosa. N Engl J Med. 2005;353:1481–8.
23. American Psychiatric Association. Diagnostic and statistical manual of mental disorders (DSM–5). 5th ed. Arlington, VA: American Psychiatric Association; 2013.
24. American Psychiatric Association. Diagnostic and statistical manual of mental disorders. 4th ed. Washington, DC: American Psychiatric Association; 2000. Text Revision
25. Bratman S. Orthorexia vs. theories of healthy eating. Eat Weight Disord. 2017;22:381–5.
26. Koven N, Abry A. The clinical basis of orthorexia nervosa: emerging perspectives. Neuropsychiatr Dis Treat. 2015;11:385–94.
27. Micali N, Solmi F, Horton NJ, Crosby RD, Eddy KT, Calzo JP, Sonneville KR, Swanson SA, Field AE. Adolescent eating disorders predict psychiatric, high-risk behaviors and weight outcomes in young adulthood. J Am Acad Child Adolesc Psychiatry. 2015;54:652–659.e1.
28. Braun H, von Andrian-Werburg J, Schänzer W, Thevis M. Nutrition status of young elite female german football players. Pediatr Exerc Sci. 2018;30:157–67.
29. Cherian KS, Sainoji A, Nagalla B, Yagnambhatt VR. Energy balance coexists with disproportionate macronutrient consumption across pretraining, during training, and posttraining among Indian junior soccer players. Pediatr Exerc Sci. 2018;30:506–15.
30. Civil R, Lamb A, Loosmore D, Ross L, Livingstone K, Strachan F, Dick JR, Stevenson EJ, Brown MA, Witard OC. Assessment of dietary intake, energy status, and factors associated with RED-S in vocational female ballet students. Front Nutr. 2019;5:136. https://doi.org/10.3389/fnut.2018.00136.
31. McCormack WP, Shoepe TC, LaBrie J, Almstedt HC. Bone mineral density, energy availability, and dietary restraint in collegiate cross-country runners and non-running controls. Eur J Appl Physiol. 2019;119:1747–56.
32. Kinoshita N, Uchiyama E, Ishikawa-Takata K, Yamada Y, Okuyama K. Association of energy availability with resting metabolic rates in competitive female teenage runners: a cross-sectional study. J Int Soc Sports Nutr. 2021;18:70.
33. Matt SA, Barrack MT, Gray VB, Cotter JA, Van Loan MD, Rauh MJ, McGowan R, Nichols JF. Adolescent endurance runners exhibit suboptimal energy availability and intakes of key nutrients. J Am Coll Nutr. 2021;41:1–8.
34. Martinsen M, Sundgot-Borgen J. Higher prevalence of eating disorders among adolescent elite athletes than controls. Med Sci Sports Exerc. 2013;45:1188–97.
35. Smink FRE, van Hoeken D, Hoek HW. Epidemiology of eating disorders: incidence, prevalence and mortality rates. Curr Psychiatry Rep. 2012;14:406–14.
36. Sundgot-Borgen J. Risk and trigger factors for the development of eating disorders in female elite athletes. Med Sci Sports Exerc. 1994;26:414–9.
37. Nichols JF, Rauh MJ, Lawson MJ, Ji M, Barkai H-S. Prevalence of the female athlete triad syndrome among high school athletes. Arch Pediatr Adolesc Med. 2006;160:137–42.
38. Thein-Nissenbaum JM, Rauh MJ, Carr KE, Loud KJ, McGuine TA. Associations between disordered eating, menstrual dysfunction, and musculoskeletal injury among high school athletes. J Orthop Sports Phys Ther. 2011;41:60–9.
39. Dryer R, Farr M, Hiramatsu I, Quinton S. The role of sociocultural influences on symptoms of muscle dysmorphia and eating disorders in men, and the mediating effects of perfectionism. Behav Med. 2016;42:174–82.
40. Eik-Nes TT, Austin SB, Blashill AJ, Murray SB, Calzo JP. Prospective health associations of drive for muscularity in young adult males. Int J Eat Disord. 2018;51:1185–93.
41. Nagata JM, Brown TA, Lavender JM, Murray SB. Emerging trends in eating disorders among adolescent boys: muscles, macronutrients, and biohacking. Lancet Child Adolesc Health. 2019;3:444–5.

42. Murray SB, Griffiths S, Nagata JM. Community-based eating disorder research in males: a call to action. J Adolesc Health. 2018;62:649–50.
43. Nagata JM, Bibbins-Domingo K, Garber AK, Griffiths S, Vittinghoff E, Murray SB. Boys, bulk, and body ideals: sex differences in weight gain attempts among adolescents in the United States. J Adolesc Health. 2019;64:450–3.
44. Nagata JM, Murray SB, Bibbins-Domingo K, Garber AK, Mitchison D, Griffiths S. Predictors of muscularity oriented disordered eating behaviors in U.S. young adults: a prospective cohort study. Int J Eat Disord. 2019;52:1380–8.
45. Bratland-Sanda S, Sundgot-Borgen J. Eating disorders in athletes: overview of prevalence, risk factors and recommendations for prevention and treatment. Eur J Sport Sci. 2013;13:499–508.
46. Reardon CL, Factor RM. Sport psychiatry: a systematic review of diagnosis and medical treatment of mental illness in athletes. Sports Med. 2010;40:961–80.
47. Karrer Y, Halioua R, Mötteli S, Iff S, Seifritz E, Jäger M, Claussen MC. Disordered eating and eating disorders in male elite athletes: a scoping review. BMJ Open Sport Exerc Med. 2020;6:e000801.
48. Beals KA. Disordered eating among athletes: a comprehensive guide for health professionals. Champaign, IL: Human Kinetics; 2004.
49. Van Durme K, Goossens L, Braet C. Adolescent aesthetic athletes: a group at risk for eating pathology? Eat Behav. 2012;13:119–22.
50. Kong P, Harris LM. The sporting body: body image and eating disorder symptomatology among female athletes from leanness focused and nonleanness focused sports. J Psychol. 2015;149:141–60.
51. Sundgot-Borgen J, Torstveit MK. Prevalence of eating disorders in elite athletes is higher than in the general population. Clin J Sport Med. 2004;14:25–32.
52. Melin A, Tornberg AB, Skouby S, Faber J, Ritz C, Sjödin A, Sundgot-Borgen J. The LEAF questionnaire: a screening tool for the identification of female athletes at risk for the female athlete triad. Br J Sports Med. 2014;48:540–5.
53. Mountjoy M, Sundgot-Borgen J, Burke L, et al. RED-S CAT. Relative energy deficiency in sport (RED-S) clinical assessment tool (CAT). Br J Sports Med. 2015;49:421–3.
54. Garner DM, Olmstead MP, Polivy J. Development and validation of a multidimensional eating disorder inventory for anorexia nervosa and bulimia. Int J Eat Disord. 1983;2:15–34.
55. Morgan JF, Reid F, Lacey JH. The SCOFF questionnaire: assessment of a new screening tool for eating disorders. BMJ. 1999;319:1467–8.
56. Garner DM, Garfinkel PE. The Eating Attitudes Test: an index of the symptoms of anorexia nervosa. Psychol Med. 1979;9:273–9.
57. Garner DM, Olmsted MP, Bohr Y, Garfinkel PE. The eating attitudes test: psychometric features and clinical correlates. Psychol Med. 1982;12:871–8.
58. Cooper Z, Fairburn C. The eating disorder examination: a semi-structured interview for the assessment of the specific psychopathology of eating disorders. Int J Eat Disord. 1987;6:1–8.
59. Mond JM, Hay PJ, Rodgers B, Owen C, Beumont PJV. Validity of the Eating Disorder Examination Questionnaire (EDE-Q) in screening for eating disorders in community samples. Behav Res Ther. 2004;42:551–67.
60. Bernhardt D, Roberts W, American Academy of Family Physicians. American Academy of Pediatrics. PPE: preparticipation physical evaluation. Elk Grove Village, IL: American Academy of Pediatrics; 2010.
61. Nazem TG, Ackerman KE. The female athlete triad. Sports Health. 2012;4:302–11.
62. Mencias T, Noon M, Hoch AZ. Female athlete triad screening in National Collegiate Athletic Association Division I athletes: is the preparticipation evaluation form effective? Clin J Sport Med. 2012;22:122–5.
63. Goldstein R, Carlson J, Tenforde A, Golden N, Fredericson M. Low-energy availability and the electronic preparticipation examination in college athletes: is there a better way to screen? Curr Sports Med Rep. 2021;20:489–93.
64. Stunkard AJ, Messick S. The three-factor eating questionnaire to measure dietary restraint, disinhibition and hunger. J Psychosom Res. 1985;29:71–83.

65. Cobb KL, Bachrach LK, Greendale G, et al. Disordered eating, menstrual irregularity, and bone mineral density in female runners. Med Sci Sports Exerc. 2003;35:711–9.
66. O'Connor PJ, Lewis RD, Kirchner EM. Eating disorder symptoms in female college gymnasts. Med Sci Sports Exerc. 1995;27:550–5.
67. Gibbs JC, Williams NI, Scheid JL, Toombs RJ, De Souza MJ. The association of a high drive for thinness with energy deficiency and severe menstrual disturbances: confirmation in a large population of exercising women. Int J Sport Nutr Exerc Metab. 2011;21:280–90.
68. Barrack MT, Rauh MJ, Barkai H-S, Nichols JF. Dietary restraint and low bone mass in female adolescent endurance runners. Am J Clin Nutr. 2008;87:36–43.
69. De Souza MJ, Hontscharuk R, Olmsted M, Kerr G, Williams N. Drive for thinness score is a proxy indicator of energy deficiency in exercising women. Appetite. 2007;48:359–67.
70. Fairburn CG. Eating disorder examination. In: Cognitive behavior therapy and eating disorders. 16th ed. New York, NY: Guilford Press; 2008. p. 265–308.
71. Martinsen M, Holme I, Pensgaard AM, Torstveit MK, Sundgot-Borgen J. The development of the brief eating disorder in athletes questionnaire. Med Sci Sports Exerc. 2014;46:1666–75.
72. Lodge MT, Ackerman KE, Garay J. Knowledge of triad and RED-S in female cross-country athletes and support staff. J Athl Train. 2021; https://doi.org/10.4085/1062-6050-0175.21.
73. Curry EJ, Logan C, Ackerman K, McInnis KC, Matzkin EG. Female athlete triad awareness among multispecialty physicians. Sports Med Open. 2015;1:38.
74. Turk JC, Prentice WE, Chappell S, Shields EW. Collegiate coaches' knowledge of eating disorders. J Athl Train. 1999;34:19–24.
75. Sherman RT, Thompson RA, Dehass D, Wilfert M. NCAA coaches survey: the role of the coach in identifying and managing athletes with disordered eating. Eat Disord. 2005;13:447–66.
76. Plateau CR, Arcelus J, McDermott HJ, Meyer C. Responses of track and field coaches to athletes with eating problems. Scand J Med Sci Sports. 2015;25:e240–50.
77. Gulliver A, Griffiths KM, Christensen H. Barriers and facilitators to mental health help-seeking for young elite athletes: a qualitative study. BMC Psychiatry. 2012;12:157.
78. Arthur-Cameselle JN, Baltzell A. Learning from collegiate athletes who have recovered from eating disorders: advice to coaches, parents, and other athletes with eating disorders. J Appl Sport Psychol. 2012;24:1–9.
79. Joy E, Kussman A, Nattiv A. 2016 update on eating disorders in athletes: a comprehensive narrative review with a focus on clinical assessment and management. Br J Sports Med. 2016;50:154–62.
80. Thompson R. Eating disorders. In: Brown G, editor. Mind, body and sport: understanding and supporting student-athlete mental wellness. Indianapolis, IN: NCAA; 2014. p. 25–8.
81. Wasserfurth P, Palmowski J, Hahn A, Krüger K. Reasons for and consequences of low energy availability in female and male athletes: social environment, adaptations, and prevention. Sports Med Open. 2020;6:44.
82. Kuikman MA, Mountjoy M, Stellingwerff T, Burr JF. A review of nonpharmacological strategies in the treatment of relative energy deficiency in sport. Int J Sport Nutr Exerc Metab. 2021;31:268–75.
83. The American College of Sports Medicine. Selected issues for nutrition and the athlete: a team physician consensus statement. Med Sci Sports Exerc. 2013;45:2378–86.
84. Rodriguez NR, DiMarco NM, Langley S, American Dietetic Association, Dietitians of Canada, American College of Sports Medicine: Nutrition and Athletic Performance. Position of the American Dietetic Association, Dietitians of Canada, and the American College of Sports Medicine: nutrition and athletic performance. J Am Diet Assoc. 2009;109:509–27.
85. Wells KR, Jeacocke NA, Appaneal R, Smith HD, Vlahovich N, Burke LM, Hughes D. The Australian Institute of Sport (AIS) and National Eating Disorders Collaboration (NEDC) position statement on disordered eating in high performance sport. Br J Sports Med. 2020;54:1247–58.
86. Carnegie C. Diagnosis of hypogonadism: clinical assessments and laboratory tests. Rev Urol. 2004;6:S3–8.
87. Patino L, Yudchak C, Barbieri D, Stramesi J, Champagne V, Ramundo M. Comparative study on the effectiveness between intensive outpatient care and partial hospitalization

treatments in patients diagnosed with eating disorders. Archiv Med. 2018;10:1. https://doi.org/10.21767/1989-5216.1000258.

88. Ruohola J-P, Laaksi I, Ylikomi T, Haataja R, Mattila VM, Sahi T, Tuohimaa P, Pihlajamäki H. Association between serum 25(OH)D concentrations and bone stress fractures in Finnish young men. J Bone Miner Res. 2006;21:1483–8.

89. USDA. National Nutrient Database for Standard Reference, Legacy Release. Ag Data Commons. https://data.nal.usda.gov/dataset/usda-national-nutrient-database-standard-reference-legacy-release. Accessed 19 Feb 2022.

90. Holick MF, Binkley NC, Bischoff-Ferrari HA, Gordon CM, Hanley DA, Heaney RP, Murad MH, Weaver CM, Endocrine Society. Evaluation, treatment, and prevention of vitamin D deficiency: an Endocrine Society clinical practice guideline. J Clin Endocrinol Metab. 2011;96:1911–30.

91. Sacheck JM, Van Rompay MI, Chomitz VR, Economos CD, Eliasziw M, Goodman E, Gordon CM, Holick MF. Impact of three doses of vitamin D3 on serum 25(OH)D deficiency and insufficiency in at-risk schoolchildren. J Clin Endocrinol Metab. 2017;102:4496–505.

92. Gordon CM, Ackerman KE, Berga SL, Kaplan JR, Mastorakos G, Misra M, Murad MH, Santoro NF, Warren MP. Functional hypothalamic amenorrhea: an endocrine society clinical practice guideline. J Clin Endocrinol Metab. 2017;102:1413–39.

93. Ackerman K, Slattery M, Singhal V, Baskaran C, Campoverde Reyes K, Toth A, Lee H, Bouxsein M, Klibanski A, Misra M. Transdermal 17-β estradiol has a beneficial effect on bone parameters assessed using hrpqct compared to oral ethinyl estradiol-progesterone combination pills in oligoamenorrheic athletes: a randomized controlled trial. Denver, CO: Wiley; 2017. p. S41.

94. Ackerman KE, Singhal V, Baskaran C, et al. Oestrogen replacement improves bone mineral density in oligo-amenorrhoeic athletes: a randomised clinical trial. Br J Sports Med. 2019;53:229–36.

95. Ozier AD, Henry BW, American Dietetic Association. Position of the American Dietetic Association: nutrition intervention in the treatment of eating disorders. J Am Diet Assoc. 2011;111:1236–41.

96. Herrin M, Larkin M. Nutrition counseling in the treatment of eating disorders. 2nd ed. New York, NY: Routledge; 2013.

97. Board Certified Specialist in Sports Dietetics (CSSD). Sports, Cardiovascular, and Wellness Nutrition Dietetic Practice Group. n.d.. https://www.scandpg.org/scan/subgroups/sports-nutrition/be-a-board-certified-sports-dietitian-cssd.

98. Karpinski C, Rosenbloom CA, editors. Sports nutrition: a handbook for professionals. 6th ed. Chicago, IL: Academy of Nutrition and Dietetics; 2017.

99. Mifflin MD, St Jeor ST, Hill LA, Scott BJ, Daugherty SA, Koh YO. A new predictive equation for resting energy expenditure in healthy individuals. Am J Clin Nutr. 1990;51:241–7.

100. Cunningham JJ. A reanalysis of the factors influencing basal metabolic rate in normal adults. Am J Clin Nutr. 1980;33:2372–4.

101. Schofield WN. Predicting basal metabolic rate, new standards and review of previous work. Hum Nutr Clin Nutr. 1985;39(Suppl 1):5–41.

102. Harris JA, Benedict FG. A biometric study of human basal metabolism. Proc Natl Acad Sci U S A. 1918;4:370–3.

103. Mangieri H. Fueling young athletes. Champaign, IL: Human Kinetics; 2017.

104. Wilson GT, Shafran R. Eating disorders guidelines from NICE. Lancet. 2005;365:79–81.

105. Varchol L, Cooper H. Psychotherapy approaches for adolescents with eating disorders. Curr Opin Pediatr. 2009;21:457–64.

106. Fogelkvist M, Gustafsson SA, Kjellin L, Parling T. Acceptance and commitment therapy to reduce eating disorder symptoms and body image problems in patients with residual eating disorder symptoms: a randomized controlled trial. Body Image. 2020;32:155–66.

107. Rosen DS, The Committee on Adolescence. Identification and management of eating disorders in children and adolescents. Pediatrics. 2010;126:1240–53.

108. Lock J. Family-based treatment for anorexia nervosa. In: Grange DL, Lock J, editors. Eating disorders in children and adolescents: a clinical handbook. New York, NY: Guilford Press; 2011. p. 223–42.
109. Couturier J, Kimber M, Szatmari P. Efficacy of family-based treatment for adolescents with eating disorders: a systematic review and meta-analysis. Int J Eat Disord. 2013;46:3–11.
110. Lock J, Le Grange D, Agras WS, Moye A, Bryson SW, Jo B. Randomized clinical trial comparing family-based treatment with adolescent-focused individual therapy for adolescents with anorexia nervosa. Arch Gen Psychiatry. 2010;67:1025–32.
111. Dalle Grave R, Calugi S, Doll HA, Fairburn CG. Enhanced cognitive behaviour therapy for adolescents with anorexia nervosa: an alternative to family therapy? Behav Res Ther. 2013;51:R9–R12.
112. Dalle Grave R, Calugi S, El Ghoch M, Conti M, Fairburn CG. Inpatient cognitive behavior therapy for adolescents with anorexia nervosa: immediate and longer-term effects. Front Psychiatry. 2014;5:14.
113. Cook BJ, Wonderlich SA, Mitchell JE, Thompson R, Sherman R, McCallum K. Exercise in eating disorders treatment: systematic review and proposal of guidelines. Med Sci Sports Exerc. 2016;48:1408–14.
114. Fernandez-del-Valle M, Larumbe-Zabala E, Villaseñor-Montarroso A, Cardona Gonzalez C, Diez-Vega I, Lopez Mojares LM, Perez Ruiz M. Resistance training enhances muscular performance in patients with anorexia nervosa: a randomized controlled trial. Int J Eat Disord. 2014;47:601–9.
115. Calogero RM, Pedrotty KN. The practice and process of healthy exercise: an investigation of the treatment of exercise abuse in women with eating disorders. Eat Disord. 2004;12:273–91.
116. National Eating Disorders Association. Coach and trainer toolkit; 2015.
117. Becker CB, McDaniel L, Bull S, Powell M, McIntyre K. Can we reduce eating disorder risk factors in female college athletes? A randomized exploratory investigation of two peer-led interventions. Body Image. 2012;9:31–42.
118. Stewart T, Kilpela LS, Becker CB, Wesley NY. The female athlete body project. NCAA.org. n.d.. https://www.ncaa.org/sports/2015/2/24/the-female-athlete-body-project.aspx. Accessed 19 Feb 2022.
119. Perelman H, Schwartz N, Yeoward-Dodson J, Quiñones IC, Murray MF, Dougherty EN, Townsel R, Arthur-Cameselle J, Haedt-Matt AA. Reducing eating disorder risk among male athletes: a randomized controlled trial investigating the male athlete body project. Int J Eat Disord. 2022;55:193–206.

Chapter 4
Sleep Considerations in the Young Athlete

Jesse Allen-Dicker and Shelby Harris

Key Points
- Many children and adolescents experience impairments in sleep, which may impede their athletic engagement and performance, as well as overall mental health.
- By working to improve their sleep habits, youth athletes may perform better, may reduce their likelihood of developing sport-related injuries, and may exhibit more adaptive affective experiences.
- Understanding and utilizing evidence-based assessments and interventions is important to the care and development of young athletes.

Sleep is at the center of human existence, but much like athletic performance, sleep varies from person-to-person and almost inevitably changes from day-to-day. At the extremes, sleep causes and maintains symptoms of mental illness. And yet, even at healthier doses, changes in sleep contribute to differences in athletic performance, mood, and socialization. These changes—as well as the science and research behind them—are integral to the understanding of athletic success.

Over the past 50 years, science and research have influenced the sport landscape. This is perhaps most evident in Major League Baseball. Tommy John surgery, a treatment for tears in the ulnar collateral ligament within the elbow, has saved the careers of numerous major league pitchers and position players [1, 2]. Before winning Rookie of the Year and back-to-back Cy Young Awards (for the best pitcher in the league), Jacob deGrom had Tommy John surgery [3]. Had this surgery not been

J. Allen-Dicker (✉)
Department of Psychiatry, Lenox Hill Hospital/Northwell Health, New York, NY, USA

S. Harris
Departments of Neurology and Psychiatry, Albert Einstein College of Medicine,
Bronx, NY, USA
e-mail: Drshelbyharris@drshelbyharris.com

available, his career trajectory likely would have looked very different. Similarly, analytics have shifted the way the game of baseball is played, from pitching to hitting to fielding, and even to base-running. Advances in the understanding of people and sport have impacted the way athletes train, perform, and recover from training. These changes are not just seen among the stars of the world, but among youth athletes as well. Given its substantial literature base in support of sleep, we should consider sleep in the list of innovations that greatly benefit the field of youth athletics.

Important Sleep Variables

In order to understand the benefits of sleep and its relationship to athletics, it is essential to appreciate some of the more pertinent variables of sleep research and behavior, such as sleep quantity and sleep quality. Sleep quantity refers to how much time a person spends sleeping in a given day. While this variable typically refers to evening sleep, it also can include time spent napping (napping is discussed more fully later in this chapter). The American Academy of Sleep Medicine recommends that children between the ages of 6 and 12 sleep between 9 and 12 h per day and recommends that adolescents between the ages of 13 and 18 obtain between 8 and 10 h of sleep per day [4]. It is encouraging that approximately 89% of children and 83% of adolescents meet these recommendations "on most weeknights" in the United States; however, that overlooks the days in which those recommendations are not met and still means that there are likely millions of children and adolescents in the United States not meeting those standards [5]. Less encouraging is the fact that a cross-sectional study of adolescent sleep between 1991 and 2012 indicates that adolescent sleep quantity has decreased over time [6]. These impairments appear consistent among youth athletes as well, as a study of high school athletes at sport-specific high schools in Sweden found that approximately 19% of the athletes surveyed slept less than 8 h per night during the week [7]. Similarly, many adolescent athletes have reported that they average less sleep than they themselves believe to be optimal [8].

Sleep quality is a more complex consideration consisting of multiple sleep variables that each describe elements of how well individuals sleep, regardless of sleep quantity. Sleep onset latency refers to how long it takes an individual to fall asleep, while mid-sleep awakenings refer to the number of times an individual wakes up in the middle of their sleep. These awakenings can be due to many factors, including environmental disturbances (e.g., noises by cell phones or family members), respiratory problems, substance use, nightmares, and urges to use the bathroom [9]. Sleep efficiency, which refers to the percent of time spent sleeping out of the total time spent attempting to sleep, integrates both sleep onset latency and mid-sleep awakenings. Overall, it is recommended that the sleep onset latency of children and adolescents be below 30 min, that children and adolescents do not have more than one awakening per sleep lasting more than 5 min, that they do not spend more than 20 min awake after falling asleep, and that their overall sleep efficiency be approximately 85% or greater [10]. These goals are obtainable, though many children and adolescents do not meet them.

In addition to considering sleep quantity and sleep quality, a recent trend in the field of sleep medicine has been to evaluate sleep timing and variability (i.e., changes in sleep across nights). In short, regularity in sleep behaviors is very important to overall sleep functioning. For example, two teenagers, John and Gabriela, both average 9 h of sleep per night. John always makes sure he gets at least 9 h of sleep, though he falls asleep and wakes up at vastly different times every night due to differences in practice times, game times, homework levels, social plans, and household structure. Gabriela on the other hand sleeps from 9:30 pm to 6:30 am almost every night due to more favorable academic and athletic scheduling and a more consistent home and social life. The consistency that Gabriela exhibits in her sleep habits may positively contribute to other areas of her life, including mental health and academic performance [11–13]. Significant changes in bedtimes and waketimes between days can be likened to the conditions leading to jetlag. In this example, John may experience what is popularly known as social jetlag which is associated with impairments in a variety of physiological and psychological variables such as anxiety, cognitive ability, and increased body mass index [14–16]. While certainly not a factor for most young athletes, traditional jetlag caused by travel for recreation or competition should also be considered when developing academic and athletic schedules as it may also negatively impact athletes [17–19].

In addition, it must be noted that impairments in these sleep variables can negatively impact individuals' abilities to adequately progress through important sleep stages (i.e., rapid eye movement (REM) and non-rapid eye movement (NREM)). Early school start times frequently infringe upon teenage sleep quantity, leading to inadequate REM sleep, which is important for factors such as memory, mood, and self-control [20–23]. Similarly, challenges in obtaining healthy NREM sleep may be of particular importance to the young athlete, as NREM sleep is integral to the development of the adolescent brain, as well as to physical skill development and memory [24].

Sleep and Athletic Performance

When used effectively, adequate sleep quantity and quality can have a positive impact on athletic performance for both competitive athletes and the general population. Sleep in children and adolescents has been well studied, particularly as it pertains to school start times, mental health, and academic performance; however, the relationship between sleep and subsequent youth athletic performance has received little focus. In an experimental study, adolescent tennis players experiencing fewer than 5 h of sleep performed worse than a control group in serving and cross-court hitting, though no differences were observed for a sprinting task [25]. In looking at the emerging adult population, which spans from approximately age 18 through the 20s, Mah et al. studied sleep and exercise performance in 11 members of the Stanford University Men's Basketball team [26, 27]. Athletic performance was assessed after each practice during the initial 2- to 4-week period in which the athletes slept from 6 to 9 h each night and then again after each practice for 5–7 weeks in which they aimed to sleep as much as they could each night, with a minimum of 10 h in bed per night. Athletic performance focused on free-throw percentage, three-point percentage, sprinting speed, and self-report on performance in practice and in games. The athletes improved in each of these areas when they exhibited greater sleep quantity. While findings are limited to a small, basketball-focused sample, they are encouraging for athletes of other sports as well. Interestingly, a study of college students who exercised regularly found that one night of complete sleep deprivation did not affect performance on an anaerobic cycling task though it did impact athlete reaction time [28]. Although additional research is needed, it may be that relatively brief impairments in sleep do not impair more intensive cardiac exercises though it may impact skills-based exercises such as serving in tennis. More prolonged sleep impairments, as seen in Mah et al.'s study, may negatively impact more intensive cardiac performance.

In observing adults in a naturalistic, nonexperimental setting, McGlinchey et al. found that on days in which individuals sleep better, they engage in longer and more intensive exercise bouts the following day [29]. For those participants that typically experienced sleep impairments, greater exercise was associated with greater sleep the night following the exercise. These findings support the bidirectional relationship between exercise and sleep. They show how individuals who typically have poor sleep may benefit from a night of improved sleep in their subsequent exercise possibly. This leads to another night of enhanced sleep. In observing college students in a real-life setting, Allen-Dicker found that neither sleep quantity, sleep onset latency, nor sleep efficiency predicts next-day exercise occurrence [30]. As such, it may be that improved sleep does not necessarily lead to individuals exercising, but for those that do exercise, improved sleep may lead to more intensive exercise. These findings may be of particular importance to adolescents as many in this age range, particularly those who are female and who are of Asian or Hispanic descent, do not meet current daily exercise recommendations [31, 32]. Moreover, as exercise engagement is more impaired among overweight and obese children and adolescents, sleep may serve as an effective area of intervention to benefit youth exercise and weight.

In addition to benefiting athletic engagement and performance, sleep may also play a role in preventing sport-related injuries. Adolescent athletes who reported averaging at least 8 h of sleep during weekdays were significantly less likely to develop injuries [7]. In general, these findings are supported by Gao et al.'s meta-analysis studying the effects of sleep impairments and adolescent injury [33]. Following injury, sleep may also aid in adolescent recovery, though further research is needed [34].

Sleep and Affective Experience

Athletes' sleep may also impact youth athletes' affective experiences, which may thus impact their relationships with teammates and coaches. For example, following nights in which adolescents reported sleeping well, they experienced higher levels of positive affect and lower levels of negative affect [35]. Interestingly, mid-sleep awakenings did not predict next-day affect levels. Similarly, Allen-Dicker found that greater sleep duration and sleep efficiency and shorter sleep onset latency may predict higher levels of positive affect, with greater sleep duration and healthier sleep efficiency also predicting lower levels of negative affect [30]. Baum et al. studied adolescents over a 3-week span [36]. During that time, baseline sleep data was gathered for a week. Participants were then limited to 6.5 h in bed per night for 5 days, and then 10 h in bed per night for 5 days. During the greater sleep period, adolescents reported less anger, more vigor, less fatigue, less confusion, less oppo-sitionality or irritability, and improved emotion regulation than during the restrictive sleep period. Impairments in these areas may lead to confrontation or worsened communication, which may negatively impact overall team performance.

Child and Adolescent Sleep Considerations

School Start Time and Athletic Scheduling

Students, particularly adolescent students, can have extraordinarily busy schedules regardless of their engagement in exercise or organized team sports. Early school start times, academic extra-help, clubs, athletic obligations, homework and study-ing, religious engagements, driver's education, and preparation for college fill their schedules, frequently leaving limited time for adequate nighttime sleep. In recent times, there has been a strong push for school start times to be delayed to benefit student sleep. Since 2014, both the American Academy of Pediatrics and the American Academy of Sleep Medicine have come out with position papers in sup-port of school start times for middle school and high school students to be delayed until at least 8:30 AM [37, 38]. They both present substantial evidence indicating that later school start times may benefit sleep, mental health, physical health, safety, and academic performance, with the American Academy of Sleep Medicine specifi-cally stating that as part of this implementation, extracurricular activities such as athletic practices should also not occur before 8:30 AM. Early morning athletic events often further limit the ability for adolescents to obtain a full night of sleep.

The timing of athletic events and exercise may also impact nighttime sleep, though there are conflicting reports on the optimal time of day to exercise [29]. Research has indicated that morning or afternoon exercise may be related to better sleep than evening exercise, especially if the exercise is intensive; however, Souissi et al. found that individuals who exercise in the evening do not appear to have worse sleep than those who do not exercise in the evening [39, 40]. Given the inconsistencies in findings, it is unclear whether evening practices and games may negatively impact youth sleep. That said, due to early school start times and the recommendations for daily sleep quantity, afternoon or early evening practices and games may overall be preferable, especially on weekdays. Strictly from a sleep perspective, given the benefits of consistency in sleep timing and regularity, weekend athletic events should follow a similar structure. While morning practices and games may be possible on the weekends, as many adolescents do not meet adequate sleep recommendations, weekend mornings may serve as an effective time for them to "catch up" on sleep within reason. For the casual athlete, intensive exercise late in the evening may also delay bedtimes and may impair overall sleep quality. As the casual athlete may have greater control over their exercise scheduling, afternoon or early evening exercise may similarly be preferable. Regardless, these athletes should monitor how exercise time-of-day impacts their overall ability to sleep at night.

Youth Napping and Athletics

Napping can have numerous benefits for individuals across the life cycle, including in areas such as mood, verbal abilities, academic performance, and cognitive processing speed [41–43]. For some adolescents facing challenging athletic and academic schedules, naps may serve as a way to reduce sleep debt (aggregate sleep loss), with the consequences and correlates listed above offering encouraging support for napping [44, 45]. That said, among sleep scholars, there is inconsistent report on what are appropriate napping habits for school-aged children and adolescents [4]. Among teenagers, one or possibly two naps in a day of 20 min or less are likely indicative of healthy sleep quality; however, it is unclear how many days in a week is healthy for teenagers to nap. Additional research is needed to understand the effects of naps lasting more than 20 min in teenagers. As for school-aged children, it is also unclear whether or not naps are healthy, though children in this age range likely should not have more than two napping days per week [4].

In terms of athletic performance, Souabni et al. [46] argue that napping for 90 min may improve athletic abilities as it has been found to improve aspects of executive functioning, though additional research is needed [46]. Interestingly, recent findings suggest that napping after exercise may improve memory consolidation among adults, which offers interesting insight into how young athletes might better learn their craft [47]. Regardless of nap duration, naps should occur earlier in the day, as evening naps may interfere with one's ability to fall asleep at night (i.e., longer sleep onset latency; [48]). As children and adolescents already have a narrow window to receive adequate sleep on school nights, poorly placed naps should be avoided. While naps can help make up for poor sleep from the previous evening, they also may lead to impaired sleep the following evening [49]. In general, youth athletes should be cognizant of the effects naps have on them as individuals. For example, if naps cause subsequent sleepiness or irritability, athletes should likely avoid napping immediately prior to practice or competition. Similarly, if naps seem to make it difficult to initiate or maintain evening sleep, athletes should either modify the timing and/or duration of their naps.

Sleep and Modern Technology

Technology use can serve as a significant obstacle to child and adolescent sleep. Children and adolescents who watch television or play video games at bed have been found to sleep 30 min less than those who do not, while children and adolescents who use their phone or computer at bed have been found to sleep 60 min less [50]. Interestingly, holding one's phone closer to one's head while lying in bed may lead to poorer sleep efficiency and sleep onset latency [51]. These findings are concerning as technology use may have increased among adolescents since the early 2000s [52]. In general, families should aspire to reduce technology use at bedtime, which may be assisted by limiting the number of technological devices in the bedrooms, ideally leading to better sleep [53]. Reading may serve as an effective alternative prior to sleep [54]. These recommendations are illustrated in Table 4.1, which shows a sample weekday and weekend schedule in which a teenage athlete follows age-specific sleep standards while meeting their familial, social, academic, and athletic obligations. In this example, the athlete maintains a relatively consistent wake and sleep schedule on weekdays and weekends while enabling themselves to reduce sleep debt without developing social jet lag by sleeping in a little later on Saturday and Sunday. Within this schedule, the athlete also follows recommendations for naps, practice and games scheduling, and technology use and is a member of a school district in which school start time recommendations are met.

Sleep and Substance Use

From a developmental perspective, impairments in sleep quantity and quality predict younger and repeated use of alcohol, marijuana, and cigarettes, with greater sleep problems predicting earlier use of other illicit drugs [55, 56]. Interestingly, social jetlag may even contribute to adolescents beginning to smoke cigarettes [14]. Use of these substances has also been shown to negatively impact sleep. Alcohol has been shown to impair subsequent sleep efficiency among adolescents, with marijuana, cocaine, nicotine, and opiate intoxication also causing sleep impairments [57, 58]. While some young athletes may only engage in occasional substance use, it is important to note that intermittent usage may also negatively impact nighttime sleep, which may then impair athletic recovery and/or performance the following

Table 4.1 Sample healthy weekday and weekend schedule for a teenage athlete

		Thursday	Friday	Saturday
Time of day	7:00 AM	**Sleep (since 10:30 PM)**	**Sleep (since 10:30 PM)**	**Sleep (since 10:30 PM)**
	7:30 AM	Wake-up + breakfast	Wake-up + breakfast	
	8:00 AM	Travel to school	Travel to school	
	8:30 AM	School	School	Wake-up + breakfast
	9:00 AM			Time with family
	9:30 AM			
	10:00 AM			
	10:30 AM			
	11:00 AM			
	11:30 AM			Travel to practice
	12:00 PM			Practice
	12:30 PM			
	1:00 PM			
	1:30 PM			
	2:00 PM			Travel to home
	2:30 PM			Lunch
	3:00 PM			**Nap for 20 min**
	3:30 PM	Leave for away game	Practice	Homework
	4:00 PM	Warm-up		
	4:30 PM	Game		
	5:00 PM			
	5:30 PM		Travel to home	
	6:00 PM		Television/social media	Dinner with friends
	6:30 PM	Travel to home	Dinner	
	7:00 PM		See friends	
	7:30 PM	Dinner		
	8:00 PM	Television/social media		
	8:30 PM	Homework		Play videogames
	9:00 PM			
	9:30 PM			
	10:00 PM	Get ready for bed/read	Get ready for bed/read	Get ready for bed/read
	10:30 PM	**Sleep**	**Sleep**	
	11:00 PM			**Sleep (until 8:30 AM)**
	11:30 PM			

day. While not typically used in a recreational manner, it is important to be wary of the fact that anabolic steroids may also worsen sleep functioning, though further research is required [59].

Sleep and Mental Illness

The role of mental health in athletics was discussed in a previous chapter; however, it must be noted that sleep plays a significant role in psychiatric functioning. Within the *Diagnostic and Statistical Manual of Mental Disorders, 5th Edition, Text Revision (DSM-5-TR)*, the preeminent psychiatric classification system within the United States, sleep disorders make up the greatest number of diagnoses [60]. In general, approximately 40% of children and adolescents may experience sleep problems, with approximately 10% of adolescents experiencing insomnia (i.e., difficulty initiating and maintaining sleep [60–62]). Given the importance of sleep within athletic functioning, insomnia likely would serve as an obstacle to the performance of a young athlete. Understanding sleep apnea (snoring, pauses in breathing multiple times per night) is also important to the care of young athletes, as it can worsen athletic and daily functioning and cause issues with excessive daytime sleepiness (not to mention many other issues such as nocturia, weight gain, and depressed mood).

Diagnostically, sleep impairments are also listed as criteria for both major depression disorder and bipolar disorder (i.e., mood disorders) within the DSM-5-TR [60]. Research on the relationship between sleep and mood abounds, with impairments in sleep both causing and responding to impairments in mood [63]. As such, in recent times, sleep-focused interventions are being used to improve mood in patients experiencing depressive episodes. For example, in treating individuals with comorbid depression and insomnia, cognitive behavior therapy for insomnia (CBT-I) has been found to not only treat insomnia but also reduce depressive symptoms [64, 65]. Similarly, interpersonal and social rhythm therapy (IPSRT), a relatively new treatment for individuals with bipolar disorder, focuses on improving sleep habits, daily routines, and relationships to stabilize mood [66, 67]. Preliminary findings support its use with adolescents with bipolar disorder [68]. While not necessarily always considered criteria for these disorders, sleep impairments are also related to symptoms and diagnoses of anxiety, obsessive-compulsive disorder, schizophrenia and psychosis, and even suicidality and self-harm [69–75].

Taken together, sleep impairments and mental illness often go hand-in-hand, though difficulties with sleep are not necessarily indicative of underlying mental illness. Caretakers, providers, and team personnel should monitor youth sleep functioning as it may serve as a strong behavioral marker for other, potentially less easily observed psychiatric symptoms. Mental illness does not necessarily impede athletic performance, as indicated by the growing number of professional athletes speaking out about their own experiences with mental health difficulties; however, for some individuals, mental illness may serve as a potential obstacle to athletic performance. More importantly though, mental illness can impair daily functioning and lead to significant events, such as medical and psychiatric hospitalization, death, and suicide. As such, it is the duty of those involved in the care of young athletes to be mindful of potential symptom development. This is especially true as early intervention for mental illness may lead to greater long-term outcomes [76–79].

Sleep Assessment

As with all medical practice, a thorough assessment must be conducted to improve and treat sleep issues. There are numerous ways to monitor and assess sleep functioning within the young athlete. Several of those to be mindful of are the following:

1. **One-time self-report measures:** One-time self-report measures are typically rather brief and require youths to answer questions about their typical sleep habits. Ji and Liu [80] provide a strong summary of self-report measures available to the assessment of child and adolescent sleep [80]. There are a number of well-researched measures, including the Children's Report of Sleep Patterns (CRSP) and Sleep Disturbance Scale for Children (SDSC; [81, 82]). Several of these measures, such as the SDSC, rely on parent report or in some instances, include questions for both children and adolescents and their parents. Other measures developed initially for adults, such as the Pittsburgh Sleep Quality Index (PSQI), may serve as good assessment tools for children and adolescents, though Ji and Liu argue that additional research on the use of the PSQI with younger populations is needed [83]. As with all self-report measures, individuals are not always able to provide accurate assessment of their sleep habits, so results from these measures should be interpreted with caution. When answered in an honest manner, these measures may serve as strong initial screeners for sleep functioning, to potentially later be complemented by more in-depth assessment and/or referral to psychiatric providers.

2. **Multiday self-report measures:** A positive addition to the field has been the development of daily assessments such as the Consensus Sleep Diary [84]. Similar to measures such as the CRSP and PSQI, the Consensus Sleep Diary is a self-report measure. It differs from these other measures in that it is administered each day for a set period of time (typically 7–14 days). As such, it gathers data about daily sleep functioning which may be a more valid indicator of youth sleep habits [85]. Multiday self-report measures also show changes in sleep between days, including between weekdays and weekends. As one-time self-report measures inquire into "typical" sleep habits, they focus on average sleep behaviors and neglect to show inconsistencies between days and overlook extremes such as "party-nights," "all-nighters," and "sleep-binges." Multiday measures require greater time commitments from youths and their families, though this commitment may be worth the improvement in validity and the increase in relevant data.

3. **Actigraphic assessment:** One-time and multiday self-report measures are subjective by nature. Actigraphs provide objective data and typically take the form of wristbands that monitor daily sleep and wake habits. Of note, actigraphic data is not necessarily favored over self-report data, but rather may add an additional layer of insight into overall sleep functioning. As such, combining the use of an actigraph and multiday self-report measure may offer a more comprehensive view of sleep functioning within child and adolescent athletes. Actigraphs do require a greater financial investment, though if used for a lengthy period of time

by an athlete or used to assess the sleep functioning of many athletes, the product may be readily worth the investment.

4. **Cell phone applications:** A number of cell phone applications have been developed to assess sleep functioning. Some of these take the form of self-report, while others are argued to be objective measures of sleep functioning. At the present time, these applications are not strongly recommended due to the lack of available research on these products. Bhat et al. [86] found that the findings of one of these apps did not correlate with the findings of polysomnography, argued by the authors to be the gold standard of sleep assessment [86].

5. **Polysomnography:** While the first three methods of assessment may serve as effective initial screeners for sleep functioning, formal sleep studies conducted within hospitals or academic settings may provide more precise assessment through use of polysomnography. These assessments are typically not warranted for the average youth athlete, as they are more expensive and in-depth, though they may offer insight into severe sleep disturbance, treatment-resistant sleep issues, and potential sleep apnea [86, 87].

Improvement, Referral, and Treatment

Impairments in sleep do not necessarily indicate "illness" but do offer insight into potential areas for intervention. There is no "one-size-fits-all" solution for athletes seeking to repair or optimize their sleep habits, but there are many steps that can be taken to help improve sleep functioning. Athletes exhibiting substantial impairments may require formal treatment. Mental health providers that have specialized sleep training can offer athletes, families, and teams assistance in these matters. Psychologists, sleep specialists, mental health social workers, and psychiatrists may help in this process. That said, not all providers in these fields have the relevant training to benefit these parties, so it is essential to inquire as to the providers' credentials for treating youths with sleep difficulties. Team personnel and healthcare providers within the sport medicine field are encouraged to develop a list of potential referrals with the proper skillset. It can be challenging to find a provider with these skillsets whose payment plans meet the financial needs of individuals and their families. Thus, having a comprehensive referral list to share may decrease the time spent before treatment initiation.

If sleep difficulties are not at a level that necessarily requires clinical care, athletes can work to identify the aspects of their sleep they seek to improve. Proper sleep hygiene and allowing for enough time routinely to obtain an adequate night of sleep is paramount (see Table 4.2). Caffeine use and energy drinks are routinely used in this population, and proper education about their negative impact on nighttime sleep should be given. Athletes should develop goals that follow the SMART goal approach. In short, these goals should be specific, measurable, achievable, relevant, and time-bound. Adherence to SMART goals, an avoidance of negative thinking, and an effective use of positive reinforcement (e.g. "If I get in bed by X

Table 4.2 Steps for the young athlete to achieve greater sleep hygiene

1. Maintain consistent bed and wake times as often as possible 7 days a week
2. Obtain between 8 and 10 h of sleep each night
3. Delay school start times to at least 8:30 AM
4. Limit weekday and weekend games to afternoons and early evenings, when possible
5. Exercise earlier in the day if evening exercise appears to disrupt subsequent sleep
6. Limit naps to 20 min at most and only nap in the morning or afternoon
7. Do not use electronics (e.g., television, cell phone, video games) while in bed
8. Minimize sound and light emitted by electronics while sleeping
9. Limit caffeine consumption within 8 h of bedtime
10. Avoid alcohol and drug use
11 Limit liquid consumption after dinner and use the bathroom prior to bed
12. Establish a daily pre-sleep routine that includes peaceful activities without the use of screens (e.g., relaxed reading and meditation)
13. Only use the bed for sleep or sex, not for relaxing or homework, etc.

pm, *Y* times this week, I will get Z") will help individuals meet their goals in a positive, healthy, and sustainable manner. In general, sleep improvements should be made gradually. There are numerous books, worksheets, websites, and cell phone apps dedicated to helping individuals meet their sleep goals. Some adolescents will be able to accomplish these goals on their own. Others may prefer or may benefit from assistance from family members, team personnel, and healthcare providers. These adults can help the athletes with goal development, follow-through, and positive reinforcement. Parents may also wish to model effective sleep hygiene within the home. Integrating regular sleep assessments into their plans for change will reinforce improvements and help athletes identify additional areas for improvement as they progress in their sleep goals.

In instances in which the child or adolescent is not initially motivated for change, it may be helpful for them to have the time and training to develop an understanding of *why* change is important for them given *their* own values and athletic goals. If the athletes and their families are not motivated to make changes, it cannot be forced upon them, as this may only lead to feelings of frustration and thoughts of failure. Stigma toward mental health and mental health services may also act as obstacles to change.

For those with more entrenched issues in obtaining adequate sleep, even when the opportunity is there for a full night's sleep, a variety of psychotherapies have been developed specifically for the treatment of children and adolescents with sleep impairments. As stated previously, CBT-I is a well-validated treatment for symptoms of insomnia and has been found to be effective in treating these symptoms within children and adolescents [88]. CBT-I can be provided by mental health providers with the proper education and experience. This treatment focuses on modifying patient thoughts and behaviors to improve sleep. Examples of these modifications include reductions in caffeine intake, softening of dysfunctional thoughts about sleep, and increased pre-sleep relaxation. Within the psychotherapy field, CBT-I is frequently considered to be the primary intervention for insomnia. IPSRT and the Youth version of the Transdiagnostic Intervention for Sleep and Circadian Dysfunction (Trans-C-Youth) build upon CBT-I through their focus on sleep timing and variability [89]. Additionally, psychotherapeutic interventions focused on non-sleep symptoms such as anxiety may additionally benefit sleep [90]. Several recent meta-analyses show that exercise may also reduce symptoms of sleep apnea, though adolescent and adult athletes are still at risk of developing the sleep disorder [91–94]. Similarly, exercise may also benefit the sleep quality of individuals with mental illness [95]. Psychotherapy has also been found to be an effective treatment for sleep impairments and can be used to improve and optimize the sleep habits of children and adolescents. In applying these treatments to young athletes, factors specific to children and adolescents such as school start times and practice and game schedules should be considered.

Inadequate allowed time for sleep during the adolescent years is currently a major issue within our society, and as noted earlier, the American Academy of Sleep Medicine and American Academy of Pediatrics have issued strong statement papers urging for school start times that are in better alignment with the natural circadian delay of adolescents. Schools and educational and athletic groups need to further support the goal for appropriate morning start times while also taking into consideration the immense demands put upon adolescents in today's times. Although school may start later as more and more school districts follow suit, there still needs to be adequate time in the evening for sports, afterschool activities, and homework—all while allowing for enough time to obtain sufficient nighttime sleep.

Conclusion

In conclusion, sleep can both serve as an obstacle to athletic performance and a tool to improve athletic performance for child and adolescent athletes. Sleep may also prevent athletic injuries and improve the affective experiences of youth athletes, which may further benefit team performance. That said, additional naturalistic and experimental research is needed particularly for youth athletes as much of the current research has focused on college students, professional athletes, and the general adult population. It is essential that families, schools, and athletic organizations consider the importance of sleep when developing athletic and academic schedules, as millions of children and adolescents likely experience sleep impairments which may cause or maintain symptoms of mental illness. Fortunately, there have been a number of positive developments in the assessment and treatment of youths experiencing sleep dysfunction, such as the Consensus Sleep Diary, actigraphic assessment, and CBT-I. While it is encouraging that schools today are focusing more on recognizing and treating both mental and physical health challenges, obtaining adequate sleep should be considered a fundamental in which many other aspects of an adolescent's life are built upon.

References

1. Landers C. Just who is Tommy John, and why does everyone talk about his surgery all the time? mlb.com. 2019. https://www.mlb.com/cut4/why-is-it-called-tommy-john-surgery.
2. Tommy John. Surgery (ulnar collateral ligament reconstruction). Johns Hopkins Medicine. n.d.. https://www.hopkinsmedicine.org/health/treatment-tests-and-therapies/tommy-john-surgery-ulnar-collateral-ligament-reconstruction.
3. Adler D. Top 10 Tommy John success stories. Mlb.com. 2020. https://www.mlb.com/news/top-10-tommy-john-surgery-success-stories-c295719048.
4. Paruthi S, Brooks LJ, D'Ambrosio C, Hall WA, Kotagal S, Lloyd RM, et al. Consensus statement of the American Academy of Sleep Medicine on the recommended amount of sleep for healthy children: methodology and discussion. J Clin Sleep Med. 2016;12(11):1549–61.
5. Friel CP, Duran AT, Shechter A, Diaz KM. U.S. children meeting physical activity, screen time, and sleep guidelines. Am J Prev Med. 2020;59(4):513–21.
6. Keyes KM, Maslowsky J, Hamilton A, Schulenberg J. The great sleep recession: changes in sleep duration among US adolescents, 1991–2012. Pediatrics. 2015;135(3):460–8.
7. von Rosen P, Frohm A, Kottorp A, Fridén C, Heijne A. Too little sleep and an unhealthy diet could increase the risk of sustaining a new injury in adolescent elite athletes. Scand J Med Sci Sports. 2017;27(11):1364–71.
8. Anderson ML, Reale RJ. Discrepancies between self-reported current and ideal sleep behaviors of adolescent athletes. Sleep Sci. 2020;13(1):18–24.
9. Camhi SL, Morgan WJ, Pernisco N, Quan SF. Factors affecting sleep disturbances in children and adolescents. Sleep Med. 2000;1(2):117–23.
10. Ohayon M, Wickwire EM, Hirshkowitz M, Albert SM, Avidan A, Daly FJ, et al. National Sleep Foundation's sleep quality recommendations: first report. Sleep Health. 2017;3(1):6–19.
11. Fuligni AJ, Hardway C. Daily variation in adolescents' sleep, activities, and psychological well-being. J Res Adolesc. 2006;16(3):353–78.
12. Bono TJ, Hill PL. Sleep quantity and variability during the first semester at university: implications for well-being and academic performance. Psychol Health Med. 2022;27(4):931–6.
13. Fuligni AJ, Arruda EH, Krull JL, Gonzales NA. Adolescent sleep duration, variability, and peak levels of achievement and mental health. Child Dev. 2018;89(2):e18–28.
14. Wittmann M, Dinich J, Merrow M, Roenneberg T. Social Jetlag: misalignment of biological and social time. Chronobiol Int. 2006;23(1–2):497–509.
15. Malone SK, Zemel B, Compher C, Souders M, Chittams J, Thompson AL, et al. Social jet lag, chronotype and body mass index in 14–17-year-old adolescents. Chronobiol Int. 2016;33(9):1255–66.
16. Díaz-Morales JF, Escribano C. Social jetlag, academic achievement and cognitive performance: understanding gender/sex differences. Chronobiol Int. 2015;32(6):822–31.
17. Lemmer B, Kern R-I, Nold G, Lohrer H. Jet lag in athletes after eastward and westward time-zone transition. Chronobiol Int. 2002;19(4):743–64.
18. Rutters F, Lemmens SG, Adam TC, Bremmer MA, Elders PJ, Nijpels G, et al. Is social jet-lag associated with an adverse endocrine, behavioral, and cardiovascular risk profile? J Biol Rhythm. 2014;29(5):377–83.
19. Hill DW, Hill CM, Fields KL, Smith JC. Effects of Jet Lag on Factors Related to Sport Performance. Can J Appl Physiol. 1993;18(1):91–103.
20. Pesonen A-K, Gradisar M, Kuula L, Short M, Merikanto I, Tark R, et al. REM sleep fragmentation associated with depressive symptoms and genetic risk for depression in a community-based sample of adolescents. J Affect Disord. 2019;245:757–63.
21. Campbell IG, Kraus AM, Burright CS, Feinberg I. Restricting time in bed in early adolescence reduces both NREM and REM sleep but does not increase slow wave EEG. Sleep. 2016;39(9):1663–70.
22. Brunet J-F, McNeil J, Doucet É, Forest G. The association between REM sleep and decision-making: supporting evidences. Physiol Behav. 2020;225:113109.

23. Boyce R, Williams S, Adamantidis A. REM sleep and memory. Curr Opin Neurobiol. 2017;44:167–77.
24. Walker M. Why we sleep: unlocking the power of sleep and dreams. New York, NY: Scribner; 2017.
25. Vitale JA, Bonato M, Petrucci L, Zucca G, La Torre A, Banfi G. Acute sleep restriction affects sport-specific but not athletic performance in junior tennis players. Int J Sports Physiol Perform. 2021;16:1–6.
26. Mah CD, Mah KE, Kezirian EJ, Dement WC. The effects of sleep extension on the athletic performance of collegiate basketball players. Sleep. 2011;34(7):943–50.
27. Arnett JJ. Emerging adulthood. A theory of development from the late teens through the twenties. Am Psychol. 2000;55(5):469–80.
28. Taheri M, Arabameri E. The effect of sleep deprivation on choice reaction time and anaerobic power of college student athletes. Asian J Sports Med. 2012;3(1):15–20.
29. McGlinchey EL, Gershon A, Eidelman P, Kaplan KA, Harvey AG. Physical activity and sleep: day-to-day associations among individuals with and without Bipolar Disorder. Ment Health Phys Act. 2014;7(3):183–90.
30. Allen-Dicker JK. Daily exercise, sleep, and affect: a micro-longitudinal study. Dissertation. 2022.
31. Chung AE, Skinner AC, Steiner MJ, Perrin EM. Physical activity and BMI in a nationally representative sample of children and adolescents. Clin Pediatr. 2012;51(2):122–9.
32. Haughton CF, Wang ML, Lemon SC. Racial/ethnic disparities in meeting 5-2-1-0 recommendations among children and adolescents in the United States. J Pediatr. 2016;175:188–94.e1.
33. Gao B, Dwivedi S, Milewski MD, Cruz AI. Chronic lack of sleep is associated with increased sports injury in adolescents: a systematic review and meta-analysis. Orthop J Sports Med. 2019;7(3 Suppl):2325967119S00132.
34. Copenhaver EA, Diamond AB. The value of sleep on athletic performance, injury, and recovery in the young athlete. Pediatr Ann. 2017;46(3):e106–e11.
35. van Zundert RMP, van Roekel E, Engels RCME, Scholte RHJ. Reciprocal associations between adolescents' night-time sleep and daytime affect and the role of gender and depressive symptoms. J Youth Adolesc. 2015;44(2):556–69.
36. Baum KT, Desai A, Field J, Miller LE, Rausch J, Beebe DW. Sleep restriction worsens mood and emotion regulation in adolescents. J Child Psychol Psychiatry. 2014;55(2):180–90.
37. Adolescent Sleep Working G, Committee On A, Council On School H, Au R, Carskadon M, Millman R, et al. School start times for adolescents. Pediatrics. 2014;134(3):642–9.
38. Watson Nathaniel F, Martin Jennifer L, Wise Merrill S, Carden Kelly A, Kirsch Douglas B, Kristo David A, et al. Delaying middle school and high school start times promotes student health and performance: an American Academy of Sleep Medicine Position Statement. J Clin Sleep Med. 2017;13(4):623–5.
39. Buman MP, Phillips BA, Youngstedt SD, Kline CE, Hirshkowitz M. Does nighttime exercise really disturb sleep? Results from the 2013 National Sleep Foundation Sleep in America Poll. Sleep Med. 2014;15(7):755–61.
40. Souissi M, Chtourou H, Zrane A, Cheikh RB, Dogui M, Tabka Z, et al. Effect of time-of-day of aerobic maximal exercise on the sleep quality of trained subjects. Biol Rhythm Res. 2012;43(3):323–30.
41. Liu J, Feng R, Ji X, Cui N, Raine A, Mednick SC. Midday napping in children: associations between nap frequency and duration across cognitive, positive psychological well-being, behavioral, and metabolic health outcomes. Sleep. 2019;42(9):zsz126.
42. Lim J, Lo JC, Chee MWL. Assessing the benefits of napping and short rest breaks on processing speed in sleep-restricted adolescents. J Sleep Res. 2017;26(2):219–26.
43. Milner CE, Cote KA. A dose-response investigation of the benefits of napping in healthy young, middle-aged and older adults. Sleep Biol Rhythms. 2008;6(1):2–15.
44. Leger D, Richard J-B, Collin O, Sauvet F, Faraut B. Napping and weekend catchup sleep do not fully compensate for high rates of sleep debt and short sleep at a population level (in a representative nationwide sample of 12,637 adults). Sleep Med. 2020;74:278–88.

45. Léger D, Roscoat ED, Bayon V, Guignard R, Pâquereau J, Beck F. Short sleep in young adults: insomnia or sleep debt? Prevalence and clinical description of short sleep in a representative sample of 1004 young adults from France. Sleep Med. 2011;12(5):454–62.
46. Souabni M, Hammouda O, Romdhani M, Trabelsi K, Ammar A, Driss T. Benefits of daytime napping opportunity on physical and cognitive performances in physically active participants: a systematic review. Sports Med. 2021;51(10):2115–46.
47. Mograss M, Crosetta M, Abi-Jaoude J, Frolova E, Robertson EM, Pepin V, et al. Exercising before a nap benefits memory better than napping or exercising alone. Sleep. 2020;43(9):zsaa062.
48. Milner CE, Cote KA. Benefits of napping in healthy adults: impact of nap length, time of day, age, and experience with napping. J Sleep Res. 2009;18(2):272–81.
49. Santos JS, Pereira SIR, Louzada FM. Chronic sleep restriction triggers inadequate napping habits in adolescents: a population-based study. Sleep Med. 2021;83:115–22.
50. Fuller C, Lehman E, Hicks S, Novick MB. Bedtime use of technology and associated sleep problems in children. Glob Pediatr Health. 2017;4:2333794X17736972-2333794X.
51. Yoshimura M, Kitazawa M, Maeda Y, Mimura M, Tsubota K, Kishimoto T. Smartphone viewing distance and sleep: an experimental study utilizing motion capture technology. Nat Sci Sleep. 2017;9:59–65.
52. Fomby P, Goode JA, Truong-Vu K-P, Mollborn S. Adolescent technology, sleep, and physical activity time in two U.S. cohorts. Youth Soc. 2019;53(4):585–609.
53. Calamaro CJ, Yang K, Ratcliffe S, Chasens ER. Wired at a young age: the effect of caffeine and technology on sleep duration and body mass index in school-aged children. J Pediatr Health Care. 2012;26(4):276–82.
54. Dube N, Khan K, Loehr S, Chu Y, Veugelers P. The use of entertainment and communication technologies before sleep could affect sleep and weight status: a population-based study among children. Int J Behav Nutr Phys Act. 2017;14(1):97.
55. Mike TB, Shaw DS, Forbes EE, Sitnick SL, Hasler BP. The hazards of bad sleep—sleep duration and quality as predictors of adolescent alcohol and cannabis use. Drug Alcohol Depend. 2016;168:335–9.
56. Wong MM, Brower KJ, Fitzgerald HE, Zucker RA. Sleep problems in early childhood and early onset of alcohol and other drug use in adolescence. Alcohol Clin Exp Res. 2004;28(4):578–87.
57. Chan JKM, Trinder J, Andrewes HE, Colrain IM, Nicholas CL. The acute effects of alcohol on sleep architecture in late adolescence. Alcohol Clin Exp Res. 2013;37(10):1720–8.
58. Gordon HW. Differential effects of addictive drugs on sleep and sleep stages. J Addict Res. 2019;3(2):1. https://doi.org/10.33140/JAR.03.02.01.
59. Venâncio DP, Tufik S, Garbuio SA, da Nóbrega ACL, de Mello MT. Effects of anabolic androgenic steroids on sleep patterns of individuals practicing resistance exercise. Eur J Appl Physiol. 2008;102(5):555–60.
60. American Psychiatric Association. Diagnostic and statistical manual of mental disorders. 5th ed. Washington, DC: American Psychiatric Association; 2022. Text Revision
61. Owens J. Insomnia in children and adolescents. J Clin Sleep Med. 2005;1(4):e454–e8.
62. Johnson EO, Roth T, Schultz L, Breslau N. Epidemiology of DSM-IV insomnia in adolescence: lifetime prevalence, chronicity, and an emergent gender difference. Pediatrics. 2006;117(2):e247–e56.
63. Talbot LS, Stone S, Gruber J, Hairston IS, Eidelman P, Harvey AG. A test of the bidirectional association between sleep and mood in bipolar disorder and insomnia. J Abnorm Psychol. 2012;121(1):39–50.
64. Clarke G, McGlinchey EL, Hein K, Gullion CM, Dickerson JF, Leo MC, et al. Cognitive-behavioral treatment of insomnia and depression in adolescents: a pilot randomized trial. Behav Res Ther. 2015;69:111–8.
65. Cunningham JEA, Shapiro CM. Cognitive behavioural therapy for insomnia (CBT-I) to treat depression: a systematic review. J Psychosom Res. 2018;106:1–12.
66. Frank E, Kupfer D, Ehlers C, Monk T. Interpersonal and social rhythm therapy for bipolar disorder: integrating interpersonal and behavioral approaches. Behav Ther. 1994;17:143.

67. Frank E, Kupfer DJ, Thase ME, Mallinger AG, Swartz HA, Fagiolini AM, et al. Two-year outcomes for interpersonal and social rhythm therapy in individuals with bipolar I disorder. Arch Gen Psychiatry. 2005;62(9):996–1004.
68. Hlastala SA, Kotler JS, McClellan JM, McCauley EA. Interpersonal and social rhythm therapy for adolescents with bipolar disorder: treatment development and results from an open trial. Depress Anxiety. 2010;27(5):457–64.
69. Alvaro PK, Roberts RM, Harris JK. A systematic review assessing bidirectionality between sleep disturbances, anxiety, and depression. Sleep. 2013;36(7):1059–68.
70. Chorney DB, Detweiler MF, Morris TL, Kuhn BR. The interplay of sleep disturbance, anxiety, and depression in children. J Pediatr Psychol. 2008;33(4):339–48.
71. Reynolds KC, Gradisar M, Alfano CA. Sleep in children and adolescents with obsessive-compulsive disorder. Sleep Med Clin. 2015;10(2):133–41.
72. Lee YJ, Cho S-J, Cho IH, Jang JH, Kim SJ. The relationship between psychotic-like experiences and sleep disturbances in adolescents. Sleep Med. 2012;13(8):1021–7.
73. Riemann D, Kammerer J, Löw H, Schmidt MH. Sleep in adolescents with primary major depression and schizophrenia: a pilot study. J Child Psychol Psychiatry. 1995;36(2):313–26.
74. Wong MM, Brower KJ, Zucker RA. Sleep problems, suicidal ideation, and self-harm behaviors in adolescence. J Psychiatr Res. 2011;45(4):505–11.
75. Hysing M, Sivertsen B, Stormark KM, O'Connor RC. Sleep problems and self-harm in adolescence. Br J Psychiatry. 2015;207(4):306–12.
76. Schimmelmann BG, Schultze-Lutter F. Early detection and intervention of psychosis in children and adolescents: urgent need for studies. Eur Child Adolesc Psychiatry. 2012;21(5):239–41.
77. Goldstein TR, Fersch-Podrat R, Axelson DA, Gilbert A, Hlastala SA, Birmaher B, et al. Early intervention for adolescents at high risk for the development of bipolar disorder: pilot study of Interpersonal and Social Rhythm Therapy (IPSRT). Psychotherapy. 2014;51(1):180–9.
78. Read H, Roush S, Downing D. Early intervention in mental health for adolescents and young adults: a systematic review. Am J Occup Ther. 2018;72(5):7205190040p1–8.
79. Dadds MR, Spence SH, Holland DE, Barrett PM, Laurens KR. Prevention and early intervention for anxiety disorders: a controlled trial. J Consult Clin Psychol. 1997;65(4):627–35.
80. Ji X, Liu J. Subjective sleep measures for adolescents: a systematic review. Child Care Health Dev. 2016;42(6):825–39.
81. Meltzer LJ, Avis KT, Biggs S, Reynolds AC, Crabtree VM, Bevans KB. The Children's Report of Sleep Patterns (CRSP): a self-report measure of sleep for school-aged children. J Clin Sleep Med. 2013;9(3):235–45.
82. Bruni O, Ottaviano S, Guidetti V, Romoli M, Innocenzi M, Cortesi F, et al. The Sleep Disturbance Scale for Children (SDSC). Construction and validation of an instrument to evaluate sleep disturbances in childhood and adolescence. J Sleep Res. 1996;5(4):251–61.
83. Buysse DJ, Reynolds CF III, Monk TH, Berman SR, Kupfer DJ. The Pittsburgh Sleep Quality Index: a new instrument for psychiatric practice and research. Psychiatry Res. 1989;28(2):193–213.
84. Carney CE, Buysse DJ, Ancoli-Israel S, Edinger JD, Krystal AD, Lichstein KL, et al. The consensus sleep diary: standardizing prospective sleep self-monitoring. Sleep. 2012;35(2):287–302.
85. Buysse DJ, Ancoli-Israel S, Edinger JD, Lichstein KL, Morin CM. Recommendations for a standard research assessment of insomnia. Sleep. 2006;29(9):1155–73.
86. Bhat S, Ferraris A, Gupta D, Mozafarian M, DeBari Vincent A, Gushway-Henry N, et al. Is there a clinical role for smartphone sleep apps? Comparison of sleep cycle detection by a smartphone application to polysomnography. J Clin Sleep Med. 2015;11(7):709–15.
87. Rundo JV, Downey R. Chapter 25 - Polysomnography. In: Levin KH, Chauvel P, editors. Handbook of clinical neurology, vol. 160. Amsterdam: Elsevier; 2019. p. 381–92.
88. Trauer JM, Qian MY, Doyle JS, Rajaratnam SMW, Cunnington D. Cognitive behavioral therapy for chronic insomnia. Ann Intern Med. 2015;163(3):191–204.
89. Harvey AG. A transdiagnostic intervention for youth sleep and circadian problems. Cogn Behav Pract. 2016;23(3):341–55.

90. Peterman JS, Carper MM, Elkins RM, Comer JS, Pincus DB, Kendall PC. The effects of cognitive-behavioral therapy for youth anxiety on sleep problems. J Anxiety Disord. 2016;37:78–88.
91. Iftikhar IH, Kline CE, Youngstedt SD. Effects of exercise training on sleep apnea: a meta-analysis. Lung. 2014;192(1):175–84.
92. Aiello KD, Caughey WG, Nelluri B, Sharma A, Mookadam F, Mookadam M. Effect of exercise training on sleep apnea: a systematic review and meta-analysis. Respir Med. 2016;116:85–92.
93. Iso Y, Kitai H, Kyuno E, Tsunoda F, Nishinaka N, Funato M, et al. Prevalence and significance of sleep disordered breathing in adolescent athletes. ERJ Open Res. 2019;5(1):29–2019.
94. Dunican IC, Walsh J, Higgins CC, Jones MJ, Maddison K, Caldwell JA, et al. Prevalence of sleep disorders and sleep problems in an elite super rugby union team. J Sports Sci. 2019;37(8):950–7.
95. Lederman O, Ward PB, Firth J, Maloney C, Carney R, Vancampfort D, et al. Does exercise improve sleep quality in individuals with mental illness? A systematic review and meta-analysis. J Psychiatr Res. 2019;109:96–106.

Chapter 5
The Psychological Effects of Injury on Youth Athletes

Michelle Codner, Caroline Ames, and Emily I. Pluhar

Key Points
- Psychosocial impacts include time loss, fear or re-injury, return to play, and increased vulnerability to mental health illnesses such as depression, anxiety, and post-traumatic stress disorder.
- The consequences of injuries to an athlete with a strong athletic identity may include difficulty coping with an injury, reduced confidence, and feelings of helplessness. When an injury gets in the way of athletic identity, it may be experienced as a loss of identity and result in psychological distress.
- Studies of quality of life in adolescents with concussions indicate that these injuries can have a lasting impact on the youth's cognitive, emotional, and social life even 5 years post-injury, regardless of whether the injury has been a mild, moderate, or severe traumatic brain injury (TBI).
- The first step in identifying mental health symptoms in injured athletes is through screening. Established tools for injured athletes measure self-efficacy, athletic identity, readiness to return to sport (RTS), and kinesiophobia, or fear and anxiety of re-injury.

M. Codner (✉)
Boston Children's Hospital, Boston, MA, USA
e-mail: michelle.codner@childrens.harvard.edu

C. Ames
New York, NY, USA

E. I. Pluhar
Division of Sports Medicine, Boston Children's Hospital, Boston, MA, USA

Division of Adolescent/Young Adult Medicine, Boston Children's Hospital, Boston, MA, USA

M. A. Christino et al. (eds.), *Psychological Considerations in the Young Athlete*,
Contemporary Pediatric and Adolescent Sports Medicine,
https://doi.org/10.1007/978-3-031-25126-9_5

- Evidence-based interventions such as mindfulness-based stress reduction (MBSR), deep diaphragmatic breathing, visualization, cognitive behavioral therapy (CBT), and acceptance and commitment therapy (ACT) have proven helpful in facilitating the post-recovery process of injured athletes.

Introduction

There has been a significant increase in sports-related injuries among student-athletes throughout the last decade. Recent statistics in the United States suggested that about 60 million youth are involved in organized sports, with an estimated 3.5 million injuries leading to time lost from sports each year [1]. Male and individuals between 5 and 24 years of age accounted for greater than 50% of all injury episodes [2]. Football, along with ice hockey and wrestling, accounts for the highest incidence of sports-related injuries in male sports [3].

Participation in sports is associated with numerous physiological and psychological benefits. In addition to the health benefits of physical activity, sports can offer youths growth opportunities and enjoyment which can help enhance self-esteem and reduce stress [1, 4, 5]. Through sports participation, youth can make friends and be part of a team and achieve higher levels of confidence and social functioning. According to Malm et al. [5], those who play sports have an increased level of physical activity later in life, and knowledge of nutrition, exercise, and health. Moreover, physical activity may enhance motor control [6] and reduce the likelihood of stress, hopelessness, anxiety, depression, suicidal ideation, suicide attempts, and substance use [1, 7, 8]. Given that adolescence is characterized by physical, cognitive, and developmental changes, it is important to consider the effect of sports participation on the brain and physical development during this period [4].

An essential developmental task in youth is to establish an autonomous self-identity. For adolescents, participation in sports during this period can help cultivate a solid athletic identity which often leads to a strong sense of self and certainty of who they are. Haraldsdottir and Watson [1] defined athletic identity as "the degree to which an individual identifies with the athlete role and looks to others for the acknowledgment of it" (p. 107). Edison et al. theorized that identity affirmation and inclusion are pursued from participation in group sports. Athletic identity is believed to occur on a spectrum that ranges from a small part of how someone identifies to a large all-encompassing part of their life [9].

Conversely, sports participation can increase the risk of injury that may threaten athletes' short- and long-term overall health. Injuries often result in pain, immobility, and disability, but more severe injuries may also lead to time lost from sports participation, absences from school, missed activities of social integration, and other developmental events [1]. When an athlete is injured, they are precipitously thrown from a high stimulation lifestyle to a sedentary and potentially mundane one. In a study by Hunt and Harris [10], boredom led the participants to engage in activities that did not aid in recovery. In a sample of urban youths who were required to rest after a sports injury, the ensuing boredom was associated with increased stress and loss of social contact [10]. Sports injuries are common in many athletes but are more prevalent in adolescent athletes with a history of disordered eating than those with healthy attitudes toward body image and eating [11]. However, elite athletes in both youth and adult samples exhibit higher eating disorder symptoms than non-elite athletes or physically active females who are not competing [11].

Consequently, the greater emphasis youth assign to their athletic role, the higher the tendency for their self-esteem, motivation, and outlook to be based on their athletic competence, performance, and achievement [9]. Athletes high in athletic identity generally have increased self-confidence and discipline and demonstrate greater involvement in exercise. Adolescents who participate in team sports can engage in more positive social interactions and establish self-concepts that foster a positive feedback loop (i.e., communication with others, including teammates, coaches, parents, and spectators) that enhances their physical and psychosocial health [1, 9].

Injuries are often an inevitable consequence of sports. The consequences of injuries to an athlete with a strong athletic identity may include difficulty coping with an injury, reduced confidence, and feelings of helplessness. Further, adolescents who only see their identity as an athlete may struggle to explore alternative career or educational opportunities if their injuries threaten their athletic career. This athletic identity is threatened when an injury ends their competitive career [1]. Studies have found more significant emotional trauma following injury among athletes 21 years or younger who identify strongly as athletes than those who don't strongly identify as athletes [1]. Contrarily, a systematic review involving youth athletes revealed that higher performance outcomes and levels of enjoyment of sports were associated with stronger athlete identity than their peers who are less invested in an athlete role [9]. In another study, lower levels of athletic identity were protective among athletes who sustained a severe injury [1].

Along with identity loss, sports participation is an escape for many athletes and provides a healthy coping mechanism for managing emotions and stress [12]. Research has, however, suggested that athletic identification though protective against lower self-esteem before the injury serves as a predisposing factor for diminished feelings of self-worth and increased mood disturbance following an injury [13]. As such, when an injury gets in the way of athletic identity, it may be experienced as a loss of identity and result in psychological distress [1].

Epidemiology of Sports Injuries

Sports injuries are frequently an inevitable corollary of athletic activity and are associated with potential risks that impact adolescent athletes in many ways. For example, it is estimated that 1.6–3.8 million people in the United States sustain a sport and recreational traumatic brain injury each year [3]. However, this estimate may be underrepresented because of underreporting to the appropriate authorities [3]. In June of 2005, there were 7.2 million students who participated in high school sports [2]. Studies have shown that high school sports accounted for two million injuries, 500,000 doctor visits, and 30,000 hospitalizations annually [2]. According to a High School Sports-Related Injury Surveillance study, the overall injury rate in all high school sports combined was 2.29 injuries per 1000 athlete exposures [14]. The High School Sports-Related Injury Surveillance data, which included nine sports (see Table 5.1) [14], showed high injury rates in both competition and practice sessions in the 2018–2019 period. In terms of economic consequences, the estimated cost is more than 8 billion dollars annually [1].

Besides the economic burden, the accompanying physical symptoms of injuries can result in time lost from school, return time to sports, social engagements, and other significant developmental events [1, 3]. The amount of time lost to injury varies. The High School Sports-Related Injury Surveillance data suggest that about 42% of injuries resulted in less than 7 days of time lost from participation, while almost 60% resulted in 7 or more days of time lost from sports participation [14]. However, one study revealed significant differences between sexes for time lost in sports, with female high school student-athletes taking longer to return than male high school student-athletes [3]. The number of consecutive injuries among high school competitive athletes seems to impact the amount of time loss from sports participation. For instance, Haraldsdottir and Watson [1] opined that every fifth injury in high school competitive athletes led to an absence from regular training of 2 months or more.

Although participation in sports predisposes adolescents to the risk of injury, the literature has primarily focused on the physical implications of those injuries. The psychosocial impact has been mostly neglected [1]. The mind-body connection has not been adequately explored and yet this connection may lead to more significant outcomes, including adverse effects on mental health, quality of life, time loss, and other psychosocial consequences.

Table 5.1 Injury rates by sport, High School Sports-Related Injury Surveillance Study, United States, 2018–2019 school year (only includes injuries resulting in ≥1 days' of time loss)

Sports	# Injuries		Injury rate per 1000 athlete-exposures
	Competition	Practice	
Overall total	2257	1712	2.29
Boys' American football	927	685	3.85
Boys' soccer	229	122	1.83
Girls' soccer	297	151	2.72
Girls' volleyball	83	134	1.34
Boys' basketball	196	146	1.61
Girls' basketball	170	130	1.95
Boys' wrestling	163	194	2.52
Boys' baseball	101	74	1.03
Girls' softball	91	76	1.43

Sports Specialization

Sports specialization, in which the athlete focuses on a single sport, has become the norm for young athletes in the context of collegiate sports, scholarships, Olympic, or professional levels [1, 12]. The prevalence rates of sport specialization among youth athletes are 17–41% and vary by factors such as athlete sex, age, sport, socioeconomic status (SES), school size, and geographic location [15]. The reasoning behind specialization differs but is related to aspirations to compete at a high level [12]. Sport specialization typically occurs before the age of 12 years but can happen as early as 5 or 6 years of age, in individual sports such as gymnastics, figure skating, and swimming or diving [12]. Specializing, grouped into low, moderate, and high levels, often requires an adolescent to devote most of their free time to a sport of choice, linking their self-esteem to their performance, and sometimes experiencing higher rates of burnout, compromised sleep, well-being, and increased susceptibility to injury [1]. Dahab et al. [16] noted that highly specialized athletes were more likely to report previous lower extremity injuries, severe overuse injuries, and knee injuries. In this same study, sport specialization was separately linked to an increased injury risk among high school athletes [16].

Single sport athletes may also be more vulnerable to psychological burnout and social isolation than nonspecialized athletes [16]. One primary aspect of sport specialization that impacts psychological distress is burnout due to overtraining, to the extent athletes no longer participate in an activity that was once pleasurable [15, 16]. Additional potential physical risks of specialization and overtraining include acute injury and illness [15]. Research has shown that while early sports specialization is often driven by a path toward succeeding in a sport, it may increase the risk of overuse injury and burnout and has not been positively related to athletic performance [1, 12].

Sports Participation and Adolescent Psychosocial Development

During adolescence, athletic participation can play a significant role in building coping repertoire, resilience, and resistance to social pressures. Adolescent athletes who sustain sports injuries may present with unique psychological challenges because they deal with developmental issues such as a balance between dependence on parental feedback, independence, identity development, and social skills acquisition [1, 17]. For early adolescents, much of their time is spent comparing themselves to peers and worrying over perceived physical differences [18]. When they are involved in sports, adolescents can listen to the opinions of peers and adults and independently weigh the consequences of their choices before engaging in decision-making [18]. Additionally, given their limited life experiences, adolescents may be vulnerable to criticism and negative comments from others, which in theory could lead to false beliefs of being hated by others, including a coach, trainer, or team-mates [18]. Given the nature of the adolescent growth spurt, youth may find it difficult to adjust in the context of their sports or physical activity-specific performance [18]. They may also encounter pressure to increase muscle bulk, weight, strength, and/or endurance to improve performance, depending on the specific sport in which they are participating and may resort to unhealthy practices (i.e., steroids, disordered eating) to achieve said goal [18].

Simultaneously, sports participation contributes to muscle mass, strength, and cardiopulmonary endurance. It improves agility skills, motor coordination, power, and speed, enhancing and developing through middle adolescence [18]. Exercise's physiological effects can include increased endorphin levels, body temperature, increased neurotransmitter production, and attenuation of the hypothalamic-pituitary-adrenal (HPA) axis response to stress [19]. Consequently, the psychological effects of exercise may include a distraction from feelings of depression and anxiety and an increase in positive feelings associated with mastery and self-efficacy [19]. On the other hand, it can be inferred that when exercise is suspended due to injury, youth may experience elevated levels of the body's stress hormone cortisol, exacerbating mental health outcomes [19].

Psychosocial Impacts of Injury

Assessment of Quality of Life

Very few studies have evaluated the relationship between adolescent sports injuries on their quality of life. One measure used to develop a greater understanding of a person's well-being is the health-related quality of life (HRQOL), a patient self-report measure that taps into the domains of physical, mental, emotional, and social health [1]. Another measure, the PedsQL, is a valid, reliable, and responsive 18–20-item generic patient-reported outcome measure that has been used to evaluate generic HRQOL in athletes [20]. Lam and Markbreiter [20], in their study on the impact of knee injury history on HRQOL in adolescent athletes who were medically cleared for full participation, suggest that, despite clearance for full sport participation, adolescent athletes with a previous knee injury were likely to experience lower HRQOL than their peers with no knee injury history, specifically in their physical, school, and social functioning. So too, these athletes may report more significant impairments in terms of pain, swelling, feeling of giving way, as well as function in the knee [20]. Further, Lam and Markbreiter posited that athletes with a knee injury may experience difficulty with activities of daily living, including walking, running, climbing stairs, and completing chores in the home [20].

Similarly, studies of quality of life in adolescents with concussions indicate that these injuries can have lasting impact on the youth's cognitive, emotional, and social life even 5 years post-injury, regardless of whether the injury has been a mild, moderate, or severe traumatic brain injury (TBI) [21]. According to the Centers for Disease Control and Prevention guidelines around concussion, concussion symptoms may present during the normal healing process as youth resume regular activities. Recovery may be impacted by several factors, including a history of previous concussions, other brain injuries, neurological or mental health disorders, learning challenges, and psychosocial stressors. Hunt et al. highlighted dizziness as one of the most frequent concussion symptoms, affecting approximately 50–90% of patients [22]. These participants reported that coping with blurred vision, lightheadedness, sensitivity to noise or light, and dizziness, relentless headaches became an added burden due to others' beliefs that the seriousness of their complaints may not be warranted [21, 22]. A study by Howell et al. suggested that following a concussion injury, greater somatic symptoms were associated with a longer symptom duration among youth [23]. Further, youth who reported moderate to severe dizziness endorsed higher concussion symptom burden and higher anxiety and depression scores than those with little to no dizziness [22]. In fact, higher acute symptom severity has been correlated with worse clinical outcomes following concussions [23].

The Iadevaia et al. [24] study showed that athletes consistently mentioned the influence of the concussion on their school attendance and activities throughout the post-concussion recovery process [24]. More specifically, this qualitative study reported reduced concentration, confusion, and feelings of forgetfulness when engaging in academic activities. Other studies have measured additional cognitive symptoms of concussions such as someone not feeling right and like they are in a fog [23]. The athletes in Iadevaia et al. [24] study also voiced other struggles with returning to pre-concussion levels of aptitude, confidence, and a sense of social ease and well-being [24]. Choudhury et al. [21] identified lower comprehension, memory, and concentration as significant contributors to social isolation, thus impacting youth academic and social functioning. While current evidence suggests that concussive injuries frequently result in psychological distress, adding prescribed isolation from peers and activities may further aggravate these adverse psychological outcomes [10]. Along the same lines, a traumatic injury, particularly one that limits or ends sports participation, may activate a new mental or emotional concern, or intensify an existing mental health condition in a young athlete [12]. The CDC brain injury basic guidelines outline recovery to foster youth return to normal activities after a concussion in the following order: rest, light activity, moderate activity, and back to regular activity [25].

When adolescent athletes are healthy, they tend to report a higher quality of life than their nonathlete counterparts. However, after injury, many athletes express heightened feelings of anxiety and stress [16]. Primarily, those who experience prolonged recovery time, i.e., symptoms for 28 days or more after the initial injury, are increasingly vulnerable to anxiety, depression, impaired school performance, and quality of life [22]. Studies have found anxiety and depression to be more prevalent among young athletes who play individual sports than team sports [8]. Other significant reasons for athletes in individual sports to be at increased risks for mental health concerns included judges determining success in individual sports, which correlate with the highest rates of anxiety in elite athletes as they may feel enormous pressure to distinguish themselves from the competition in the pursuit of perfection and a judge's approval [8]. Specifically, Dahab et al. found that Olympic rhythmic gymnasts who increased their training volume at an earlier age reported having less fun in their sport and lower perceived health quality when compared to non-Olympic elite rhythmic gymnasts [16].

Time Loss

In a study by Bretzin et al. [3], time loss was defined as "the days between the sports-related concussion (SRC) injury date and the authorized date of return to sport participation." Investigators have demonstrated that high school and collegiate student-athletes missed an average of 5–6 school days following a concussive injury [3]. The highest clinical incidence for time loss in male sports included football 3.9 and ice hockey 3.3, and one-way ANOVA revealed noteworthy differences between sexes [3]. For instance, female student-athletes were more susceptible to lingering recovery time than male student-athletes from SRC symptoms in collegiate athletics, which led to greater time loss from participation [3]. The sex differences may be attributed to nondisclosure, which may also explain the differences in time loss between male and female athletes and the increased number of missed school days by females [3].

Researchers have indicated a wide range of time loss (2–25 days) from athletics following concussion in football [10]. Meanwhile, athletes involved in club sports had a higher proportion of prior time-loss musculoskeletal (MSK) injuries and injuries requiring imaging, injection, a cast, a brace, or crutches [16]. In addition to the number of days lost, other factors that determine the severity of musculoskeletal injuries include the nature of the injury, duration of treatment, absence from school, and cost of treatment [2]. Furthermore, about 50% of MSK injuries result in warranted medical care and may result in permanent disability [2].

Time lost due to prescribed cognitive rest after a sport-related concussion can have significant psychological effects; "cognitive rest disengages adolescents from academic and social activities, thus resulting in isolation from peers" [10]. For males, when the athlete is removed from sports due to prescribed cognitive rest, added social support or interventions to sustain contact with the teammates, coaches, and peers are indicated [10]. Athletes who were interviewed identified a familial bond with their teammates, which led to a feeling of void when they could no longer participate due to their concussions [10]. Nippert and Smith [13] reasoned that cognitive appraisal determines how athletes react emotionally to injury and ultimately dictates their behavioral responses to injury and rehabilitation.

Return to Play and Fear of Re-injury

Often pressing in the minds of injured high school athletes is whether they can return to play and how long they will have to wait to return to play. The overall return to play (RTP) rate after sports injury has, over the years, remained stable between 50% and 80%, with very few studies noting rates higher than the mid-80% [9]. Gennarelli et al. [26] posited kinesiophobia and fear of re-injury as two of the most important psychological factors that impact an athlete's ability to return to pre-injury activity level. In addition, negative psychological responses to injury, including anxiety, low self-esteem, and depression, are negatively associated with RTP [26]. Historically, physical performance tests (PPTs) that assess sport-specific skills concurrently with an assessment of pain, range of motion, and strength have been used to assess athletes' recovery from injury and readiness to return to play (RTP) [26]. Measures for return to play include the Y-Balance Test (YBT). This functional RTP assessment is considered a reliable and repeatable evaluation that uses side-to-side differences and measures the operative and nonoperative limb based on normative data [27]. A higher proportion of club sport athletes reported a history of injury since club sports are generally considered more competitive than nonclub sports [16].

In a study of athletes who had undergone ACL reconstruction, Ellis et al. found that psychosocial factors, such as coping resources, social support, and fear of re-injury, had vital roles in the recovery process following the ACL surgery [27]. In fact, an athlete's psychological response to the injury and the recovery process impacted RTP. The authors suggested that psychological factors can put an athlete at risk for not returning to their previous level of activity following injury. Furthermore, Ellis et al. opined that increased emotional distress negatively impacts an athlete's overall recovery progress and return to action [27]. In their study, patients with a greater fear or fear of re-injury following both an ACL injury and ACL reconstruction were more likely to have poor performance and function, lower RTP rates, and increased frequency of repeated injuries [27].

Another important consideration in an athlete's return to play is the discrepancy in the patient's understanding of recovery compared to the medical determination of recovery [21]. Explorations of concussion recovery suggest "feelings of isolation, depression, devastation, hopelessness, and loss of independence are mitigating factors to recovery" [10]. Ellis et al. maintained that athletes might use imagery, relaxation training, and coping skill development to reduce fear of re-injury and improve psychological readiness and self-efficacy as they attempt to return to play [27].

Mental Health Outcomes

For some athletes, the psychological response to injury can impose tremendous physical and mental health sequelae, including depression, anxiety, disordered eating, trauma responses, and substance use [28, 29]. The ability to engage in sports is related to positive psychological benefits. Psychological responses to injury may lead to long-term effects and differ from normal reactions of sadness, isolation, frustration, and disengagement to injury. Depression, anxiety, and fear generally occur in the context of a repeated sense of vulnerability [21]. Athletes differ in how they may respond to injuries, but also the type of sport may impact the incidence of mental health disorders. For example, in looking at depression in athletes, those competing in individual sports such as gymnastics, track and field, figure skating, and dance were at increased risk for depressive symptoms when compared to athletes involved in team sports [12]. Likewise, in their study, Pluhar et al. found that individual sports athletes had a greater tendency to report anxiety and depression than team sports athletes [8]. Moreover, the presence of anxiety in the preseason is associated with an elevated risk of injury compared to student-athletes without anxiety [29]. Askow et al. noted that adolescent concussions may be particularly problematic as early exposure to repetitive head impacts can predispose patients to mental health problems later including anxiety, cognitive decline, decision-making difficulties, and other concerns.

Statistics from the National Institute of Mental Health, SAMHSA 2020 data, estimated the rate of a major depressive episode as 17.0% of the US population aged 12–17 years, with females having a higher prevalence than males (25.2% vs. 9.2%) [30]. In a study that reviewed the literature on depression in young athletes after an injury, Palisch and Merritt found that athletes with ACL injuries reported seven times greater levels of depression at 11 days after injury than uninjured athletes, while concussed athletes showed three times more depression at 4 days after the injury than control participants [12]. Daley et al. [28] found patients with more symptoms of depression reported worse perceived knee function after surgery and were more likely to report postoperative complications [28]. In terms of gender differences, according to Palisch and Merritt, female athletes experienced greater post-injury depression symptom severity compared to male athletes [12].

In addition to the mental health effects of sports injuries, participation in athletics, specifically in aesthetic sports like gymnastics, figure skating, and dance, may put health at increased risk through intense pressure to change their weight to improve performance or personal appearance. Due to this competitive pressure, adolescent athletes may engage in negative behaviors including dieting and restrictive and disordered eating tendencies, which can result in serious eating disorders [11]. To illustrate, Ravi et al. used a web-based study with 846 female athletes from 67 different sports [11]. Results indicated that 25%, 18%, and 32% of the athletes endorsed restrictive eating, eating disorders, and menstrual dysfunction, respectively. Additionally, restrictive eating, eating disorders, and menstrual dysfunction were higher among lean sport athletes than non-lean sports athletes, which predisposed them to greater risks. While no differences were noted between elite and non-elite athletes, younger athletes reported higher rates of menstrual dysfunction and a lower lifetime prevalence of eating disorders [11]. Ravi et al. also highlighted distinctions between younger and older athletes, where younger athletes reported lower rates of current or previous eating disorders, while the prevalence of menstrual dysfunction was lower in the older athletes [11]. Lean sports athletes (i.e., those with increased desire and external social pressures to be thin) endorsed more restrictive eating, eating disorders, and menstrual dysfunction than non-lean sports athletes; however, more non-lean sports athletes had sustained at least one injury during the preceding year than lean sport athletes [11]. Moreover, athletes with restrictive eating or current or past eating disorder had a greater tendency to report a sports-related injury than those with no restrictive eating or eating disorder [11].

For some youth athletes, a sports injury can precipitate suicidal ideation or other acute mental health crises. Miller et al. documented an association between reporting a sport- or physical activity-related concussion and "having seriously considered attempting suicide, having made a suicide plan, and having attempted suicide was significant and remained significant even after they controlled for sex, grade level, and race/ethnicity" [19]. Miller et al. also found frequent substance use disorders among adults and adolescent athletes who sustained a moderate or severe traumatic brain injury [7]. Finally, a study involving athletes 21 years of age and younger who suffered ACL ruptures showed high rates of post-traumatic stress disorder (PTSD) symptoms, including avoidance, hyperarousal, and intrusion [1].

Mental Health Treatments for Athletic Injuries

Studies have found that pain and other physiological effects from injury may lead to anxiety, depression, isolation, anger, and frustration [31, 32]. Leddy et al. found that 51% of injured collegiate athletes met the criteria for mild or more severe depressive symptoms, with 12% experiencing moderate depressive symptoms [33]. In addition, studies have shown that depressive symptoms may be linked to worse recovery outcomes. Garcia et al. found that after orthopedic surgical repair, including hand surgery and total knee arthroplasties, there was an inverse relationship between depressive symptoms and patient-reported outcomes [34]. Given the impact injury may have on mental health, recent research has focused on the benefits of screening for mental health concerns and interventions to reduce mental health symptoms and improve recovery outcomes, including education, goal setting, meditation, guided imagery, and cognitive behavioral therapy (CBT) and third wave CBT treatments such as acceptance and commitment therapy (ACT) [13, 26, 35, 36]. At this point, the majority of research on these interventions has been focused on subject pools of injured adults rather than youth. In the following exploration of treatment options and outcomes, we are extrapolating from adult research to inform the basis for best practices for injured youth.

A first step in identifying mental health symptoms in injured athletes is through screening. Established tools for injured athletes measure constructs such as self-efficacy, athletic identity, readiness to return to sport (RTS), and kinesiophobia, or fear and anxiety of re-injury [28, 37]. Although mental health professionals are likely to be the best qualified to perform most screening and assessment tools, the first line of defense for many athletes is via their sports med physician or athletic trainer (AT). Screening tools can be made available for use by athletic trainers. However, many ATs may lack training or feel uncomfortable administering the questionnaires. Athletic trainers can, however, initiate the conversation by asking their patients how they are coping with recovery emotionally and refer patients to psychologists as needed. Having this discussion can help to minimize the stigma of mental health struggles among athletes and develop trust between the patient and

AT [28]. However, it is important for these professionals to keep in mind that building rapport may take multiple sessions before an athlete feels comfortable enough to disclose any negative emotions. This could be due to fluctuating feelings surrounding their injury at different points in recovery, or due to feeling uncomfortable admitting negative feelings initially [28, 33]. Especially for younger athletes who are experiencing some of these challenging emotions for the first time, it may be even more difficult for them to communicate their mental health symptoms with an AT. As a result, it is important for all providers to implement thorough assessment and re-evaluations throughout the recovery process.

In addition to screening, educating injured athletes on their treatment plan and recovery timeline is important for managing expectations throughout rehabilitation. In a qualitative study looking at individuals with a mean age of 29 recovering from ACL injury, athletes who did not have clear expectations for the recovery process, or falsely believed they would be able to recovery more quickly than the minimum time to recover indicated to them, endorsed feeling frustrated and guilty that they were not recovering "on time." Due to these challenges in recovery, some athletes noted feeling hopeless, which reduced their motivation to persevere through the recovery process [38]. In a study by Maddison et al., athletes with a mean age of 30 recovering from ACL surgery were either given a modeling video to watch, which explained the expectations for the 2 weeks prior to the operation through 6-week post-operation or were placed in the no video control group [39]. Those who were given the modeling videos had lower expectations for pain and increased rehabilitation self-efficacy [39]. Further, in a study by Francis et al., athletes with a mean age of 27 without thorough information about their injury endorsed more negative emotions, a lack of motivation toward recovery, and higher anxiety [40, 41]. An interdisciplinary medical team consisting of mental health professionals, team physicians, and ATs can help injured athletes by setting achievable goals together. This can increase the athlete's sense of control over their injury and improve motivation and adherence to the treatment [28, 42].

Another option for athletes recovering from injury is Mindfulness-Based Stress Reduction (MBSR), an evidence-based intervention that has been shown to be effective with individuals struggling from stress, anxiety, depression, and pain [32, 43]. MBSR was developed in 1979 by Dr. Jon Kabat-Zinn at the University of Massachusetts Medical Center's Stress Reduction Clinic. The intervention is comprised of activities such as mindfulness exercises, body scans, gentle yoga, and sitting mediation in order to help individuals recognize their own behavior patterns, learn to respond thoughtfully to stressful situations, and increase pain tolerance. Individuals typically complete an 8-week series of weekly sessions ranging from 90-min to 3 h [44, 45]. In a study by Mohammed et al., MBSR was implemented in conjunction with physical therapy for injured athletes ages 21–36 and helped these athletes increase pain tolerance and mindful awareness over the course of the program [45]. In a small study conducted by Pappous et al., all six athletes (mean age 28.9) interviewed noted that the MBSR intervention had a positive impact on their psychological state during the rehabilitation, improved their pain tolerance and mindfulness, and helped them manage negative emotions [32]. The impact of improved pain tolerance among injured athletes may have additional positive consequences, such as feeling motivated by the ability to successfully manage a larger workload due to a reduction in pain, and progress through physical therapy more quickly as a result.

In addition to MBSR, other mindfulness-based interventions have also facilitated injury recovery and improved mental health symptoms of injured athletes. In studies by Johnson and Cupal and Brewer, deep diaphragmatic breathing helped injured athletes focus on accomplishing a task while limiting distraction from anxieties that may accompany the challenge at hand [36, 46]. Injured athletes have also been aided by guided imagery, or the process of visualizing some experience related to the rehabilitation of their injury and imagining the successful completion [47]. In a study by Johnson, athletes were asked to connect with their injured body part through guided imagery and specifically imagine it functioning properly without pain. This activity resulted in the improvement of the athlete's mood post-visualization [46, 47].

Kinesiophobia and fear of re-injury have both been shown to play a role in impeding the successful recovery from athletic injury and RTS. A meta-analysis by Ardern et al. showed that kinesiophobia prevented 19% of patients recovering from ACL surgery from returning to pre-injury levels of sport [48]. A study by Hsu et al. showed that fear of re-injury may have in impact on injury recovery and prevent a successful return to sport [4]. In another study by Kvist et al., among athletes recovering from ACL reconstruction surgery, 53% returned to their pre-injury activity level, and those who did not reported higher levels of fear of re-injury [49].

In addition to anxiety-related symptoms, adolescent athletes in particular commonly endorse feelings of psychological distress and PTSD as a result of injury, which can result in less successful coping methods [50]. Cognitive behavioral therapy (CBT) can help patients develop awareness of their behaviors and unlearn maladaptive tendencies and has been found to be particularly helpful among injured athletes experiencing mood disorder symptoms such as fear, anxiety, and kinesiophobia. For the injured population, the primary pillars of CBT focused on include education, goal setting, challenging negative thoughts, and exposure [28]. In particular, CBT has helped improve pain tolerance among patients dealing with injury or chronic pain, given it is common for these individuals to develop maladaptive thought patterns regarding their pain [51]. CBT helps to reconceptualize pain and allows individuals to see pain as a part of recovery rather than a barrier to it [52].

Acceptance and commitment therapy (ACT), a third behavior therapy, is focused on accepting challenging or difficult emotions to change previously maladaptive responses or behaviors and improve mindfulness and psychological flexibility [47, 53]. Studies have shown that individuals can use psychological flexibility, or the ability to be present and have awareness of their body and mind, to increase parasympathetic activity, which can in turn help injury rehabilitation as well as improve mental health symptoms [35]. Additionally, Mahoney and Hanrahan reported an adapted four-session ACT intervention on four injured athletes in addition to their physician rehabilitation [54]. ACT helped these athletes face challenges during their recovery process and taught them valuable skills to help them persevere to reach a point where they would be able to return to their sport.

While there are many treatment and intervention options to help injured athletes reduce negative mental health symptoms and improve recovery outcomes, it is imperative that all athletes are first screened for possible symptoms, educated about their recovery, and work with their care team to develop a series of rehabilitation goals. Patients should be monitored for new or existing mental health symptoms and make referrals to mental health professionals as needed. Mental health professionals should work together with their clinicians to provide a multidisciplinary approach to patient care and discuss treatment progression and the possible onset of new symptoms through the ups and downs of the rehabilitation process. Especially for younger athletes who may not have experience communicating their needs to adults that aren't their parents or guardians, cohesion among the treatment team is critical. Mental health professionals can also integrate mindfulness-based practices, CBT, or ACT based on their patient's symptoms. An approach that integrates the mental health support with their clinical care will help the athlete to be adequately prepared for their rehabilitation process, feel supported by their AT, and motivated within their treatment process in order to improve mental health symptoms and ensure that they do not negatively impact recovery [28, 41].

Mitigating the Mental Health Consequences of Sports Injuries

Healthcare providers can help to reduce the mental health effect of sports injuries by monitoring students for signs of depression after a concussion, providing education, and encouraging parents to watch for the symptoms [7]. The CDC's HEADS UP concussion education and awareness campaign is one attempt to increase parents' awareness of the impact and healing process. Similarly, through the process of education, parents, caregivers, and coaches of adolescent athletes can seek medical and mental health support services when signs of depression and suicidality are observed [7]. Further, annual screening in child and adolescent patients for emotional and behavioral problems, such as depression at age 12 years and major depressive disorder for adolescents ages 12 through 18 using either the Patient Health Questionnaire for Adolescents or the primary care versions of the Beck Depression Inventory, can facilitate early intervention [12]. Also, implementing comprehensive suicide prevention strategies, such as those included in CDC's Preventing Suicide: A Technical Package of Policy, Programs, and Practices, may also reduce the risk of suicide among student-athletes [7].

Conclusion

Sports participation plays an essential role in the lives of many adolescents with tremendous benefits in the areas of sense of self, interpersonal, physical, and psychological health. Injuries sustained during athletic activity may disrupt these athletes' day-to-day functioning, interfere with their engagement in developmentally appropriate activities, and even lead to negative mental health outcomes. Though there are limited studies on the psychosocial impacts of sports-related injury among youth athletes, the studies that do exist suggest that there can be mental health sequelae associated with physical injuries. Given the literature in this study and the developmental trajectory of the adolescence period, which is characterized by rapid physical, psychological, social, and emotional growth, it becomes imperative that the effects of sports-related injuries' psychosocial functioning be considered. Sports-related injuries result in time loss, reduced quality of life, re-injury risk, delayed return to play, and identity threats and may lead to mental health problems. However, screening for mental health concerns such as anxiety, depression, and suicidality and providing education on mental health and recovery to coaches, athletes, and parents may help to minimize the physical and psychological effects of sports-related injury. Psychosocial interventions including relaxation, cognitive behavioral therapy, guided imagery, and mindfulness can facilitate post-recovery injury in athletes. Future research should focus on resources, medical and psychological interventions, and reintegration techniques for return to play, which will help to minimize the developmental and psychological consequences of sports-related injury on adolescents.

Acknowledgements   We are grateful to Jill Kavanaugh for her guidance and assistance with database searches. We also appreciate Joan Axelrod's assistance with editing the paper.

References

1. Haraldsdottir K, Watson AM. Psychosocial impacts of sports-related injuries in adolescent athletes. Curr Sports Med Rep. 2021;20(20):104–8.
2. Patel DR, Yamasaki A, Brown K. Epidemiology of sports-related musculoskeletal injuries in young athletes in United States. Transl Pediatr. 2017;6(3):160–6.
3. Bretzin AC, Covassin T, Fox ME, Petit KM, Savage JL, Walker LF, et al. Sex differences in the clinical incidence of concussions, missed school days, and time loss in high school student-athletes: part 1. Am J Sports Med. 2018;46(9):2263–9.
4. Howell DR, Kirkwood MW, Laker S, Wilson JC. Collision and contact sport participation and quality of life among adolescent athletes. J Athl Train. 2020;55(11):1174–80.

5. Malm C, Jakobsson J, Isaksson A. Physical activity and sports—real health benefits: a review with insight into the public health of Sweden. Sports. 2019;7(5):127.
6. Walker GA, Seehusen CN, Armento A, Provance AJ, Wilson JC, Howell DR. Family affluence relationship to sports specialization in youth athletes. Clin Pediatr (Phila). 2021;60(1):50–5.
7. Miller GF, DePadilla L, Jones SE, Bartholow BN, Sarmiento K, Breiding MJ. The association between sports- or physical activity–related concussions and suicidality among US high school students, 2017. Sports Health. 2021;13(2):187–97.
8. Pluhar E, McCracken C, Griffith KL, Christino MA, Sugimoto D, Meehan WP III. Team sport athletes may be less likely to suffer anxiety or depression than individual sport athletes. J Sports Sci Med. 2019;18(3):490–6.
9. Edison BR, Christino MA, Rizzone KH. Athletic identity in youth athletes: a systematic review of the literature. Int J Environ Res Public Health. 2021;18(14):7331.
10. Hunt TN, Harris LL. Psychological impact of cognitive rest following sport-related concussion on low socioeconomic status adolescent patients. J Allied Health. 2017;46(4):e81–3.
11. Ravi S, Ihalainen JK, Taipale-Mikkonen RS, Kujala UM, Waller B, Mierlahti L, et al. Self-reported restrictive eating, eating disorders, menstrual dysfunction, and injuries in athletes competing at different levels and sports. Nutrients. 2021;13(9):3275.
12. Palisch AR, Merritt LS. Depressive symptoms in the young athlete after injury: recommendations for research. J Pediatr Health Care. 2018;32(3):245–9.
13. Nippert AH, Smith AM. Psychologic stress related to injury and impact on sport performance. Phys Med Rehabil Clin N Am. 2008;19(2):399–418, x.
14. Comstock RD, Currie DW, Pierpoint LA. National high school sports-related injury surveillance study report. National Center for Health Statistics, 2018–2019. n.d.. https://coloradosph.cuanschutz.edu/docs/librariesprovider204/default-document-library/2018-19.pdf?sfvrsn=d26400b9
15. Jayanthi NA, Post EG, Laury TC, Fabricant PD. Health consequences of youth sport specialization. J Athl Train. 2019;54(10):1040–9.
16. Dahab K, Potter MN, Provance A, Albright J, Howell DR. Sport specialization, club sport participation, quality of life, and injury history among high school athletes. J Athl Train. 2019;54(10):1061–6.
17. Manuel JC, Shilt JS, Curl WW, Smith JA, Durant RH, Lester L, et al. Coping with sports injuries: an examination of the adolescent athlete adolescents athletes coping depression emotional outcomes sports injuries. J Adolesc Health. 2002;31(5):391–3.
18. Brown KA, Patel DR, Darmawan D. Participation in sports in relation to adolescent growth and development. Transl Pediatr. 2017;6(3):150–9.
19. Mikkelsen K, Stojanovska L, Polenakovic M, Bosevski M, Apostolopoulos V. Exercise and mental health. Maturitas. 2017;106:48–56.
20. Lam KC, Markbreiter JG. The impact of knee injury history on health-related quality of life in adolescent athletes. J Sport Rehabil. 2019;28(2):115–9.
21. Choudhury R, Kolstad A, Prajapati V, Samuel G, Yeates KO. Loss and recovery after concussion: adolescent patients give voice to their concussion experience. Health Expect. 2020;23(6):1533–42.
22. Hunt DL, Oldham J, Aaron SE, Tan CO, Meehan WP III, Howell DR. Dizziness, psychosocial function, and postural stability following sport-related concussion. Clin J Sport Med. 2021;32:361.
23. Howell DR, Kriz P, Mannix RC, Kirchberg T, Master CL, Meehan WP. Concussion symptom profiles among child, adolescent, and young adult athletes. Clin J Sport Med. 2019;29(5):391–7.
24. Iadevaia C, Roiger T, Zwart MB. Qualitative examination of adolescent health-related quality of life at 1 year postconcussion. J Athl Train. 2015;50(11):1182–9.
25. Centers for Disease Control and Prevention (CDC). Brain basics: recovery from concussion. 2019. Updated 2019 February 12. https://www.cdc.gov/headsup/basics/concussion_recovery.html. Accessed 8 Mar 2022.

26. Gennarelli SM, Brown SM, Mulcahey MK. Psychosocial interventions help facilitate recovery following musculoskeletal sports injuries: a systematic review. Phys Sportsmed. 2020;48(4):370–7.
27. Ellis HB, Sabatino M, Nwelue E, Wagner KJ, Force E, Wilson P. The use of psychological patient reported outcome measures to identify adolescent athletes at risk for prolonged recovery following an ACL reconstruction. J Pediatr Orthop. 2020;40(9):e844–52.
28. Daley MM, Griffith K, Milewski MD, Christino MA. The mental side of the injured athlete. J Am Acad Orthop Surg. 2021;29(12):499–506.
29. Sutcliffe JH, Greenberger PA. Identifying psychological difficulties in college athletes. J Allergy Clin Immunol Pract. 2020;8:2216–9.
30. National Institute of Mental Health. Major depression. 2022. Updated 2022 January. https://www.nimh.nih.gov/health/statistics/major-depression. Accessed 8 Mar 2022.
31. Walker N, Heaney C. Relaxation techniques in sport injury rehabilitation. In: Arvinen-Barrow M, Walker N, editors. The psychology of sport injury and rehabilitation. London: Routledge; 2013. p. 105–21.
32. Pappous A, Mohammed WA, Sharma D. (2021). Perceptions of injured athletes after eight weeks of mindfulness based stress reduction program. J Psychol Res. 2021;3(2):35–44.
33. Leddy MH, Lambert MJ, Ogles BM. Psychological consequences of athletic injury among high-level competitors. Res Q Exerc Sport. 1994;65(4):347–54.
34. Garcia GH, Wu H-H, Park MJ, Tjoumakaris FP, Tucker BS, Kelly JD, Sennett BJ. Depression symptomatology and anterior cruciate ligament injury: incidence and effect on functional outcome—a prospective cohort study. Am J Sports Med. 2016;44(3):572–9.
35. Cecil S. Less control, more flexibility: using acceptance and commitment therapy with injured athletes. In: Wadey R, editor. Sport injury psychology: cultural, relational, methodological, and applied considerations. London: Routledge; 2020. p. 197–205.
36. Cupal DD, Brewer BW. Effects of relaxation and guided imagery on knee strength, reinjury anxiety, and pain following anterior cruciate ligament reconstruction. Rehabil Psychol. 2001;46(1):28–43.
37. Hsu C-J, Meierbachtol A, George SZ, Chmielewski TL. Fear of reinjury in athletes: implications for rehabilitation. Sports Health. 2017;9(2):162–7.
38. Heijne A, Axelsson K, Werner S, Biguet G. Rehabilitation and recovery after anterior cruciate ligament reconstruction: patients' experiences. Scand J Med Sci Sports. 2008;18(3):325–35.
39. Maddison R, Prapavessis H, Clatworthy M. Modeling and rehabilitation following anterior cruciate ligament reconstruction. Ann Behav Med. 2006;31(1):89–98.
40. Francis SR, Andersen MB, Maley P. Physiotherapists' and male professional athletes' views on psychological skills for rehabilitation. J Sci Med Sport. 2000;3(1):17–29.
41. Santi G, Pietrantoni L. Psychology of sport injury rehabilitation: a review of models and interventions. J Sport Health Sci. 2013;8(4):1029–44.
42. Arvinen-Barrow M, Massey WV, Hemmings B. Role of sport medicine professionals in addressing psychosocial aspects of sport-injury rehabilitation: professional athletes' views. J Athl Train. 2013;49(6):764–72.
43. Kabat-Zinn J. Full catastrophe living, revised edition: how to cope with stress, pain, and illness using mindfulness meditation. London: Piatkus; 2013.
44. Institute for Mindfulness Based Approaches. What is MBSR?. 2022. Updated 2022. https://www.institute-for-mindfulness.org/offer/mbsr/what-is-mbsr. Accessed 8 Mar 2022.
45. Mohammed W, Pappous A, Sharma D. Effect of Mindfulness Based Stress Reduction (MBSR) in increasing pain tolerance and improving the mental health of injured athletes. Front Psychol. 2018;9:722.
46. Johnson U. Short-term psychological intervention: a study of long-term-injured competitive athletes. J Sport Rehabil. 2000;9(3):207–18.
47. Schwab Reese LM, Pittsinger R, Yang J. Effectiveness of psychological intervention following sport injury. J Sport Health Sci. 2012;1(2):71–9.

48. Ardern CL, Taylor NF, Feller JA, Whitehead TS, Webster KE. Psychological responses matter in returning to preinjury level of sport after anterior cruciate ligament reconstruction surgery. Am J Sports Med. 2013;41(7):1549–58.
49. Kvist J, Ek A, Sporrstedt K, Good L. Fear of re-injury: a hindrance for returning to sports after anterior cruciate ligament reconstruction. Knee Surg Sports Traumatol Arthrosc. 2005;13(5):393–7.
50. Christino MA, Fantry AJ, Vopat BG. Psychological aspects of recovery following anterior cruciate ligament reconstruction. J Am Acad Orthop Surg. 2015;23(8):501–9.
51. Smeets RJ, Vlaeyen JW, Kester AD, Knottnerus JA. Reduction of pain catastrophizing mediates the outcome of both physical and cognitive-behavioral treatment in chronic low back pain. J Pain. 2006;7(4):261–71.
52. Riddle DL, Keefe FJ, Nay WT, McKee D, Attarian DE, Jensen MP. Pain coping skills training for patients with elevated pain catastrophizing who are scheduled for knee arthroplasty: a quasi-experimental study. Arch Phys Med Rehabil. 2011;92(6):859–65.
53. Gardner FL, Moore ZE. A mindfulness-acceptance-commitment-based approach to athletic performance enhancement: theoretical considerations. Behav Ther. 2004;35(4):707–23.
54. Mahoney J, Hanrahan SJ. A brief educational intervention using acceptance and commitment therapy: four injured athletes' experiences. J Clin Sport Psychol. 2011;5(3):252–73.

Chapter 6
Psychological Consequences of Concussion

Mary M. Daley, Jamie Shoop, and William P. Meehan III

Key Points
- Sport-related concussion is associated with psychological symptoms including depression, anxiety, and behavioral problems.
- Activity restrictions, isolation from friends and teammates, academic consequences of cognitive symptoms, sleep-related difficulties, and other sequelae of concussion can contribute to psychological symptoms.
- Keys to promoting emotional well-being after concussion include setting positive expectations, routinely discussing and screening for mental health concerns, and providing resources commensurate to each patient's needs, including appropriate referrals when indicated.

M. M. Daley (✉)
Division of Sports Medicine, Department of Orthopedic Surgery, Children's Hospital of Philadelphia, Philadelphia, PA, USA

Pediatrics, Perelman School of Medicine at the University of Pennsylvania, Philadelphia, PA, USA
e-mail: daleym2@chop.edu

J. Shoop
Minds Matter Concussion Program, Department of Child and Adolescent Psychiatry and Behavioral Sciences, Children's Hospital of Philadelphia, Philadelphia, PA, USA
e-mail: shoopj@chop.edu

W. P. Meehan III
Division of Sports Medicine, Department of Orthopedic Surgery, The Micheli Center for Sports Injury Prevention, Boston Children's Hospital, Boston, MA, USA

Pediatrics and Orthopedics, Harvard Medical School, Boston, MA, USA
e-mail: William.Meehan@childrens.harvard.edu

© The Author(s), under exclusive license to Springer Nature   117
Switzerland AG 2023
M. A. Christino et al. (eds.), *Psychological Considerations in the Young Athlete*,
Contemporary Pediatric and Adolescent Sports Medicine,
https://doi.org/10.1007/978-3-031-25126-9_6

Introduction

Definitions and Pathophysiology

Sport-related concussion (SRC) is a condition in which a physical trauma results in a combination of physical, cognitive, and emotional symptoms. The 2017 Concussion in Sport Group (CISG) consensus statement defines SRC as a traumatic brain injury induced by biomechanical forces caused by a direct or indirect blow with a linear and/or rotational force transmitted to the head, typically resulting in the rapid onset of short-lived impairment of neurological function, which in some cases evolves over a number of minutes to hours. They further define SRC as a largely functional disturbance rather than a gross structural injury, resulting in a range of clinical signs and symptoms that typically follow a sequential course of recovery [1, 2].

This functional disturbance is best understood as a consequence of axonal changes resulting in significant alterations in intracellular and extracellular glutamate, potassium, and calcium concentrations [2]. This triggers a cascade in which a widespread release of neurotransmitters (particularly excitatory amino acids such as glutamate) causes further cellular depolarization and ultimately an influx of calcium ions into the cells [3]. The calcium influx disrupts mitochondrial function, increasing oxidative stress and creating a metabolic imbalance in which energy demand essentially exceeds the neuronal capacities, rendering neurons vulnerable to additional stress or insult, which in turn can result in further damage or possibly cell death [2, 3].

Epidemiology

A large 2016 cross-sectional study of adolescents in the United States found that an estimated 19.5% had sustained at least one concussion in their lifetime, and 5.5% had sustained two or more [4]. A follow-up study by the same group found that by 2020, approximately 24.6% of adolescents had been diagnosed with at least one lifetime concussion, representing an increase in prevalence of more than 1% per year; and 6.8% had sustained two or more [5]. These trends may be due, in part, to efforts to educate the general population about the effects of concussion, resulting in increased reporting and recognition.

Clinical Manifestations

Several systems are affected by concussion, likely with overlapping contributions to the wide array of clinical manifestations. Disturbance of the autonomic nervous system, which is responsible for regulating the internal organs including the cerebrovascular, cardiorespiratory, and gastrointestinal systems, may contribute to nausea, dysautonomia, and lightheadedness. Disruptions of the vestibular and oculomotor systems can result in difficulty with balance, dizziness, eye tracking, and visual function including convergence and accommodation.

The cognitive effects of concussion include impairments in concentration, memory, and attention, with cognitive strain commonly identified as a cause of headaches and other symptoms. The sleep-wake cycle is also affected to varying degrees, often resulting in fatigue and changes in duration and quality of sleep.

Finally, there are substantial psychological and emotional consequences of concussion, including but not limited to depression, anxiety, and irritability. Just as with all clinical manifestations of concussion, there is variation in the extent to which each patient experiences these psychological symptoms.

Depression is characterized by feelings of sadness or hopelessness; decreased interest in activities (anhedonia); fatigue; changes in appetite, weight, or sleep patterns; feelings of worthlessness or guilt; difficulty concentrating; irritability; and in some cases thoughts of self-harm or suicide. According to the *Diagnostic and Statistical Manual of Mental Health Disorders fifth edition (DSM-5)*, a diagnosis of major depressive disorder requires the presence of at least five of these symptoms that persist for at least 2 weeks [6]. Anxiety disorders are characterized by marked fear and/or excessive worry often resulting in significant distress, avoidance, sleep disturbance, difficulty concentrating, irritability, and impairments in social function [6]. While many patients experience depression and anxiety after sustaining a concussion, not all will meet criteria for a clinical diagnosis.

Psychological Sequelae of Concussion

Risk Factors for Post-concussive Psychological Symptoms

The strongest predictor of post-concussive mental health outcomes is a history of mental health problems, which accounts for an estimated 38.4–65% of the variance seen between patients [7, 8]. According to a 2021 meta-analysis, psychological and emotional symptoms were reported after concussion by 19.3–40% of patients with no psychiatric history, compared to 50–60% of patients with preexisting mental health conditions [7]. A study of division I collegiate athletes found that following a concussion, those with preexisting depression symptoms were 4.6 times more likely to experience depression and 3.4 times more likely to experience anxiety after sustaining a concussion when compared with athletes who had no depression symptoms at baseline [9].

Older children and adolescents seem to be at greater risk for internalizing symptoms such as depression, anxiety, and withdrawal, whereas younger children more commonly exhibit externalizing symptoms, including impulsive or disruptive behaviors. Women and girls are more likely to experience depression, anxiety, and other internalizing symptoms following a concussion compared to their male counterparts, but this is true in the general population and unlikely to represent a pattern unique to post-concussive syndrome [7, 10, 11]. Potential protective factors include a positive family environment and psychological resilience, both of which are associated with better quality of life and lower rates of depression, anxiety, and attention deficit/hyperactivity symptoms after a concussion [7, 12].

In addition to increased incidence and severity of psychological and emotional symptoms after concussion, preexisting depression and anxiety are also associated with prolonged recovery [13]. A prospective multicenter cohort study of children and adolescents age 5–18 years found that persistent post-concussion syndrome, defined as symptoms lasting more than 4 weeks after the injury, occurred in 53–57% of patients with pre-injury depression, and in 37–66% with preexisting anxiety, compared to about 29% of patients with no history of depression or anxiety [14]. Still, it is important to recognize that while preexisting mental health problems may contribute to post-concussive symptoms, many children and adolescents who experience depression and anxiety in the aftermath of concussion have no prior history of psychiatric or neurodevelopmental disorders [15]. Additional pre-injury factors associated with prolonged post-concussive syndrome include a history of learning and behavioral problems [16–18] and low psychological resilience, as measured by the degree to which one is able to successfully adapt to adverse life events [12, 16].

Acute Post-concussive Symptoms

Many athletes present with symptoms of depression within the first week of sustaining a concussion. While this may be due in part to the neuronal injury and resultant alterations in neurotransmitter release, some studies have found comparable rates of depression in the aftermath of non-concussion sport-related injuries such as anterior cruciate ligament (ACL) injuries, the latter of which are actually associated with a longer duration of depression symptoms [8, 19]. Others have found that children and adolescents have significantly higher rates of behavioral and emotional problems within the first 2 weeks after concussion compared with patients with other orthopedic injuries [15].

Behavioral and emotional problems occurring in the acute post-injury phase may provide early indicators of those at risk for experiencing prolonged symptoms, but generally these symptoms improve significantly within a few months of the injury [15]. Early recognition, education, and provision of appropriate resources to address psychological symptoms in the aftermath of concussion can be instrumental in supporting patients and families through the recovery process.

Persistent Post-concussive Symptoms

Existing literature suggests an inverse relationship between age and symptom duration. Approximately 85% of professional American football players return to play within 7 days of injury, and the median time to full return to play among collegiate athletes ranges from 1 to 2 weeks [20, 21]. However, symptom duration in children and particularly in adolescents can be substantially longer [22]. On average, symptomatic improvement in younger children (age 5–7 years) occurs within approximately 2 weeks after the injury, whereas the majority of older children (age 8–12 years) and adolescents can be expected to recover within 4 weeks after the injury, with female adolescents being most susceptible to symptom duration exceeding 4 weeks [23].

Persistent post-concussive syndrome in children and adolescents (symptoms persisting beyond 4 weeks after the initial injury) occurs in an estimated 11–31% of this age group [15]. This can include visual, vestibular, cognitive, and/or sleep-related symptoms, but the presence of ongoing psychological and emotional symptoms more than 4 weeks after the injury often requires a nuanced approach to evaluation and management. It is important to remember that the symptoms of concussion are nonspecific and, therefore, the presence of prolonged symptoms does not necessarily mean the presence of persistent concussion pathophysiology. Failure to recognize this might result in the misattribution of symptoms and a missed opportunity to treat contributing etiologies. As such, we recommend consideration of other potential contributing etiologies for patients with prolonged concussion symptoms while simultaneously managing for the possibility of prolonged concussion physiology.

Internalizing Symptoms

The broad classification of internalizing symptoms includes depression, anxiety, withdrawal, and post-traumatic stress. Whether there is a known history of mental health problems, or symptoms are first recognized in the acute post-concussive period, both are associated with prolonged recovery. Though most likely reflective of emergence or uncovering of underlying conditions as opposed to a causal relationship, up to one third of young patients will have a new psychiatric diagnosis after sustaining a concussion [7]. Psychological and emotional symptoms after concussion seem to persist over the course of the recovery, taking longer to resolve than many other post-concussive symptoms in children and adolescents [7].

The reason for this is likely multifactorial. In addition to the pathophysiological impact, concussion is a unique injury in that signs and symptoms are not readily apparent to others in the way that musculoskeletal injuries might require crutches, casting, or the like. This creates an experience for patients in which the degree of the injury is not necessarily evident to family members, teachers, or peers. As such, concussion is sometimes referred to as an "invisible injury," creating feelings of loneliness and frustration, made worse as the athlete is withheld from sports and socially isolated from friends and teammates. Many patients also experience provocation of symptoms with cognitive activity and stimulating environments, resulting in time away from school and often missing out on social events.

Additionally, even absent a concussive injury, depression, and anxiety can result in somatic symptoms such as headaches, stomachaches, and even dizziness. Therefore, the association of psychological symptoms with prolonged recovery is likely a reciprocal relationship, as prolonged headaches and/or other somatic, vestibular, or sleep-related symptoms can certainly contribute to feelings of sadness or depression as well.

Anxiety is often the result of uncertainty or unpredictable circumstances creating a fear response. Although a sequential resolution of symptoms can be expected after concussion, there are no definitive means by which the duration of symptoms and return to sport can be reliably predicted. Prolonged post-concussive symptoms can also result in mounting academic pressures, and absence from school and sports can have implications for college prospects, scholarship opportunities, and the like. In addition to these stressors that occur as a direct result of the injury, many athletes and their families express concern about the potential for them to sustain recurrent injuries going forward, and if so, what the long-term consequences might be. These questions likely further contribute to heightened anxiety in the aftermath of concussion.

Externalizing Symptoms

Externalizing symptoms include aggression, disruptive or impulsive behaviors, hyperactivity, and risk-taking behaviors [7, 15]. These behavioral symptoms are more common in younger children and can be explained by a variety of factors. Symptoms of inattention can be caused by the cognitive impacts of concussion, while aggression and other disruptive behaviors may be reflective of internal distress such as fear or anxiety. Further, just as with depression and anxiety, preexisting attention deficits, hyperactivity, and behavioral problems can all be exacerbated by concussion as well.

While these symptoms are generally temporary, often with substantial improvement if not complete resolution within weeks or months of the injury, they can nonetheless have significant implications [15]. Regardless of whether they occur in the setting of concussion, disruptive behaviors can have tremendous impact not only on the child's ability to function in school and social settings but also on their relationships with parents, siblings, teachers, classmates, and others. This can lead to self-esteem problems, feelings of shame or guilt, and increased anxiety both for the child and their family. Early education for families pertaining to the behavioral components of recovery can help parents and teachers to moderate expectations accordingly and may allow them to better support the child.

Treatment

Psychological interventions can be extremely beneficial in the aftermath of concussion, particularly for those with comorbid mental health needs or with symptoms of concussion that persist beyond expected time frames. However, brief interventions in the acute post-injury period may also promote positive outcomes and prevent the development of persistent symptoms. Researchers and clinicians increasingly call for a biopsychosocial approach to concussion care in which biological (e.g., pathophysiology of injury, genetics), psychological (e.g., emotional and behavioral response to injury or treatment, premorbid mental health needs), and social/contextual factors (e.g., parent support, other life stressors) are understood to impact recovery [24]. Within this framework, providers can practice psychologically informed care to prevent and respond to complications that arise throughout the recovery process. This section describes the emerging evidence base for psychological treatments of persistent post-concussion symptoms and comorbid mental health needs. It also highlights barriers to psychological care and strategies to promote psychological resilience following injury.

Cognitive Behavioral Therapy

Research increasingly suggests that cognitive behavioral therapy (CBT), which targets unhelpful beliefs and behaviors, can support youth following concussion. Table 6.1 describes how CBT can be applied in the setting of concussion. One multisite pilot study demonstrated that a brief, six-session CBT-based intervention significantly reduced concussion symptoms in children and adolescents who were on average 64 days from injury at the time of enrollment [25]. The intervention consisted of common CBT modules including psychoeducation, sleep hygiene, activity scheduling and pacing, relaxation skills, and cognitive coping. In addition to reductions in post-concussion symptoms, they found that symptoms of anxiety and depression decreased with this intervention as well. Overall quality of life and functional outcomes (e.g., sleep quality, exercise frequency) also improved following treatment. Another study demonstrated that a collaborative care intervention

Table 6.1 Potential applications of cognitive behavioral therapy after concussion

Thoughts	Feelings	Behaviors
• Identify negative or unhelpful thoughts	• Understand physiological components of emotions	• Implement specific guidelines for activity pacing
• Identify false beliefs	• Identify and express emotions about injury and post-concussion symptoms	• Use schedules to balance required and preferred activities
• Identify injury-related "thinking traps" (e.g., catastrophizing, overgeneralizing, or dichotomous thinking)	• Improve self-validation around emotional response to injury	• Increase healthy habits (e.g., sleep, exercise, hydration)
		• Practice relaxation strategies (e.g., diaphragmatic breathing, progressive muscle relaxation)

consisting of CBT as well as case management and access to psychiatric consultation was effective in reducing post-concussion symptoms, suicidal ideation, and sleep disturbance, over and above care as usual in a group of youth with symptoms lasting 1 month or longer [26]. Participants in the study group took part in 8.4 sessions of CBT on average, consisting of psychoeducation and skill building in pain management, relaxation, sleep, emotion regulation, problem-solving, family communication, and mindfulness. Despite requiring a greater number of sessions in the collaborative care intervention (i.e., increased treatment burden), treatment satisfaction scores were significantly higher compared to the group who underwent care as usual, suggesting that patients are eager to participate in additional services to support their recoveries. Although both concussion symptoms and suicidal ideation decreased following the collaborative care intervention, symptoms of anxiety and depression did not significantly differ compared to those receiving usual care. Interestingly, over half of patients received all CBT sessions via telehealth, indicating that these types of interventions do not need to be delivered face-to-face to be effective [26].

Other research has examined whether well-established CBT interventions for insomnia and post-traumatic stress disorder (PTSD) are as effective for youth with concussion as they are in those without concussion. In a sample of adolescents with insomnia and persistent post-concussion symptoms, a 6-week course of CBT for insomnia (CBT-I) was associated with clinically significant improvements in insomnia and sleep quality, with benefits comparable to those seen in non-concussed patients [27]. Similarly, in a study comparing the effects of CBT for PTSD in youth with and without concussion, symptoms of PTSD were significantly reduced following the intervention regardless of concussion status [28]. Both of these studies found that improvements in the target symptoms (insomnia and post-traumatic stress symptoms) were also accompanied by reductions in post-concussion symptoms, highlighting the potential role for psychological interventions after concussion regardless of comorbid mental health needs. Although more research is clearly needed, these early findings join a sizeable and well-established body of literature showing the benefits of CBT for pediatric chronic headache, one of the most common symptoms of concussion [29].

Utilizing a biopsychosocial lens, psychological treatments such as CBT also address modifiable factors that impact concussion recovery. For example, although sleep disturbance may be related to biological processes following concussion, particularly in the early post-injury phase, behavioral, emotional, and social factors also impact sleep [30]. Many patients develop poor sleep hygiene behaviors (e.g., using electronics before bed, napping after school) and/or experience unhelpful sleep-related thoughts and emotions (e.g., thinking "I'll never be able to fall asleep" or feeling frustrated or worried about continued tossing and turning). Caregivers may experience uncertainty about appropriate sleep guidelines in the aftermath of concussion, including what limits to set around sleep and how to implement these effectively. Given that even a 1-h sleep restriction for several nights negatively impacts emotion regulation and attention in children, addressing the behavioral, emotional, and social factors that contribute to difficulties in this domain is critical following concussion [31]. CBT can help youth and their caregivers understand the role of sleep following concussion, develop a behavior plan to improve sleep hygiene, learn specific relaxation strategies to support sleep onset, and challenge unhelpful sleep-related thought processes using cognitive coping skills. These strategies can be similarly applied to other relevant behaviors following concussion, including physical activity and compliance with recommended therapies or home exercises.

While there is a growing body of literature highlighting the role of CBT in managing psychological sequelae of concussion, more research is needed to better inform the optimal timing and duration of treatment and how best to identify appropriate candidates for these interventions. For example, an intensive course of CBT with a qualified mental health professional may be indicated for patients with pre-existing mental health diagnoses or symptoms that rise above the diagnostic threshold for a psychiatric disorder. However, patients with subthreshold symptoms of anxiety, depression, or post-traumatic stress may respond to brief, less intensive forms of CBT targeting overall concussion recovery. There is some evidence to suggest that even providing written psychoeducation to children and families on brief CBT-based coping strategies can minimize symptom duration and severity when provided soon after injury [32]. Table 6.2 provides suggestions for appropriate ways to support the mental health needs of all patients.

Table 6.2 Suggested approaches to providing appropriate psychological care

Most patients
• Discuss emotional symptoms and screen for mental health needs
• Set positive expectations for recovery
• Encourage stress reduction and appropriate activity pacing
• Review sleep hygiene
• Provide resources to promote emotional resilience, including handouts, books, and/or web resources on relaxation techniques and stress management
Patients with persistent symptoms
• Provide resources for CBT-based coping strategies that families can implement at home
• Refer for formal CBT to support healthy coping mechanisms and to promote adherence to medical recommendations (e.g., sleep, exercise)
• Identify patients who may require additional mental health referrals beyond concussion-focused CBT
Patients with identified mental health needs
• Continue existing mental health services, if any
• If no services are in place, refer for further mental health evaluation
• Consider "bridging" with interim treatment while waiting to establish long-term care

Other Evidence-Based Psychological Treatments

In addition to CBT, other psychological treatments may be useful in supporting youth following concussion. One such intervention is acceptance and commitment therapy (ACT), which emphasizes the importance of values-driven behavior while accepting the presence of symptoms. Although not yet studied in pediatric concussion, research in youth with chronic pain has demonstrated that ACT can significantly improve functioning and comorbid symptoms of depression [33]. Notably, these effects held regardless of whether the intervention was offered in an individual- or group-based treatment model. Other work has similarly suggested that ACT may be effective at reducing disability and comorbid mental health needs among those with migraine headaches [34]. In light of these findings, clinicians and researchers have highlighted the potential merits of ACT for patients recovering from concussion [35, 36].

Another psychological intervention likely to be helpful for youth recovering from concussion both with and without comorbid mental health needs is motivational interviewing (MI). MI aims to enhance a person's readiness to change and has been shown to effectively support health-related behavior change across a range of pediatric conditions [37]. In adults with concussion, MI has been linked to reduced likelihood of developing persistent post-concussion symptoms and comorbid mental health needs following injury [38]. In pediatric populations with headache or other pain, MI can support patient and parent readiness to engage in non-pharmacological pain management and utilize active coping strategies [39].

Preventative Interventions

Although not a formal psychological intervention, provider language during the acute post-injury phase may have the power to promote positive outcomes. Concussion management guidelines often highlight the importance of setting positive recovery expectations early in care, consistent with findings that the majority of youth who experience concussion will recover quickly and fully without the need for specialized treatments or supports [40]. Setting positive expectations for recovery leverages psychological and cognitive science by minimizing what has been called "the nocebo effect," referring to the power of expectations to negatively impact symptom experience through information processing or attentional biases [41]. Other research has highlighted the potential risks of overloading patients with information early in recovery, particularly if that information could lead to negative recovery expectations, increased attention to symptoms, heightened injury-related stress, or misattribution of normative processes as pathological [42].

Implementation of psychologically informed care can also be achieved with the help of resources available through the CDC HEADS UP educational initiative, which provides several strategies parents can use to support the emotional well-being of their child after injury. This includes identifying opportunities to lessen stress, encouraging ongoing connection with friends, practicing relaxation exercises such as deep breathing, and reminding them that most people feel better soon after a concussion. Discussing emotional symptoms with all patients in the early stages of post-concussion management can normalize conversations about mental health, effectively opening the door for patients and families to share concerns that develop at any point throughout recovery.

Ultimately, all providers working with youth and families in the aftermath of concussion can promote resilience by adopting a psychologically informed approach to care when considering the content and timing of information provided to patients and families.

Promoting Access to Psychological Treatments After Concussion

Access to mental health resources is limited both by provider shortages and an ever-increasing demand for services, particularly in the setting of escalating mental health needs associated with the COVID-19 pandemic [43]. However, insufficient availability of providers is not the only barrier to care.

First and foremost, identifying the psychological needs of youth can be challenging, particularly in the aftermath of concussion. Providers working with youth after concussion are tasked with assessing many different facets of the injury and may lack the time or resources to adequately screen for mental health needs. Moreover, despite increasing attention to the psychological aspects of injury, many providers may not be aware of the emerging evidence highlighting the importance of identifying and treating mental health needs following concussion [44].

Recent studies suggest that even in the absence of anxiety, depression, or other mental health symptoms, psychological interventions such as CBT can help to reduce post-concussion symptoms. Although CBT is a well-established treatment for headache management, one in three primary care physicians is not aware of the benefits of CBT for headaches, and only one in ten has ever referred a headache patient for CBT [45]. As a result of many providers being unfamiliar with the potential role for CBT, together with having limited time and resources, some patients who would benefit from psychological treatment are likely going undetected.

Given the importance of addressing mental health concerns early in recovery, implementation of routine screening measures should be considered.

Validated screening tools such as the Patient Health Questionnaire (PHQ) or Generalized Anxiety Disorder-7 (GAD-7) may be useful in identifying patients with clinically significant symptoms of anxiety, depression, or other emotional symptoms that warrant intervention. In a prospective study of adolescents presenting to an outpatient concussion clinic within 1 month of injury, initial scores on the PHQ and GAD-7 significantly predicted self-perceived recovery at 3-month follow up, above and beyond the predictive value of injury characteristics or time since injury

[46]. Another study of adolescents with SRC presenting within 2 weeks of injury found that for every 1-point increase on the GAD-7, there was a 1.4 times greater chance of protracted recovery, defined as symptoms persisting for 30 days or more [47]. Of note, this study used a receiver operating characteristic (ROC) curve analysis to determine a GAD-7 score of 3 was the optimal cutoff in this context. However, classic interpretation of the GAD-7 classifies a score of 0–4 as indicative of *minimal anxiety*, whereas a score of 10 or greater is considered the cutoff for identifying likely cases of generalized anxiety disorder. These findings suggest that even subtle elevations in anxiety can carry increased risk for prolonged recovery, which may have significant clinical implications. Further study is needed to determine how best to interpret these screening tools in the context of concussion, and how they might inform appropriate mental health referrals or other psychological interventions, particularly for patients with scores that fall below the established diagnostic thresholds.

Mental health stigma is another key barrier to psychological care following concussion. Stigma can impact not only patient willingness to participate in treatment but also whether providers proactively assess psychological needs after injury, and even whether researchers study psychological treatments for patients with concussion [24]. Although a sizeable barrier to acceptance requires solutions at the societal level, individual providers can take steps to reduce stigma around psychological care following concussion. One approach to reducing stigma involves normalizing the emotional impact of concussion and associated stressors, such as missed school or sports, by talking about these factors early and often throughout recovery [24]. Implementing standardized screening processes throughout the recovery process can help to normalize conversations about emotional health as well. Other potential strategies include highlighting the mind-body connection and the potential benefits of practicing relaxation strategies and other coping skills to alleviate the physical, cognitive, and emotional symptoms following injury [48].

Barriers to care are greater among youth and families from diverse or disadvantaged backgrounds, with racial and ethnic disparities in healthcare being described as "extensive, pervasive, and persistent" [49, 50]. Research shows that concussion care for youth and their families is no exception, and most of the interventions described in this chapter have been studied on predominantly white samples [51]. Given these realities, future research is sorely needed to address the unique psychological needs of youth from diverse backgrounds following concussion. This requires the use of more representative study populations and a focus on developing novel approaches to care that promote health equity.

Breaking Down Barriers to Care

One potential avenue for reducing the myriad barriers to psychological treatment is the use of integrated care models. Integrated care models embed psychologists or other licensed mental health providers within multidisciplinary teams where they provide both direct patient care and ongoing consultation with other team members.

This allows mental health providers to be readily accessible to patients in the same facility, and often on the same day or even within the same appointment as other providers on their healthcare team. In addition to decreasing barriers related to time or convenience, integrated care models can also help to reduce stigma [52]. Mental health professionals might also enhance care in this setting by administering and/or responding to mental health screenings and providing immediate, brief interventions when indicated, without requiring patients and families return for a separate appointment. Research suggests that integrated care models are associated with improved overall accessibility and utilization of mental health services and increased patient and provider satisfaction [53]. Further, integrated care models are associated with improved access to care for patients from diverse backgrounds and may be one strategy for reducing healthcare inequities [54].

Self-paced web modules, smartphone applications, and workbooks may also play a role in increasing access to psychological care following concussion. One study found that an interactive, online CBT module helped to reduce postsurgical pain and fear of movement in adults undergoing ACL repair, with effects similar to therapist-guided CBT interventions within this population [55]. Other studies have demonstrated that self-help workbooks and other nontraditional methods can improve mental health in adolescents [56, 57]. Although these interventions are likely not sufficient for youth with clinically significant mental health needs, they represent a viable means by which patients and families can start to learn and develop healthy coping skills while waiting for traditional treatment. These modalities might also offer utility for those with subclinical symptoms, or even potentially serve as preventative interventions.

Summary of Approaches to Treatment

Psychological interventions including cognitive behavioral therapy (CBT), acceptance and commitment therapy (ACT), and motivational interviewing (MI) can reduce post-concussion symptoms as well as clinical or subclinical symptoms of anxiety, depression, and post-traumatic stress. Appropriate psychological treatments implemented in the acute post-injury period may prevent more significant complications later in recovery. These approaches can also be used to inform care throughout concussion recovery, including provider messaging and recommendations to support healthy coping skills. Although promising, these findings need to be replicated in larger and more diverse samples to promote equitable outcomes following concussion. In addition, novel care models need to be developed and examined. Stepped-care models, for example, would provide varying degrees of therapeutic interventions commensurate to the severity of symptoms and/or phase of recovery. Beyond investigating the most efficacious treatment methods and modalities, existing barriers to care should be addressed in a meaningful way in order to ensure that all patients have access to appropriate mental healthcare based on their individual needs.

Addressing Concerns About Long-Term Effects

As concussion awareness has increased in the last several years, questions pertaining to the potential for long-term irreversible consequences have captured the attention of the media and medical community alike [58]. Chronic traumatic encephalopathy (CTE) is defined as a neurodegenerative disease characterized by the "phosphorylated tau aggregates in neurons, astrocytes, and cell processes around small vessels in an irregular pattern at the depths of the cortical sulci." [59] As it is a pathological diagnosis, it can only be made postmortem. Many experts have raised concerns that misrepresentations of the degree of scientific certainty regarding the prevalence, etiology, and progressive nature of the illness may have unintended harmful consequences for athletes of all ages [60]. Furthermore, while signs and symptoms are regularly attributed to the pathological condition by the lay media, the connection between the pathology and symptoms remains uncertain [1, 60–62].

Underscoring the importance of risk perception, existing literature suggests that patients who believe concussion will result in serious negative consequences are at increased risk for worse outcomes, including prolonged recovery [63, 64]. A survey study of collegiate football players found that one in ten believed that they would go on to develop dementia, Alzheimer's disease, or CTE as a result of having sustained sport-related concussions [65]. In light of these findings, it is essential for providers to have informed discussions with patients and their families about what is known on the subject.

Most experts agree that a single sport-related concussion is unlikely to result in long-term consequences [1, 58]. For many patients and families, concern for the potential development of long-term neuropsychological sequelae tends to increase with recurrent concussions [65]. Much of the existing research is indeed based largely on postmortem neuropathological findings in former combat and/or collision sport athletes such as boxers and American football players and others with a history of repetitive head injuries. Neuropathological findings are then correlated with retrospective reports of concussion history and development of mood and behavioral changes, subjecting findings to both sampling and recall bias. Additional limitations include the lack of appropriate control subjects and the potential for selection bias, as families with loved ones who suffered what they believe were the detrimental and sometimes catastrophic effects of multiple head injuries sustained during sports may be more likely to donate their brains to this type of research. While this remains a valid hypothesis worthy of further investigation, misleading coverage by the media on this topic may result in unnecessary and undue anxiety for some patients and, therefore, should be discouraged [58, 60].

Conclusion

Psychological consequences of concussion such as depression and anxiety can have tremendous implications for recovery and are most common in those with preexisting mental health issues and/or prolonged recoveries. Females are also at greater risk, but this is consistent with findings in the general population and might not be unique to concussion. While psychological symptoms may be due to the pathophysiology of the concussion itself, it is perhaps more likely that they arise from a combination of factors, including activity restrictions, changes in exercise patterns, isolation from friends and teammates, sleep disruption, and other sequelae of injury. Regardless of the specific etiology, early recognition and targeted treatment can significantly improve patient outcomes.

References

1. McCrory P, Meeuwisse W, Dvořák J, Aubry M, Bailes J, Broglio S, et al. Consensus statement on concussion in sport—the 5th international conference on concussion in sport held in Berlin, October 2016. Br J Sports Med. 2017;51(11):838–47.
2. Herring S, Ben KW, Putukian M, Solomon GS, Boyajian-O'Neill L, Dec KL, et al. Selected issues in sport-related concussion (SRC|mild traumatic brain injury) for the team physician: a consensus statement. Br J Sports Med. 2021;55(22):1251–61.
3. Signoretti S, Lazzarino G, Tavazzi B, Vagnozzi R. The pathophysiology of concussion. PM R. 2011;3(10 Suppl 2):359–68.
4. Veliz P, McCabe SE, Eckner JT, Schulenberg JE. Prevalence of concussion among US adolescents and correlated factors. J Am Med Assoc. 2017;318(12):1180–2.
5. Veliz P, McCabe SE, Eckner JT, Schulenberg JE. Trends in the Prevalence of Concussion Reported by US Adolescents, 2016-2020. J Am Med Assoc. 2021;325(17):1789–91.
6. American Psychiatric Association. Diagnostic and statistical manual of mental disorders (5th ed.). 2013. https://doi.org/10.1176/appi.books.9780890425596.
7. Gornall A, Takagi M, Morawakage T, Liu X, Anderson V. Mental health after paediatric concussion: a systematic review and meta-analysis. Br J Sports Med. 2021;55(18):1048–58.
8. Solomon GS, Kuhn AW, Zuckerman SL. Depression as a modifying factor in sport-related concussion: a critical review of the literature. Phys Sportsmed. 2016;44(1):14–9.
9. Yang J, Peek-Asa C, Covassin T, Torner JC. Post-concussion symptoms of depression and anxiety in division i collegiate athletes. Dev Neuropsychol. 2015;40(1):18–23.
10. Ghandour RM, Sherman LJ, Vladutiu CJ, Ali MM, Lynch SE, Bitsko RH, et al. Prevalence and treatment of depression, anxiety, and conduct problems in US children. J Pediatr. 2019;206:256–267.e3.
11. Mojtabai R, Olfson M, Han B. National trends in the prevalence and treatment of depression in adolescents and young adults. Pediatrics. 2016;138(6):e20161878.
12. Laliberté C, Durish K, Yeates KO, Brooks BL. Psychological resilience as a predictor of symptom severity in adolescents with poor recovery following concussion. J Int Neuropsychol Soc. 2019;25(4):346–54.
13. Iverson GL, Williams MW, Gardner AJ, Terry DP. Systematic review of preinjury mental health problems as a vulnerability factor for worse outcome after sport-related concussion. Orthop J Sport Med. 2020;8(10):1–12.
14. Zemek R, Barrowman N, Freedman SB, Gravel J, Gagnon I, McGahern C, et al. Clinical risk score for persistent postconcussion symptoms among children with acute concussion in the ED. J Am Med Assoc. 2016;315(10):1014–25.
15. Gornall A, Takagi M, Clarke C, Babl FE, Davis GA, Dunne K, et al. Behavioral and emotional difficulties after pediatric concussion. J Neurotrauma. 2020;37(1):163–9.

16. Cairncross M, Brooks BL, Virani S, Silverberg ND. Fear avoidance behavior in youth with poor recovery from concussion: measurement properties and correlates of a new scale. Child Neuropsychol. 2021;27(7):911–21.
17. Bernard C, Ponsford J, McKinlay A, McKenzie D, Krieser D. Predictors of post-concussive symptoms in young children: injury versus non-injury related factors. J Int Neuropsychol Soc. 2016;22(8):793–803.
18. Zemek R, Farion K, Sampson M, McGahern C. Prognosticators of persistent symptoms following pediatric concussion: a systematic review. JAMA Pediatr. 2013;167(3):259–65.
19. Yrondi A, Brauge D, Lemen J, Arbus C, Pariente J. Depression and sports-related concussion: a systematic review. Presse Med. 2017;46:890. https://doi.org/10.1016/j.lpm.2017.08.013. Accessed 4 Sep 2022.
20. Broglio SP, McAllister T, Katz B, LaPradd M, Zhou W, McCrea M. The natural history of sport-related concussion in collegiate athletes Findings from the NCAA-DoD. CARE Consortium. Sports Med. 2021;52:403.
21. Casson IR, Viano DC, Powell JW, Pellman EJ. Concussions involving 7 or more days out in the National Football League. Sports Health. 2011;3(2):130–44.
22. Meehan WP, Taylor AM, Proctor M. The pediatric athlete: younger athletes with sport-related concussion. Clin Sports Med. 2011;30(1):133–44. https://doi.org/10.1016/j.csm.2010.08.004.
23. Ledoux AA, Tang K, Yeates KO, Pusic MV, Boutis K, Craig WR, et al. Natural progression of symptom change and recovery from concussion in a pediatric population. JAMA Pediatr. 2019;173(1):1–19.
24. Kapadia M, Scheid A, Fine E, Zoffness R. Review of the management of pediatric post-concussion syndrome—a multidisciplinary, individualized approach. Curr Rev Musculoskelet Med. 2019;12:57–66.
25. Simpson T, Peterson R, Patrick K, Forster J, McNally K. Concussion symptom treatment and education program: a feasibility study. J Head Trauma Rehabil. 2020;36(2):E79.
26. McCarty C, Zatzick D, Marcynyszyn L, Wang J, Hilt R, Jinguji T, et al. Effect of collaborative care on persistent postconcussive symptoms in adolescents: a randomized clinical trial. JAMA Netw Open. 2021;4(2):1–14.
27. Tomfohr-Madsen L, Madsen J, Bonneville D, Virani S, Plourde V, Barlow K, et al. A pilot randomized controlled trial of cognitive-behavioral therapy for insomnia in adolescents with persistent postconcussion symptoms. J Head Trauma Rehabil. 2020;35(2):E103.
28. Shorer M, Segev S, Rassovsky Y, Fennig S, Apter A, Peleg T. Efficacy of psychological intervention for children with concurrent posttraumatic stress disorder and mild traumatic brain injury. J Trauma Stress. 2020;33:330–7.
29. Kroon Van Diest A, Powers S. Cognitive behavioral therapy for pediatric headache and migraine: why to prescribe and what new research is critical for advancing biobehavioral care. Headache. 2019;59(2):289–97.
30. McNally K, Bangert B, Dietrich A, Nuss K, Rusin J, Wright M, et al. Injury versus non-injury factors as predictors of post-concussive symptoms following mild traumatic brain injury in children. Neuropsychology. 2013;27(1):1–12.
31. Vriend J, Davidson F, Corkum P, Rusak B, Chambers C, McLaughlin E. Manipulating sleep duration alters emotional functioning and cognitive performance in children. J Pediatr Psychol. 2013;38(10):1058–69.
32. Ponsford J, Willmott C, Rothwell A, Cameron P, Ayton G, Nelms R, et al. Impact of early intervention on outcome after mild traumatic brain injury in children. Pediatrics. 2001;108(6):1297–303.
33. Kanstrup M, Wicksell R, Kemani M, Lipsker C, Lekander M, Holmstrom L. A clinical pilot study of individual and group treatment for adolescents with chronic pain and their parents: effects of acceptance and commitment therapy on functioning. Children. 2016;3(30):1–18.
34. Smitherman T, Wells R, Ford S. Emerging behavioral treatments for migraine. Curr Pain Headache Rep. 2015;19(4):13.
35. Faulkner J, Snell D, Theadom A, Mahon S, Barker-Collo S. The role of psychological flexibility in recovery following mild traumatic brain injury. Rehabil Psychol. 2021;66(4):479–90.

36. King L, Prescott L. Acceptance and commitment therapy for people with mild traumatic brain injury and post-concussion symptoms. In: Curvis W, Methley A, editors. Acceptance and commitment therapy and brain injury: a practical guide for clinicians. London: Routledge; 2022. p. 40–52.

37. Gayes L, Steele R. A meta-analysis of motivational interviewing interventions for pediatric health behavior change. J Consult Clin Psychol. 2014;82(3):521–35.

38. Bell K, Temkin N, Powell J, Fraser R, Esselman P, Barber J, et al. The effect of telephone counseling on reducing post-traumatic symptoms after mild traumatic brain injury: a randomized trial. J Neurol Neurosurg Psychiatry. 2008;79:1275–81.

39. Knestrick K, Gibler R, Reidy B, Powers S. Psychological interventions for pediatric headache disorders: a 2021 update or research progress and needs. Curr Pain Headache Rep. 2022;26(1):85–91.

40. Silverberg N, Iaccarino M, Panenka W, Iverson G, McCulluch K, Dams-O'Connor K, et al. Management of concussion and mild traumatic brain injury: a synthesis of practice guidelines. Arch Phys Med Rehabil. 2020;101(2):382–93.

41. Kirkwood M, Howell D, Brooks B, Wilson J, Meehan W. The nocebo effect and pediatric concussion. J Sport Rehabil. 2021;30(6):837–43.

42. Yang CC, Chiu HC, Xiao SH, Tsai YH, Lee YC, Ku YT, et al. Iatrogenic effect? Cautions when utilizing an early health education for post-concussion symptoms. Arch Clin Neuropsychol. 2018;33(2):131–42.

43. Storch E, Ding E. Addressing the unfolding children's mental health crisis. Child Psychiatry Hum Dev. 2022;53(1):1–2.

44. Bloom G, Trbovich A, Caron J, Kontos A. Psychological aspects of sport-related concussion: an evidence-based position paper. J Appl Sport Psychol. 2020;34:495.

45. Langenbahn D, Matsuzawa Y, Lee Y, Fraser F, Penzien D, Simon N, et al. Underuse of behavioral treatments for headache: a narrative review examining society and cultural factors. J Gen Intern Med. 2021;36(10):3103–12.

46. Wright B, Wilmoth K, Juengst S, Didehbani N, Maize R, Cullum C. Perceived recovery and self-reported functioning in adolescents with mild traumatic brain injury: the role of sleep, mood, and physical symptoms. Dev Neurorehabil. 2021;24(4):237–43.

47. Wilmoth K, Curcio N, Tarkenton T, Meredith-Duliba T, Tan A, Didehbani N, et al. Utility of brief psychological measures for prediction of prolonged symptom clearance in concussed student athletes. Arch Clin Neuropsychol. 2021;36:430–6.

48. Ernst M, O'Brien H, Powers S. Cognitive-behavioral therapy: how medical providers can increase patient and family openness and access to evidence-based multimodal therapy for pediatric migraine. Headache. 2015;55(10):1382–96.

49. Graaf G, Snowden L. Public health coverage and access to mental health care for youth with complex behavioral healthcare needs. Adm Policy Ment Heal Serv Res. 2020;47:395–409.

50. Flores G. Technical report—racial and ethnic disparities in the health and healthcare of children. Pediatrics. 2010;125(4):e979–1020.

51. Copley M, Jimenez N, Kroshus E, Chrisman S. Disparities in use of subspecialty concussion care based on ethnicity. J Racial Ethn Health Disparities. 2020;7(3):571–6.

52. Miller-Matero L, Khan S, Thiem R, DeHondt T, Dubaybo H, Moore D. Integrated primary care: patient perceptions and the role of mental health stigma. Prim Health Care Res Dev. 2018;20:1–4.

53. Ward W, Smith A, Munns C, Bai S. The process of integrating psychology into medical clinics: pediatric psychology as an example. Clin Child Psychol Psychiatry. 2021;26(2):323–41.

54. Bridges A, Villalobos B, Anastasia E, Dueweke A, Gregus S, Cavell T. Need, access, and the reach of integrated care: a typology of patients. Fam Syst Health. 2017;35(2):193–206.

55. Brewer BW, Van Raalte JL, Cornelius AE. An interactive cognitive-behavioural multimedia program favourably affects pain and kinesiophobia during rehabilitation after anterior cruciate ligament surgery: an effectiveness trial. Int. J Sport Exerc Psychol. 2021;20:1133.

56. Muto T, Hayes S, Jeffcoat T. The effectiveness of acceptance and commitment therapy bibliotherapy for enhancing the psychological health of Japanese college students living abroad. Behav Ther. 2011;42(2):323–35.

57. Cohen K, Stiles-Shields C, Winquist N, Lattie E. Traditional and nontraditional mental healthcare services: usage and preferences among adolescents and younger adults. J Behav Health Serv Res. 2021;48:537–53.
58. Mannix R, Meehan WP, Pascual-Leone A. Sports-related concussions-media, science and policy. Nat Rev Neurol. 2016;12(8):486–90. https://doi.org/10.1038/nrneurol.2016.99.
59. Bieniek KF, Cairns NJ, Crary JF, Dickson DW, Folkerth RD, Keene CD, et al. The Second NINDS/NIBIB Consensus Meeting to define neuropathological criteria for the diagnosis of chronic traumatic encephalopathy. J Neuropathol Exp Neurol. 2021;80(3):210–9.
60. Stewart W, Allinson K, Al-Sarraj S, Bachmeier C, Barlow K, Belli A, et al. Primum non nocere : a call for balance when reporting on CTE. Lancet Neurol. 2018;18(3):231–3. https://doi.org/10.1016/S1474-4422(19)30020-1.
61. Lobue C, Schaffert J, Cullum CM. Chronic traumatic encephalopathy: understanding the facts and debate. Curr Opin Psychiatry. 2020;33:130–5.
62. Moon K, Theodore N. Football and chronic traumatic encephalopathy: how much evidence actually exists? World Neurosurg. 2016;89:720–1.
63. Whittaker R, Kemp S, House A. Illness perceptions and outcome in mild head injury: a longitudinal study. J Neurol Neurosurg Psychiatry. 2007;78(6):644–6.
64. Snell DL, Siegert RJ, Hay-Smith EJC, Surgenor LJ. Associations between illness perceptions, coping styles and outcome after mild traumatic brain injury: preliminary results from a cohort study. Brain Inj. 2011;25(11):1126–38.
65. Baugh CM, Kroshus E, Kiernan PT, Mendel D, Meehan WP. Football players' perceptions of future risk of concussion and concussion-related health outcomes. J Neurotrauma. 2017;34(4):790–7.

Chapter 7
Psychological Considerations for Surgical Outcomes in the Pediatric and Adolescent Athlete

Aneesh G. Patankar, Matthew D. Milewski, and Melissa A. Christino

Key Points
- Athletes undergoing surgery can have significant psychological responses to their injury and recovery.
- Understanding how to mitigate negative psychological responses and enhance positive coping strategies can help with postoperative pain response, surgical outcomes, adherence to rehabilitation, and return to sport.
- A multidisciplinary care approach to athletes undergoing surgery can improve outcomes.

Introduction

Orthopedic surgery can be a traumatic experience for a patient, and this may be especially true in the pediatric population [1]. Surgeries in the pediatric population are common, with nearly 500,000 pediatric surgeries being performed annually [2] and close to 5% of all pediatric patients undergoing surgical procedures [3]. The

A. G. Patankar
Rutgers Robert Wood Johnson Medical School, New Brunswick, NJ, USA
e-mail: ap1350@rwjms.rutgers.edu

M. D. Milewski · M. A. Christino (✉)
Division of Sports Medicine, Department of Orthopedic Surgery, Boston Children's Hospital, Boston, MA, USA
e-mail: matthew.milewski@childrens.harvard.edu;
melissa.christino@childrens.harvard.edu

M. A. Christino et al. (eds.), *Psychological Considerations in the Young Athlete*, Contemporary Pediatric and Adolescent Sports Medicine, https://doi.org/10.1007/978-3-031-25126-9_7

pediatric orthopedic literature has reported greater than 30,000 cases in a single year, including surgeries for particular types of trauma and scoliosis [4]. Additionally, in pediatric sports medicine, one study found a surgical rate of 1.45 per 10,000 athlete exposures among high school athletes [5]. The psychological impact of these procedures can be significant, with systematic reviews and large database analyses finding that young patients experienced greater rates of post-traumatic stress disorder (PTSD) and other mental health disorders following surgery [1, 6, 7].

Sports participation in young athletes continues to be on the rise [8]. Sports-related traumatic injuries, such as anterior cruciate ligament (ACL) injuries, and subsequent surgeries have also been increasing over the past 20 years [9]. Because of these increasing rates, understanding factors that affect postoperative outcomes in young patients is particularly important.

While most of the literature focuses on the physical and functional aspects of rehabilitation following sports medicine surgery in the pediatric population, studies on the psychological aspects of postoperative outcomes are more limited but are also extremely important. This chapter aims to describe the current literature regarding how psychological considerations impact postoperative outcomes in pediatric and adolescent athletes. Figure 7.1 summarizes psychological factors that have been associated with postoperative pain experience, surgical outcomes, adherence to rehabilitation, and return to sport.

	Positive Contributing Factors	Negative Contributing Factors
Pain	• Self-confidence • Optimism • Resilience • Self-efficacy • Motivation • Realistic expectations • Decreased anxiety	• Preoperative anxiety (child or parents) • Anticipated pain • Pain catastrophizing • Preoperative mental health disorders (e.g., depression, anxiety) • Kinesiophobia • Low self-efficacy
Surgical Outcomes	• Self-efficacy • Self-esteem • Motivation • Optimistic and realistic expectations • Confidence • Readiness for operation • Transient decrease in athletic identity • Coping skills • Knowledge of injury • Coordination of care between athlete, coaches, and parents • Parental encouragement of supportive environment • Appropriate response to pain	• Preoperative mental health disorders (e.g., depression, anxiety) • Strong athletic identity • Low acceptance of injuries • Pain catastrophizing • Symptoms of post-traumatic stress disorder • Early age of first surgery • Larger number of surgeries • Parental misjudgment of child's psychological status
Adherence to Rehabilitation	• Strong athletic identity (adolescents) • Self-motivation (adult athletes) • Social support (adult athletes)	• Postoperative anxiety • Postoperative pain • Low self-efficacy • Kinesiophobia • Low psychological readiness • Weak athletic identity
Return to Sport	• High psychological readiness • Positive outlook on recovery course • Male sex • Young age • Short interval between injury and surgery • Increased preinjury sports participation • Gender-specific differences in recovery and motivational themes • High coping skills (i.e., "Concentration" and "Peaking Under Pressure" scores) • Positive reframing • Education of injury • Rapport with care team • Individualized therapeutic approach • Self-efficacy	• Fear of reinjury • Kinesiophobia • Less confidence with playing sport with limb • More frustration with injured extremity • Low coping skills • Postoperative pain and anxiety, pain catastrophizing • Decreased self-efficacy • Fear avoidance • Frustration with recovery speed • Uncertainty of recovery • Lack of motivation • Comparison to others • Loss of athletic identity • Preoperative mental health disorders (e.g., depression, anxiety)

Fig. 7.1 Summary of psychological factors that are associated with postoperative experience and recovery

Postoperative Pain and Mental Health

Effects of Postoperative Pain on the Young Athlete

Pain following a procedure is one of the most feared aspects of surgery, regardless of patient age [10]. However, adolescent athletes have been shown to experience higher levels of pain [11], increased rates of chronic postsurgical pain [12, 13], and persistent opioid use [14], compared to their adult counterparts. In addition to the effects that a high level of pain can have on a young athlete's overall quality of life—negatively impacting mood, sleep patterns, appetite, social skills, and performance in both academics and athletics—excessive pain can also affect mental health [15–17]. This can manifest as decreased likelihood of full return-to-sport [18] due to increased levels of fear avoidance (engaging in behaviors to avoid pain- or fear-related emotions) [19] and pain catastrophizing (magnification of thoughts about pain and its associated threat level) [11, 20]. Young athletes that suffer from postoperative pain can also experience persistent symptoms from the initial injury, decreased overall activity levels, and poor rehabilitation compliance [21]. Following orthopedic surgery, postoperative pain can also exacerbate preexisting depression, anxiety, and other psychological disorders from which athletes may already suffer [11, 21].

Factors That Exacerbate Postoperative Pain

While pain following a sports medicine surgery can exacerbate existing psychological disorders, many psychological factors have been shown to affect an adolescent athlete's perception of his/her pain postoperatively.

Numerous studies and systematic reviews have shown that adolescent athletes who have higher levels of preoperative anxiety and who anticipate significant pain actually experience elevated levels of postoperative pain [12, 22–26]. A study by Logan and Rose showed that adolescents' preoperative characteristics, such as anxiety and anticipated pain, increased their perceived pain and predicted their postoperative pain scores, patient-controlled analgesia use, and other quantifiers of pain [22]. A review by William et al. further demonstrated that young athletes who experienced high levels of preoperative anxiety were also more likely to develop chronic postsurgical pain, which was defined as significant, often debilitating postoperative pain not attributable to another cause is experienced at least 3 months following the initial procedure [27–29].

Research has also shown that parental pain catastrophizing regarding the procedure can contribute to the child's anxiety and subsequently the increased postoperative pain that is experienced by the young patient [11, 12, 21, 23, 24, 29]. Tripp et al., in a study of adolescent athletes after ACL reconstruction surgery, suggested that the constant worry about the procedure by the child's parents can cause the young athlete to ruminate and feel helpless, inadvertently worsening the pain that the child experiences [11]. Similar associations of parental pain catastrophizing and postsurgical pain were seen in other adolescent and adult populations [19, 30–33]. Noel et al. found that adolescent patients who experienced higher levels of self-induced and parental pain catastrophizing prior to surgery continued to experience persistent pain memories associated with the procedure many months after surgery [30]. Preoperative pain [12] and sleep patterns [23, 24] have also been associated with the intensity of postoperative pain experienced by nonathlete adolescents.

Similar findings have been seen in adult patients undergoing arthroscopy for femoroacetabular impingement. Studies show that preoperative depression, anxiety, and other mental health disorders are associated with elevated levels of postoperative pain [34–37]. Gillies et al. [38] found that adult femoroacetabular impingement patients that reported high levels of pain also had higher rates of kinesiophobia—the fear of movement and activity due to worry of painful reinjury [39]—and low self-efficacy—the belief in one's own ability to succeed [40]. Similarly, adult orthopedic sports medicine patients and adolescent surgical patients with a history of depression reported higher levels of pain and utilized more opioid medications to control their pain than those without a psychological history [38, 41]. Though these studies are not necessarily specific to young athletes undergoing sports medicine procedures, these findings continue to support a link between psychological distress and pain experience.

Factors That Mitigate Postoperative Pain

While postoperative pain can be challenging for the young athlete, optimizing expectations and the psychological environment can help mitigate the severity of pain experienced. A review by Herring et al. found that adolescent athletes that have higher levels of "self-confidence, optimism, resilience, self-efficacy … and motivation to recover" have been shown to report lower levels of postoperative pain [21]. Expectations are also important. In a study of 58 athletes following ACL reconstruction, the study group was shown modeling videos describing the expected course of recovery and demonstrating functional movements in the setting of rehabilitation before their surgery [42]. Athletes who watched the modeling videos reported significantly lower levels of pain postoperatively among other beneficial functional outcomes compared to those who did not watch the videos.

Many studies recommend a multimodal, multidisciplinary approach to treating postsurgical pain in young athletes [12, 14, 29, 43–47]. In addition to standard pharmacologic and physical therapy techniques, recommendations to mitigate postsurgical levels of pain include decreasing patient anxiety during the perioperative period through the use of child-life specialists [43], guided imagery [44–46], and relaxation techniques [45]. Williams et al. recommended the use of cognitive-behavioral therapy (CBT) augmented by relaxation techniques, biofeedback, sleep management, and pain education for the patient, parent, and coaches to further address the psychological component of pain [29]. Rabbitts and Kain also supported the use of deep breathing, self-regulation techniques, and other cognitive strategies to help reduce anxiety and modify thoughts and beliefs about pain and recovery [14]. Other strategies, such as stress inoculation therapy alongside physical therapy, have been found to improve pain, anxiety, and muscle function in adult patients, but this has been less studied in younger patients [47]. Therapeutic techniques addressing self-efficacy and kinesiophobia in these adolescent athletes should also be explored, as addressing these issues in the perioperative period may help to promote a more favorable recovery.

Mood and Behavioral Factors That Affect Surgical Outcomes

Factors That Negatively Impact Surgical Outcomes

The stress of surgical procedures can not only manifest as increased pain but can also exacerbate existing psychological disorders or cause symptoms that have negative effects on postoperative recovery [40, 48]. Some of these complicating symptoms include depression, mood disturbances, anxiety, and post-traumatic stress disorder (PTSD) and these have all been found to have negative effects on surgical outcomes.

Rates of depression have increased in the pediatric population in general from 2.2% in the early 2000s to rates as high as 13.3% in 2019 [49–54]. Even higher rates (21%) have been observed in adolescents following ACL reconstruction [55] and adult athletes following similar sport surgeries (42%) [56, 57]. Udry et al. found that adolescents reported higher levels of overall mood disturbance than adult athletes with ACL injury, when taking into account negative mood states like "tension" and "anger" from the short-form Profile of Mood States (POMS-SF) [58]. Because mental and emotional health has been shown to correlate with quality-of-life and functional measures of recovery in young athletes, mood disturbance following sports medicine surgery are a prevalent and important issue to consider [59].

Preoperative psychological characteristics of young athletes can influence the mood disturbances they experience postoperatively. Manuel et al. found that adolescent athletes with stronger athletic identity—the extent of self-identity derived from participation and achievement in sports [60]—had higher rates of depression following orthopedic surgery than those with weaker athletic identity [61]. In adults, Baranoff et al. found that patients that had lower acceptance of their injuries also tended to have greater depressive symptoms 6 weeks following their procedure [31]. The authors also found that athletes with higher pain catastrophizing scores continued to report depressive symptoms at 6 months postoperatively, even after controlling for preoperative depression and athletic identity [31]. A history of depression alone has been correlated with more intense levels of postoperative pain, and acute postoperative pain correlated with postoperative depressive episodes in adults who had undergone non-orthopedic procedures [38, 41, 62]. Ghoneim and O'Hara suggest that pain may contribute to depression by damaging regions of the brain and signaling pathways associated with serotonin, offering a potential mechanism behind this observed association [62].

Just as depressive symptoms can be exacerbated in the postoperative period, so too can an athlete's anxiety. A review by LaMontagne et al. of children hospitalized for orthopedic surgeries found that higher preoperative anxiety levels in both the patient and their parents correlated with higher postoperative anxiety levels [63]. The authors suggested that this anxiety stems from separation from the patient's parents, loss of control, and the unknowns associated with the surgery and postoperative recovery course. Similarly, parental pain catastrophizing has also been shown to increase postoperative anxiety in the young athlete [64]. Because anxiety can negatively impact rehabilitation, as anxious children may not tolerate or adhere to the weight-bearing and range-of-motion progressions that are recommended, reducing postoperative anxiety may help with the recovery process following surgery in young athletes.

Symptoms of PTSD have also been shown to influence postoperative outcomes in young patients. Preoperatively, Padaki et al. found that over 75% of adolescent athletes that suffered ACL injuries reported symptoms of posttraumatic stress disorder (PTSD), with symptoms being more severe in athletes 15–21 years old compared to athletes 14 years old or younger [65]. The authors also reported that athletes with higher levels of athletic identity trended toward having more severe symptoms, though this finding was not statistically significant. This suggests that children who more strongly identify themselves as athletes may be more affected by injuries that interfere with their athletic progress.

The traumatic nature of orthopedic surgery and its effect on the psyche and behavior of children is further illustrated in the study by Matsumoto et al. [66] Using the Child Behavior Checklist to evaluate behavioral categories such as Aggression, Rule-breaking, and Conduct, the authors found that in adolescent patients with early-onset scoliosis (a disease often requiring multiple, invasive spinal surgeries), those that underwent more surgeries reported more abnormal behaviors. In addition, the younger a patient was at the time of his/her first scoliosis surgery, the worse the Child Behavior Checklist score [66]. Other studies exploring the emotional and behavioral disturbances in children undergoing numerous surgeries for early-onset scoliosis also found higher rates of behavioral issues and increased risk of psychiatric disorders within 5 years of the child's initial surgery [66–69].

In addition, parents were found to be poor reporters of their child-athlete's psychological status. In high school athletes who underwent ACL reconstruction, Matsumoto et al. found that parents consistently underestimated the young athlete's physical functioning and overestimated their general and mental health compared to self-reports by the athletes [70]. This disconnect in accurately gauging their child's health may prevent parents from addressing their postoperative concerns and can contribute to the psychological effects of sports medicine surgery on the young athlete. These findings suggest that the mood disturbances that can occur after surgery can exacerbate or trigger maladaptive symptoms, which have negative effects on pain response and outcomes.

Factors That Positively Impact Surgical Outcomes

Psychological factors can also have very favorable effects on postoperative outcomes. Higher levels of self-efficacy, self-esteem, and having more realistic expectations have been associated with better outcomes.

Adolescent athletes have been found to have higher rates of self-efficacy than their adult counterparts [71]. Studies by Thomee et al. found that athletes who underwent ACL reconstruction who reported higher levels of self-efficacy—both preoperatively and during the rehabilitation process—had higher rates of return to sport, greater knee-related quality-of-life, and better functional outcomes at 1 year after their surgery [72, 73]. Self-efficacy has also been associated with increased recovery of muscle function and quality of life in adult athletes [71, 74].

A higher level of self-esteem has been shown to positively affect postoperative outcomes. In a study of 27 athletes who had undergone ACL reconstruction, Christino et al. found that the athletes that returned to playing sports at a competitive level reported higher self-esteem than their non-returning counterparts [40]. The authors also found that greater self-esteem was associated with higher knee-related quality of life, subjective knee function, and general health scores.

Being motivated and having a positive outlook during the postoperative recovery course is associated with better outcomes as well. A prospective study by Sonesson et al. of 65 athletes following ACL reconstruction found that higher motivation during rehabilitation was associated with greater rates of return to sport [75]. Similarly, Henn et al. [76] found that adult athletes undergoing rotator cuff repair who had more positive preoperative expectations for their postoperative course experienced greater recovery of function. These findings support the conclusions drawn by Ardern et al. in their systematic review of psychological factors associated with return to sport in athletes following injury [77]. The authors found that athletes with greater levels of motivation, confidence, and optimism of the recovery course were both more likely and more quickly able to return to preinjury levels of sports participation. Just as negative expectations and anxiety of postoperative outcomes can lead to poor recovery, a positive outlook can lead to better postsurgical outcomes.

In order to optimize postoperative recovery, strategies to improve athletes' levels of self-efficacy can be explored. Maddison et al. found that watching modeling videos that demonstrate functional tasks associated with rehabilitation improved athletes' self-efficacy, pain levels, and subjective knee scores [42]. Athletes who endorsed being ready for their operation and focused on the tangible, modifiable aspects of recovery showed better functional and psychological outcomes compared to those who focused on the emotions or had no focus during the postoperative period [70, 78]. These athletes with better outcomes showed increased readiness for their operation and recovery. Other studies suggest strategies such as goal-setting [79], guided imagery/relaxation, and microcounseling [80] can improve various aspects of an athletes' psychological outlook and enhance postoperative outcomes. Additional specific psychological interventions and treatment options to improve outcomes are further discussed in other chapters in this text.

Physicians and the rest of the care team should also look to address the impact of patient and parental preoperative anxiety in order to prevent the negative impact it can have on postoperative anxiety. Physicians can aim to mitigate some of these worries by providing more detailed information to both the patient and the parents, keeping the parents in the room during induction of anesthesia if possible, and having the child participate in preoperative or perioperative therapy [63, 81]. These adaptations can help make pediatric surgery less psychologically harmful for the patient. In addition, Christino et al. suggested that athletes that suffer an injury and undergo orthopedic surgery may naturally deidentify with the role of an athlete in order to protect their ego and self-esteem from the possibility of performing below their previous baseline level of athleticism [40]. If this process is normalized for families, this self-preserving change in athletic identity may be more flexible and less stressful, leading to improved outcomes, but this deserves further study.

A consensus statement described athletes' typical psychological responses to injury and sports medicine surgery (e.g., anger, sadness, fear, feelings of isolation, lack of motivation), and the fact that these responses can be influenced by antecedent psychological factors [21]. Mitigating interventions described by the authors that may yield more favorable outcomes include promoting and monitoring coping skills that temper emotional responses; encouragement to seek mental health care as part of comprehensive plan; educating athletes, coaches, and parents about the injury and the expected recovery course; and promoting the use of social support. In this way, athletes can be more comprehensively cared for, and the care team can help to optimize the effects of psychological factors on the athlete's postoperative recovery (e.g., reducing anxiety in the patient and parents, managing expectations of recovery and the level of athletic identity of the individual, referring the athlete to psychological therapy as needed).

A review by Gornitzky and Diab further suggested ways that parents can facilitate their child's postoperative recovery [82]. The authors advised parents to avoid projecting their feelings of anxiety onto the child, instead encouraging the projection of confidence in the athlete's recovery process. They suggest that parents should optimize the safety, stability, and comfort of the child's environment, including providing a robust social support with family and friends as well as learning about and ideally teaching their child appropriate responses to pain (e.g., minimizing the use of opioids).

Factors That Affect Adherence to Rehabilitation

Adherence to rehabilitation has been extensively associated with more favorable outcomes and return to sport after injury [40, 83, 84]. In addition to sociodemographic variables that have been shown to affect pediatric patient compliance with postoperative rehabilitation, several psychological factors have also been shown to play a role in the athlete's adherence to rehabilitation [85]. Matsuzaki et al. found that adolescent patients that experienced elevated levels of postoperative anxiety and pain had decreased success with rehabilitation, likely due to their inability to tolerate weight-bearing exercises and hesitancy to complete range-of-motion progression [64]. Additionally, young athletes with low self-efficacy have been found to report poor adherence to rehabilitation programs and decreased activity [21].

Conversely, athletes with high levels of motivation were more likely to comply with their rehabilitation program, leading to faster return to sport and functionality at levels prior to the injury [86]. Brewer et al. revealed that athletes with increased self-motivation had increased rates of home-exercise completion [43]. They also found that a gamut of psychological factors (e.g., self-motivation, social support, and athletic identity) were associated with improvements in rehabilitation outcomes (e.g., increased functional ability, decreased subjective symptoms, and decreased knee laxity). However, they found that these psychological factors did not produce these outcomes via increased rehabilitation adherence (e.g., attendance rate, home exercise completion), suggesting that another aspect of rehabilitation is being improved through these positive psychological factors.

In a subsequent study, Brewer et al. again found that increased self-motivation and athletic identity correlated with increased adherence to home exercise and cryotherapy completion during rehabilitation [87]. However, the authors also found that age was a moderator of these interactions, observing different factors that affected adherence to rehabilitation. Adolescent athletes showed an association between athletic identity and home rehabilitation completion whereas older athletes showed an association between self-motivation and social support with home rehabilitation completion. The care team can potentially enhance these psychological factors to impact an adolescent athlete's recovery more favorably.

Return to Sport

Return to sport after injury can be an especially challenging time for young athletes. Concerns about skill proficiency, performance, or reinjury can all affect how an athlete responds to progression back to full activity. This section will discuss some of the key literature associated with return to sport.

Psychological Readiness to Return to Sport

Psychological readiness to return to sport is an important construct that has been shown to predict a young athlete's ability to return to preinjury levels of sports participation following ACL reconstruction [86, 88]. The ACL-Return to Sport after Injury (ACL-RSI) scale has been used to quantify an athlete's psychological readiness to return to sport, with higher scores indicating greater psychological readiness. Kitaguchi et al. found that an ACL-RSI score of greater than 55 at 6 months predicted adolescent athletes' frequency of return to sport at 1 year [88]. Conversely, the authors found that athletes who did not return to sport had significantly lower ACL-RSI scores at the 6-month time point. Another study of psychological readiness by Ardern et al. found that each point increase in the ACL-RSI score was associated with twice the odds of returning to preinjury levels of activity [89].

Not only do 6-month and 1-year ACL-RSI scores correlate with return to sport, but preoperative and early recovery levels of psychological readiness have also been shown to be predictive of ultimate return to sport. A study by Ardern et al. [90] of 187 adolescent athletes following ACL reconstruction found that only 31% of athletes had returned to their original levels of sports participation 12 months postoperatively. Of those that returned, factors including psychological readiness to return to sport, fear of reinjury, and the athlete's outlook on the recovery course contributed to their ability to return to preinjury levels of sports participation. They also found that preoperative and 4-month psychological readiness scores predicted eventual return to sport.

Similarly, in a study by McPherson et al., adolescent athletes who had ACL surgery were assessed with the ACL-RSI scale at an average of 12 months after their surgery and were then followed for 2 years postoperatively [91]. The authors found that athletes who suffered a subsequent ACL injury had significantly lower ACL-RSI scores at the 12-month time point, indicating less psychological readiness than their peers. Further, patients 20 years old or younger who reinjured their ACL graft were found to have less improvement in their ACL-RSI score during the first year of their recovery, compared to those who did not reinjure their graft. The injured group also noted more nervousness, less confidence, and more frustration with their knee compared to those who did not go on to reinjury [92].

Some studies have looked at predictive factors associated with psychological readiness to return to sport. A study by Webster et al. analyzed various factors that contributed to later return to sport in a cohort of 635 athletes who had undergone ACL reconstruction surgery [93]. Male sex, young age, a short interval between injury and surgery, and higher preinjury sports participation were among the factors associated with greater rates of return to baseline sports participation while female sex was the only factor significantly associated with not returning to sport.

Coping Strategies

Coping strategies have been reportedly linked to return to sport as well. Lisee et al. found gender-specific differences in themes endorsed by the young athletes throughout their journey to return to sport after an ACL reconstruction [94]. The authors found that male athletes were motivated by a focus on the physical limitations of their injury, were frustrated by the slow speed and length of recovery, and used positive reinforcement and internal loci of control during their recovery and rehabilitation. Conversely, female athletes were motivated by a focus on staying in shape, were better able to monitor their emotions, and utilized a balance of internal and external loci of control. These gender-specific findings may help explain the differences that are seen in psychological readiness to return to sport between the genders, with males reporting higher ACL-RSI scores and higher rates of return to sport than females [86, 93]; however, these gender differences could also be the result of varied reporting styles among males versus females, and further study is warranted to understand differences between genders.

Preoperative coping scores have also been associated with ultimate return to sport. One study looked at 68 adolescent athletes and assessed psychological metrics longitudinally during recovery from ACL reconstruction [95]. Young athletes' coping skills were evaluated using the Athletic Coping Skills Inventory-28 (ACSI-28) which assesses multiple domains of coping. Those who had low preoperative scores on the ACSI-28, and particularly those who scored lower in the "Coachability" and "Coping with Adversity" subscales, were more likely to have a delayed recovery during postoperative rehabilitation. In fact, participants that scored less than 58 (scale range 0–84) on their preoperative ACSI-28 took 2 months longer to recover than participants that scored higher. Further, young athletes who had higher scores in the "Concentration" and "Peaking Under Pressure" subscales at the 6-month time point were found to have faster rates of recovery. One could surmise that an athlete with the determination that is required to "peak under pressure" in conjunction with high levels of concentration would be an ideal combination that may lead to more consistency and motivation with the rehabilitation process and working hard to return to sport. Higher preoperative coping scores predicting ultimate return to sport in patients after ACL surgery may also be reflective of individual differences that are important to consider for patient-centered care.

Kinesiophobia and Fear of Reinjury

As the young athlete continues to recover from the acute postoperative period, attention is turned to strengthening and regaining functionality to work toward returning to their baseline athletic function. Kinesiophobia, often cited as one of the most common factors preventing an athlete from return to sport, refers to fear of movement, and is commonly linked to fear of reinjury. Increased postoperative pain and anxiety can cause an athlete to hesitate upon performing rehabilitation exercises or limit their exertion and use of the injured extremity. This fear can interfere with an athlete's rate of return to sport by slowing recovery of strength and functional progression [64]. In a study by McCullough et al., half of all high school and collegiate athletes did not return to play their sport following ACL reconstruction due to fear of reinjury [96]. Similarly in a study by Kitaguchi et al., 78% of adolescent athletes who did not return to sport cited the same, with fear as their primary concern about returning to sport [88]. Coronado et al. replicated these findings, observing that adolescent athletes with higher levels of kinesiophobia, elevated pain catastrophizing, and decreased levels of self-efficacy were less likely to return to sport [97]. Similar findings were also seen in adult athletes undergoing hip arthroscopy for femoroacetabular impingement; the athletes who reported higher levels of pain catastrophizing and kinesiophobia also had lower rates of returning to preinjury levels of sports participation [98].

Young athletes that engage in behaviors to avoid pain- or fear-related emotions, called fear avoidance [19], have been found to have lower odds of return to sport, decreased knee function, and lower quality-of-life [97]. A study by Paterno et al. also found that adolescent athletes who suffered a second ACL injury following recovery from their first ACL reconstruction reported higher levels of kinesiophobia and decreased functional capabilities [99]. In addition, those that scored 19 or higher on the Tampa Scale of Kinesiophobia, indicating higher levels of kinesiophobia, were 13 times more likely to suffer a second ACL tear within 2 years of returning to their sport.

Other Psychological Factors Associated with Return to Sport

Other psychological factors (e.g., frustration with recovery speed, uncertainty of recovery, and lack of motivation) and social factors (e.g., direct comparison to others and loss of athletic identity) were identified as barriers to return to sport in adolescent athletes [94]. Mood disturbances, such as depression, have also been associated with decreased rates of returning to baseline levels of athletic activity in adult athletes [100].

A psychological strategy that can potentially be used by adolescent athletes to improve their postoperative recovery and achieve a faster return to sport is the use of positive reframing. Positive reframing, or thinking about a negative situation or outcome with a more optimistic lens, was the only coping strategy in a study by Everhart et al. that increased rates of return to sport while also decreasing kinesiophobia in athletes younger than 20 years old [101]. Athletes can receive postsurgical training in this skill in order to better encourage their rehabilitation progress. Additional applicable mental skills interventions will be discussed in other chapters.

Additionally, DiSanti et al. found that educating the patient with knowledge of the injury, building a trusting relationship between the entire care team and the patient, and developing an individualized therapeutic approach all help to support the young athlete during his/her rehabilitation journey [94]. Many studies have also found an association between increased self-efficacy and faster return to sport [21, 71, 74, 94], and enhancing self-efficacy in postoperative patients may be a helpful augment to the recovery process.

Conclusion

Psychological factors can affect every aspect of a young athlete's postoperative recovery: acute postoperative pain, the rehabilitation process, return to sport, and reinjury. By targeting modifiable aspects preoperatively or early in the postoperative course and educating the patient and parents of behaviors and psychological resources that can improve outcomes for the young athlete, the healthcare team can give the athlete the best chance at a successful postoperative recovery.

References

1. Turgoose DP, Kerr S, De Coppi P, et al. Prevalence of traumatic psychological stress reactions in children and parents following paediatric surgery: a systematic review and meta-analysis. BMJ Paediatr Open. 2021;5:e001147. https://doi.org/10.1136/bmjpo-2021-001147.
2. Tzong KY, Han S, Roh A, et al. Epidemiology of pediatric surgical admissions in US children: data from the HCUP kids inpatient database. J Neurosurg Anesthesiol. 2012;24:391–5. https://doi.org/10.1097/ANA.0b013e31826a0345.
3. Rabbitts JA, Groenewald CB. Epidemiology of pediatric surgery in the United States. Pediatr Anesth. 2020;30:1083–90. https://doi.org/10.1111/pan.13993.
4. Gutman IM, Niemeier TE, Gilbert SR. National databases in pediatric orthopaedic surgery: a comparison of demographics, procedures, and outcomes. J Pediatr Orthop. 2019;39:e636–40. https://doi.org/10.1097/bpo.0000000000001204.
5. Rechel JA, Collins CL, Comstock RD. Epidemiology of injuries requiring surgery among high school athletes in the United States, 2005 to 2010. J Trauma. 2011;71:982–9. https://doi.org/10.1097/TA.0b013e318230e716.
6. Stanzel A, Sierau S. Pediatric Medical Traumatic Stress (PMTS) following surgery in childhood and adolescence: a systematic review. J Child Adolesc Trauma. 2021;15:795. https://doi.org/10.1007/s40653-021-00391-9.
7. Chandler JM, Chan KS, Han R, et al. Mental health outcomes in pediatric trauma patients: a 10 year real world analysis using a large database approach. J Pediatr Surg. 2022;57:291–6. https://doi.org/10.1016/j.jpedsurg.2021.09.049.
8. Eime RM, Harvey JT, Charity MJ, et al. Population levels of sport participation: implications for sport policy. BMC Public Health. 2016;16:752. https://doi.org/10.1186/s12889-016-3463-5.
9. Dodwell ER, Lamont LE, Green DW, et al. 20 years of pediatric anterior cruciate ligament reconstruction in New York State. Am J Sports Med. 2014;42:675–80. https://doi.org/10.1177/0363546513518412. 20140129.

10. Ruhaiyem ME, Alshehri AA, Saade M, et al. Fear of going under general anesthesia: a cross-sectional study. Saudi J Anaesth. 2016;10:317–21. https://doi.org/10.4103/1658-354x.179094.
11. Tripp DA, Stanish WD, Reardon G, et al. Comparing postoperative pain experiences of the adolescent and adult athlete after anterior cruciate ligament surgery. J Athl Train. 2003;38:154–7.
12. Rabbitts JA, Fisher E, Rosenbloom BN, et al. Prevalence and predictors of chronic postsurgical pain in children: a systematic review and meta-analysis. J Pain. 2017;18:605–14. https://doi.org/10.1016/j.jpain.2017.03.007. 20170329.
13. Batoz H, Semjen F, Bordes-Demolis M, et al. Chronic postsurgical pain in children: prevalence and risk factors. A prospective observational study. Br J Anaesth. 2016;117:489–96. https://doi.org/10.1093/bja/aew260.
14. Rabbitts JA, Kain Z. Perioperative care for adolescents undergoing major surgery: a biopsychosocial conceptual framework. Anesth Analg. 2019;129:1181–4. https://doi.org/10.1213/ane.0000000000004048.
15. Rabbitts JA, Palermo TM, Zhou C, et al. Pain and health-related quality of life after pediatric inpatient surgery. J Pain. 2015;16:1334–41. https://doi.org/10.1016/j.jpain.2015.09.005.
16. Mekonnen ZA, Melesse DY, Kassahun HG, et al. Prevalence and contributing factors associated with postoperative pain in pediatric patients: a cross-sectional follow-up study. Perioperat Care Operat Room Manag. 2021;23:100159. https://doi.org/10.1016/j.pcorm.2021.100159.
17. Drendel AL, Kelly BT, Ali S. Pain assessment for children: overcoming challenges and optimizing care. Pediatr Emerg Care. 2011;27:773–81. https://doi.org/10.1097/PEC.0b013e31822877f7.
18. Betsch M, Hoit G, Dwyer T, et al. Postoperative pain is associated with psychological and physical readiness to return to sports one-year after anterior cruciate ligament reconstruction. Arthrosc Sports Med Rehabil. 2021;3:e1737–43. https://doi.org/10.1016/j.asmr.2021.08.001.
19. Fischerauer SF, Talaei-Khoei M, Bexkens R, et al. What is the relationship of fear avoidance to physical function and pain intensity in injured athletes? Clin Orthop Relat Res. 2018;476:754–63. https://doi.org/10.1007/s11999.0000000000000085.
20. Quartana PJ, Campbell CM, Edwards RR. Pain catastrophizing: a critical review. Expert Rev Neurother. 2009;9:745–58. https://doi.org/10.1586/ern.09.34.
21. Herring SA, Kibler WB, Putukian M, et al. Psychological issues related to illness and injury in athletes and the team physician: a consensus statement—2016 update. Curr Sports Med Rep. 2017;16:1043.
22. Logan DE, Rose JB. Is postoperative pain a self-fulfilling prophecy? Expectancy effects on postoperative pain and patient-controlled analgesia use among adolescent surgical patients. J Pediatr Psychol. 2005;30:187–96. https://doi.org/10.1093/jpepsy/jsi006.
23. Rabbitts JA, Groenewald CB, Tai GG, et al. Presurgical psychosocial predictors of acute postsurgical pain and quality of life in children undergoing major surgery. J Pain. 2015;16:226–34. https://doi.org/10.1016/j.jpain.2014.11.015. 20141222.
24. Rabbitts JA, Palermo TM, Zhou C, et al. Psychosocial predictors of acute and chronic pain in adolescents undergoing major musculoskeletal surgery. J Pain. 2020;21:1236–46. https://doi.org/10.1016/j.jpain.2020.02.004. 20200615.
25. Chieng YJ, Chan WC, Klainin-Yobas P, et al. Perioperative anxiety and postoperative pain in children and adolescents undergoing elective surgical procedures: a quantitative systematic review. J Adv Nurs. 2014;70:243–55. https://doi.org/10.1111/jan.12205. 20130719.
26. Lamontagne LL, Hepworth JT, Salisbury MH. Anxiety and postoperative pain in children who undergo major orthopedic surgery. Appl Nurs Res. 2001;14:119–24. https://doi.org/10.1053/apnr.2001.24410.
27. Macrae WA. Chronic post-surgical pain: 10 years on. Br J Anaesth. 2008;101:77–86. https://doi.org/10.1093/bja/aen099. 20080422.
28. Werner MU, Kongsgaard UE. I. Defining persistent post-surgical pain: is an update required? Br J Anaesth. 2014;113:1–4. https://doi.org/10.1093/bja/aeu012. 20140218.

29. Williams G, Howard RF, Liossi C. Persistent postsurgical pain in children and young people: prediction, prevention, and management. Pain Rep. 2017;2:e616. https://doi.org/10.1097/pr9.0000000000000616.
30. Noel M, Rabbitts JA, Tai GG, et al. Remembering pain after surgery: a longitudinal examination of the role of pain catastrophizing in children's and parents' recall. Pain. 2015;156:800–8. https://doi.org/10.1097/j.pain.0000000000000102.
31. Baranoff J, Hanrahan SJ, Connor JP. The roles of acceptance and catastrophizing in rehabilitation following anterior cruciate ligament reconstruction. J Sci Med Sport. 2015;18:250–4. https://doi.org/10.1016/j.jsams.2014.04.002. 20140413.
32. Kain ZN, Mayes LC, Weisman SJ, et al. Social adaptability, cognitive abilities, and other predictors for children's reactions to surgery. J Clin Anesth. 2000;12:549–54. https://doi.org/10.1016/s0952-8180(00)00214-2.
33. Kain ZN, Mayes LC, O'Connor TZ, et al. Preoperative anxiety in children. Predictors and outcomes. Arch Pediatr Adolesc Med. 1996;150:1238–45. https://doi.org/10.1001/archpedi.1996.02170370016002.
34. Dick AG, Smith C, Bankes MJK, et al. The impact of mental health disorders on outcomes following hip arthroscopy for femoroacetabular impingement syndrome: a systematic review. J Hip Preserv Surg. 2020;7:195–204. https://doi.org/10.1093/jhps/hnaa016. 20200402.
35. Cunningham DJ, Lewis BD, Hutyra CA, et al. Early recovery after hip arthroscopy for femoroacetabular impingement syndrome: a prospective, observational study. J Hip Preserv Surg. 2017;4:299–307. https://doi.org/10.1093/jhps/hnx026. 20170724.
36. Stone AV, Malloy P, Beck EC, et al. Predictors of persistent postoperative pain at minimum 2 years after arthroscopic treatment of femoroacetabular impingement. Am J Sports Med. 2019;47:552–9. https://doi.org/10.1177/0363546518817538.
37. Jochimsen KN, Noehren B, Mattacola CG, et al. Preoperative psychosocial factors and short-term pain and functional recovery after hip arthroscopy for femoroacetabular impingement syndrome. J Athl Train. 2021;56:1064–71. https://doi.org/10.4085/1062-6050-139-20.
38. Gillies ML, Smith LN, Parry-Jones WL. Postoperative pain assessment and management in adolescents. Pain. 1999;79:207–15. https://doi.org/10.1016/s0304-3959(98)00178-x.
39. Kori S. Kinisophobia: a new view of chronic pain behavior. Pain Manage. 1990;35–43.
40. Christino MA, Fantry AJ, Vopat BG. Psychological aspects of recovery following anterior cruciate ligament reconstruction. J Am Acad Orthop Surg. 2015;23:501–9. https://doi.org/10.5435/jaaos-d-14-00173.
41. Moutzouros V, Jildeh TR, Khalil LS, et al. A multimodal protocol to diminish pain following common orthopedic sports procedures: can we eliminate postoperative opioids? Arthroscopy. 2020;36:2249–57. https://doi.org/10.1016/j.arthro.2020.04.018. 20200428.
42. Maddison R, Prapavessis H, Clatworthy M. Modeling and rehabilitation following anterior cruciate ligament reconstruction. Ann Behav Med. 2006;31:89–98. https://doi.org/10.1207/s15324796abm3101_13.
43. Brewer BW, Van Raalte JL, Cornelius AE, et al. Psychological factors, rehabilitation adherence, and rehabilitation outcome after anterior cruciate ligament reconstruction. Rehabil Psychol. 2000;45:20–37. https://doi.org/10.1037/0090-5550.45.1.20.
44. Cupal DD, Brewer BW. Effects of relaxation and guided imagery on knee strength, reinjury anxiety, and pain following anterior cruciate ligament reconstruction. Rehabil Psychol. 2001;46:28–43. https://doi.org/10.1037/0090-5550.46.1.28.
45. Maddison R, Prapavessis H, Clatworthy M, et al. Guided imagery to improve functional outcomes post-anterior cruciate ligament repair: randomized-controlled pilot trial. Scand J Med Sci Sports. 2012;22:816–21. https://doi.org/10.1111/j.1600-0838.2011.01325.x. 20110512.
46. Davidson F, Snow S, Hayden JA, et al. Psychological interventions in managing postoperative pain in children: a systematic review. Pain. 2016;157:1872–86. https://doi.org/10.1097/j.pain.0000000000000636.

47. Ross MJ, Berger RS. Effects of stress inoculation training on athletes' postsurgical pain and rehabilitation after orthopedic injury. J Consult Clin Psychol. 1996;64:406–10. https://doi.org/10.1037//0022-006x.64.2.406.

48. Daley MM, Griffith K, Milewski MD, et al. The mental side of the injured athlete. J Am Acad Orthop Surg. 2021;29:499–506. https://doi.org/10.5435/jaaos-d-20-00974.

49. Costello EJ, Mustillo S, Erkanli A, et al. Prevalence and development of psychiatric disorders in childhood and adolescence. Arch Gen Psychiatry. 2003;60:837–44. https://doi.org/10.1001/archpsyc.60.8.837.

50. Merikangas KR, Nakamura EF, Kessler RC. Epidemiology of mental disorders in children and adolescents. Dialogues Clin Neurosci. 2009;11:7–20. https://doi.org/10.31887/DCNS.2009.11.1/krmerikangas.

51. Lewinsohn PM, Rohde P, Seeley JR. Major depressive disorder in older adolescents: prevalence, risk factors, and clinical implications. Clin Psychol Rev. 1998;18:765–94. https://doi.org/10.1016/s0272-7358(98)00010-5.

52. Bitsko RH, Holbrook JR, Ghandour RM, et al. Epidemiology and impact of health care provider-diagnosed anxiety and depression among US children. J Dev Behav Pediatr. 2018;39:395–403. https://doi.org/10.1097/dbp.0000000000000571.

53. Mojtabai R, Olfson M, Han B. National trends in the prevalence and treatment of depression in adolescents and young adults. Pediatrics. 2016;138:20161114. https://doi.org/10.1542/peds.2016-1878.

54. Administration SAaMHS. Key substance use and mental health indicators in the United States: results from the 2019 National Survey on Drug Use and Health. n.d.. https://www.samhsa.gov/data/sites/default/files/reports/rpt29393/2019NSDUHFFRPDFWHTML/2019NSDUHFFR090120.htm (2020, 2022).

55. McArdle S. Psychological rehabilitation from anterior cruciate ligament-medial collateral ligament reconstructive surgery: a case study. Sports Health. 2010;2:73–7. https://doi.org/10.1177/1941738109357173.

56. Wu HH, Liu M, Dines JS, et al. Depression and psychiatric disease associated with outcomes after anterior cruciate ligament reconstruction. World J Orthop. 2016;7:709–17. https://doi.org/10.5312/wjo.v7.i11.709. 20161118.

57. Garcia GH, Wu HH, Park MJ, et al. Depression symptomatology and anterior cruciate ligament injury: incidence and effect on functional outcome--a prospective cohort study. Am J Sports Med. 2016;44:572–9. https://doi.org/10.1177/0363546515612466. 20151201.

58. Udry E, Donald Shelbourne K, Gray T. Psychological readiness for anterior cruciate ligament surgery: describing and comparing the adolescent and adult experiences. J Athl Train. 2003;38:167–71.

59. Boykin RE, McFeely ED, Shearer D, et al. Correlation between the Child Health Questionnaire and the International Knee Documentation Committee score in pediatric and adolescent patients with an anterior cruciate ligament tear. J Pediatr Orthop. 2013;33:216–20. https://doi.org/10.1097/BPO.0b013e3182745439.

60. Houle JLW, Brewer BW, Kluck AS. Developmental trends in athletic identity: a two-part retrospective study. J Sport Behav. 2010;33:146–59.

61. Manuel JC, Shilt JS, Curl WW, et al. Coping with sports injuries: an examination of the adolescent athlete. J Adolesc Health. 2002;31:391–3. https://doi.org/10.1016/s1054-139x(02)00400-7.

62. Ghoneim MM, O'Hara MW. Depression and postoperative complications: an overview. BMC Surg. 2016;16:5. https://doi.org/10.1186/s12893-016-0120-y. 20160202.

63. Lamontagne LL, Hepworth JT, Byington KC, et al. Child and parent emotional responses during hospitalization for orthopaedic surgery. MCN Am J Matern Child Nurs. 1997;22:299–303. https://doi.org/10.1097/00005721-199711000-00004.

64. Matsuzaki Y, Chipman DE, Hidalgo Perea S, et al. Unique considerations for the pediatric athlete during rehabilitation and return to sport after anterior cruciate ligament reconstruction.

Arthrosc Sports Med Rehabil. 2022;4:e221–30. https://doi.org/10.1016/j.asmr.2021.09.037. 20220128.

65. Padaki AS, Noticewala MS, Levine WN, et al. Prevalence of posttraumatic stress disorder symptoms among young athletes after anterior cruciate ligament rupture. Orthop J Sports Med. 2018;6:2325967118787159. https://doi.org/10.1177/2325967118787159. 20180726.

66. Matsumoto H, Williams BA, Corona J, et al. Psychosocial effects of repetitive surgeries in children with early-onset scoliosis: are we putting them at risk? J Pediatr Orthop. 2014;34:172–8. https://doi.org/10.1097/BPO.0b013e3182a11d73.

67. Sanders AE, Andras LM, Iantorno SE, et al. Clinically significant psychological and emotional distress in 32% of adolescent idiopathic scoliosis patients. Spine Deform. 2018;6:435–40. https://doi.org/10.1016/j.jspd.2017.12.014.

68. Flynn JM, Matsumoto H, Torres F, et al. Psychological dysfunction in children who require repetitive surgery for early onset scoliosis. J Pediatr Orthop. 2012;32:594–9. https://doi.org/10.1097/BPO.0b013e31826028ea.

69. Lee SB, Chae HW, Kwon JW, et al. Is there an association between psychiatric disorders and adolescent idiopathic scoliosis? A large-database study. Clin Orthop Relat Res. 2021;479:1805–12. https://doi.org/10.1097/corr.0000000000001716.

70. Matsumoto H, Vitale MG, Hyman JE, et al. Can parents rate their children's quality of life? Perspectives on pediatric orthopedic outcomes. J Pediatr Orthop B. 2011;20:184–90. https://doi.org/10.1097/BPB.0b013e328343184c.

71. Beischer S, Hamrin Senorski E, Thomeé C, et al. How is psychological outcome related to knee function and return to sport among adolescent athletes after anterior cruciate ligament reconstruction? Am J Sports Med. 2019;47:1567–75. https://doi.org/10.1177/0363546519843073.

72. Thomeé P, Währborg P, Börjesson M, et al. Self-efficacy, symptoms and physical activity in patients with an anterior cruciate ligament injury: a prospective study. Scand J Med Sci Sports. 2007;17:238–45. https://doi.org/10.1111/j.1600-0838.2006.00557.x. 20060615.

73. Thomeé P, Währborg P, Börjesson M, et al. Self-efficacy of knee function as a pre-operative predictor of outcome 1 year after anterior cruciate ligament reconstruction. Knee Surg Sports Traumatol Arthrosc. 2008;16:118–27. https://doi.org/10.1007/s00167-007-0433-6. 20071123.

74. Thomeé P, Währborg P, Börjesson M, et al. A randomized, controlled study of a rehabilitation model to improve knee-function self-efficacy with ACL injury. J Sport Rehabil. 2010;19:200–13. https://doi.org/10.1123/jsr.19.2.200.

75. Sonesson S, Kvist J, Ardern C, et al. Psychological factors are important to return to pre-injury sport activity after anterior cruciate ligament reconstruction: expect and motivate to satisfy. Knee Surg Sports Traumatol Arthrosc. 2017;25:1375–84. https://doi.org/10.1007/s00167-016-4294-8. 20160825.

76. Henn RF III, Kang L, Tashjian RZ, et al. Patients' preoperative expectations predict the outcome of rotator cuff repair. J Bone Joint Surg Am. 2007;89:1913–9. https://doi.org/10.2106/jbjs.F.00358.

77. Ardern CL, Taylor NF, Feller JA, et al. A systematic review of the psychological factors associated with returning to sport following injury. Br J Sports Med. 2013;47:1120–6. https://doi.org/10.1136/bjsports-2012-091203.

78. LaMontagne LL, Johnson JE, Hepworth JT, et al. Attention, coping, and activity in children undergoing orthopaedic surgery. Res Nurs Health. 1997;20:487–94. https://doi.org/10.1002/(sici)1098-240x(199712)20:6<487::aid-nur3>3.0.co;2-i.

79. Brinkman C, Baez SE, Genoese F, et al. Use of goal setting to enhance self-efficacy after sports-related injury: a critically appraised topic. J Sport Rehabil. 2020;29:498–502. https://doi.org/10.1123/jsr.2019-0032. 20191002.

80. Schwab Reese LM, Pittsinger R, Yang J. Effectiveness of psychological intervention following sport injury. J Sport Health Sci. 2012;1:71–9. https://doi.org/10.1016/j.jshs.2012.06.003.

81. Kain ZN, Mayes LC, Caramico LA, et al. Parental presence during induction of anesthesia: a randomized controlled trial. Anesthesiology. 1996;84:1060–7. https://doi.org/10.1097/00000542-199605000-00007.
82. Gornitzky A, Diab M. Coping skills in children: an introduction to the biopsychosocial model of pain control as a tool to improve postoperative outcomes. JPOSNA. 2021;3:1.
83. Brewer BW, Cornelius AE, Van Raalte JL, et al. Rehabilitation adherence and anterior cruciate ligament reconstruction outcome. Psychol Health Med. 2004;9:163–75. https://doi.org/10.1080/13548500410001670690.
84. Han F, Banerjee A, Shen L, et al. Increased compliance with supervised rehabilitation improves functional outcome and return to sport after anterior cruciate ligament reconstruction in recreational athletes. Orthop J Sports Med. 2015;3:2325967115620770. https://doi.org/10.1177/2325967115620770. 20151210.
85. Metz AK, Hart-Johnson T, Blackwood RA, et al. Sociodemographic factors associated with decreased compliance to prescribed rehabilitation after surgical treatment of knee injuries in pediatric patients. Orthop J Sports Med. 2021;9:23259671211052021. https://doi.org/10.1177/23259671211052021.
86. Vutescu ES, Orman S, Garcia-Lopez E, et al. Psychological and social components of recovery following anterior cruciate ligament reconstruction in young athletes: a narrative review. Int J Environ Res Public Health. 2021;18:20210902. https://doi.org/10.3390/ijerph18179267.
87. Brewer BW, Cornelius AE, Van Raalte JL, et al. Age-related differences in predictors of adherence to rehabilitation after anterior cruciate ligament reconstruction. J Athl Train. 2003;38:158–62.
88. Kitaguchi T, Tanaka Y, Takeshita S, et al. Importance of functional performance and psychological readiness for return to preinjury level of sports 1 year after ACL reconstruction in competitive athletes. Knee Surg Sports Traumatol Arthrosc. 2020;28:2203–12. https://doi.org/10.1007/s00167-019-05774-y. 20191102.
89. Ardern CL, Österberg A, Tagesson S, et al. The impact of psychological readiness to return to sport and recreational activities after anterior cruciate ligament reconstruction. Br J Sports Med. 2014;48:1613–9. https://doi.org/10.1136/bjsports-2014-093842. 20141007.
90. Ardern CL, Taylor NF, Feller JA, et al. Psychological responses matter in returning to preinjury level of sport after anterior cruciate ligament reconstruction surgery. Am J Sports Med. 2013;41:1549–58. https://doi.org/10.1177/0363546513489284. 20130603.
91. McPherson AL, Feller JA, Hewett TE, et al. Psychological readiness to return to sport is associated with second anterior cruciate ligament injuries. Am J Sports Med. 2019;47:857–62. https://doi.org/10.1177/0363546518825258. 20190212.
92. McPherson AL, Feller JA, Hewett TE, et al. Smaller change in psychological readiness to return to sport is associated with second anterior cruciate ligament injury among younger patients. Am J Sports Med. 2019;47:1209–15. https://doi.org/10.1177/0363546519825499.
93. Webster KE, Nagelli CV, Hewett TE, et al. Factors associated with psychological readiness to return to sport after anterior cruciate ligament reconstruction surgery. Am J Sports Med. 2018;46:1545–50. https://doi.org/10.1177/0363546518773757. 20180502.
94. DiSanti J, Lisee C, Erickson K, et al. Perceptions of rehabilitation and return to sport among high school athletes with anterior cruciate ligament reconstruction: a qualitative research study. J Orthop Sports Phys Ther. 2018;48:951–9. https://doi.org/10.2519/jospt.2018.8277. 20180622.
95. Ellis HB, Sabatino M, Nwelue E, et al. The use of psychological patient reported outcome measures to identify adolescent athletes at risk for prolonged recovery following an ACL reconstruction. J Pediatr Orthop. 2020;40:e844–52. https://doi.org/10.1097/bpo.0000000000001624.
96. McCullough KA, Phelps KD, Spindler KP, et al. Return to high school- and college-level football after anterior cruciate ligament reconstruction: a Multicenter Orthopaedic Outcomes Network (MOON) cohort study. Am J Sports Med. 2012;40:2523–9. https://doi.org/10.1177/0363546512456836.

97. Coronado RA, Bley JA, Huston LJ, et al. Composite psychosocial risk based on the fear avoidance model in patients undergoing anterior cruciate ligament reconstruction: cluster-based analysis. Phys Ther Sport. 2021;50:217–25. https://doi.org/10.1016/j.ptsp.2021.05.012. 20210602.

98. Browning RB, Clapp IM, Alter TD, et al. Pain catastrophizing and kinesiophobia affect return to sport in patients undergoing hip arthroscopy for the treatment of femoroacetabular impingement. Arthrosc Sports Med Rehabil. 2021;3:e1087–95. https://doi.org/10.1016/j.asmr.2021.03.014.

99. Paterno MV, Flynn K, Thomas S, et al. Self-reported fear predicts functional performance and second ACL injury after ACL reconstruction and return to sport: a pilot study. Sports Health. 2018;10:228–33. https://doi.org/10.1177/1941738117745806. 20171222.

100. Parvaresh KC, Wichman D, Rasio J, et al. Return to sport after femoroacetabular impingement surgery and sport-specific considerations: a comprehensive review. Curr Rev Musculoskelet Med. 2020;13:213–9. https://doi.org/10.1007/s12178-020-09617-z.

101. Everhart JS, DiBartola AC, Blough C, et al. Positive reframing: an important but underutilized coping strategy in youth athletes undergoing sports-related knee surgery. J Athl Train. 2021;56:1334–9. https://doi.org/10.4085/1062-6050-0618.20. 20210526.

Chapter 8
Pain and Mind-Body Interactions

Samantha P. Bento, Michael B. Millis, and Christine B. Sieberg

Key Points
- All young athletes will experience pain and regardless of injury or extent of tissue damage, a significant subset of youth will experience chronic pain or persistent postsurgical pain.
- Pain should always be considered within its biopsychosocial context. Every physical injury has psychosocial sequelae.
- Multidisciplinary interventions that address psychosocial elements of pain are more effective than purely mechanistic therapy.

S. P. Bento (✉)
Department of Psychosocial Oncology & Palliative Care, Dana-Farber Cancer Institute, Boston, MA, USA

Cancer and Blood Disorders Center, Boston Children's Hospital, Boston, MA, USA

Harvard Medical School, Boston, MA, USA
e-mail: Samantha.bento@childrens.harvard.edu

M. B. Millis
Orthopaedic Surgery, Harvard Medical School, Boston, MA, USA

Child and Adult Hip Program, Boston Children's Hospital, Boston, MA, USA
e-mail: Michael.millis@childrens.harvard.edu

C. B. Sieberg
Biobehavioral Pain Innovations Lab, Department of Psychiatry & Behavioral Sciences, Boston Children's Hospital, Boston, MA, USA

Department of Anesthesiology, Critical Care, & Pain Medicine, Pain & Affective Neuroscience Center, Boston Children's Hospital, Boston, MA, USA

Department of Psychiatry, Harvard Medical School, Boston, MA, USA
e-mail: Christine.sieberg@childrens.harvard.edu

© The Author(s), under exclusive license to Springer Nature
Switzerland AG 2023
M. A. Christino et al. (eds.), *Psychological Considerations in the Young Athlete*,
Contemporary Pediatric and Adolescent Sports Medicine,
https://doi.org/10.1007/978-3-031-25126-9_8

> *Taylor was a high achieving high school athlete on her elite soccer team. She was at the top of her class and in the process of being recruited by the best college teams when during a pre-season practice, she suffered a severe inversion injury of her right ankle that required surgical intervention and caused her to miss the first several weeks of the season. While she seemingly had recovered well objectively from her acute lateral ankle ligament repair and engaged in consistent physical therapy as recommended, she continued to experience impairing pain.*
>
> *Taylor returned to her surgeon and PT multiple times for follow-up, but objective evaluations revealed no structural causes that would explain her ongoing pain. Taylor's inability to return to soccer at the intended and expected pace only grew her frustrations and anxiety. Her orthopedic team had exhausted all typical pain treatment options, yet all of their attempts seemed to have little to no impact on her overall pain and functioning.*
>
> *Several months following her surgery, Taylor continued to struggle. She ended up missing her entire soccer season due to pain flares that were only increasing in intensity and frequency over time. She also began to experience more frequent headaches accompanied by photophobia and dizziness. She missed a significant amount of school and as a result, her grades suffered.*
>
> *The combination of missing her season and poor grades placed her potential college soccer scholarship in jeopardy, which only increased her overall level of distress. Further, she experienced increased social isolation, guilt surrounding not being able to be present and support her team, anxiety about her future, and low mood. Stress at home only exacerbated her frustrations and overall pain. Taylor and her family were at a loss with how to proceed with treatment.*

While the majority of injured athletes will go on to recover as expected and return to their chosen sport, Taylor's story is not an unfamiliar one to many sports medicine and orthopedic providers. Many young athletes encounter difficult courses of recovery following injury and subsequent surgery, complicated by pain, significant functional impairment, and increased risk of developing other conditions such as osteoarthritis and sports-related stress injuries [1]. With an estimated 69–75% of youth in the United States participating in athletics [2], the experience of injury and acute injury-related pain is an all-too-common occurrence. Given the high risk of injury and the fact that injury is one of the most common precipitating factors for the development of chronic pain [3], it is not surprising that many athletes go on to experience persistent, or chronic pain. In fact, the rates of chronic pain among youth in general are surprisingly high, with an estimated 1 in 4 youth experiencing pain that lasts at least 3 months or longer [4, 5].

Persistent pain after orthopedic surgery is also not an uncommon problem among young athletes. In long-term follow-up studies of young athletes who underwent meniscus surgery, over 50% of patients reported the development of knee osteoarthritis, along with associated pain and functional impairment [6–8]. In general, chronic postsurgical pain (CPSP) is a significant and highly prevalent (impacting approximately 20–55% of youth) postsurgical complication [9]. CPSP is defined as pain that [10]:

1. Develops after a surgical procedure.
2. Is persistent (i.e., lasts for at least 3–6 months after surgery).
3. Is a continuation of acute postsurgical pain or develops after an asymptomatic period
4. Is localized to the surgical site and/or projected to a referred area.
5. Is not caused by other factors.
6. Significantly impacts quality of life.

Chronic pain can occur without injury; however, in the case of injury, pain persists once an injury has seemingly fully healed, hence why chronic pain is frequently referred to as a "false alarm." The brain cannot differentiate this false alarm from an actual alarm (i.e., tissue damage from an acute injury) and therefore, will respond to this alarm as though there is an injury or tissue damage.

Ultimately, this is a protective response when it comes to acute pain or injuries, but when pain becomes chronic, this response is no longer protective. This is demonstrated in the case with Taylor. While she initially sustained an injury during soccer that required surgical intervention, her long-term pain lasting well beyond the expected healing time from injury and surgery is indicative of an overactive, or hypersensitive, nervous system response.

It is important to discuss chronic pain as primarily a disorder of the central nervous system. Central sensitization is a phenomenon that helps explain how the "false alarm"-associated central nervous system hypersensitivity develops (for a more detailed review, please see a review by Woolf [11]). As outlined in Fig. 8.1, pain can be triggered by innocuous stimuli (otherwise known as allodynia) or worsened in response to noxious stimuli (otherwise known as hyperalgesia). This also explains why many youth with chronic pain experience pain not just at the site of the injury, but in other areas of their bodies as well (otherwise known as secondary hyperalgesia). In fact, muscle hyperalgesia, referred pain, referred hyperalgesia, and widespread hyperalgesia all play a significant role in chronic musculoskeletal pain [12]. Since chronic pain is reflective of a hypersensitive nervous system, pain or other symptoms (i.e., nausea, dizziness, photophobia, phonophobia) can be more frequently experienced.

Chronic pain, like acute pain, is **always** real. The pain signals sent to the brain by the body are interpreted as threatening or dangerous, even though no physical harm or damage is present in the body. However, using strategies that are traditionally applied to acute pain in the context of chronic pain typically worsens and maintains chronic pain, further contributing to disability and functional impairment. Pain has more than just physical (or biological) components and as such, to treat chronic

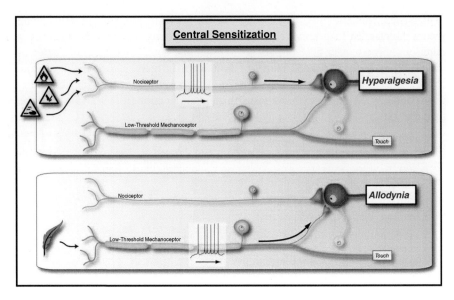

Fig. 8.1 Central sensitization. (Reprinted from Woolf CJ. Central sensitization: implications for the diagnosis and treatment of pain. *Pain*. 2011;152(3 Suppl):S2–S15. https://doi.org/10.1016/j.pain.2010.09.030)

pain, one must take a biopsychosocial approach. Given the multitude of complex biopsychosocial factors contributing to the maintenance and exacerbation of chronic pain, an interdisciplinary treatment approach is considered the gold standard of care.

This chapter will focus on outlining these biopsychosocial factors as well as treatment considerations, with a focus on the mind-body connection, for the athlete living with chronic pain. Specifically, we will review models of pain, outline biopsychosocial factors known to influence the development and maintenance of chronic pain, delve into psychological factors impacting the pain experience, and discuss assessment and treatment of chronic pain. To further illustrate key concepts, Taylor's case study will be referenced throughout.

Models of Pain

Pain is often described as a complex and multidimensional phenomenon that has neural, sensory-discriminative, affective, and motivational components. In their most recently updated definition, the *International Association for the Study of Pain* (IASP) describes pain as "an unpleasant sensory and emotional experience associated with, or resembling that associated with, actual or potential tissue damage" [13]. However, pain used to be traditionally understood through the biomedical model, which viewed pain as a sensation meant to warn the individual of physical harm or a more serious underlying problem [14, 15]. Notably, the biomedical model neglected the influence of psychosocial factors on the pain experience itself. More recent holistic theories consider the influence of cognitive and emotional factors in addition to pain sensation and intensity. Melzack and Wall's Gate Control Theory of Pain [16] posits that pain signals must pass through a neurological gate in order to influence pain perception. In addition to positive and negative feedback mechanisms that inhibit or facilitate transmission (i.e., "open" or "close" the gate), the gate control system is influenced by the "central control trigger," or a mechanism in the central nervous system that activates specific cognitive properties in the brain that modulate sensory input [17, 18]. This top-down process recognizes the influence of emotions, attention, and even past experiences with pain on the transmission of pain signals, and consequently, pain perception.

The biopsychosocial model of pain is the most comprehensive model that thoroughly integrates the biological, psychological, social, cultural, and behavioral aspects that contribute to the experience and maintenance of chronic pain [19]. Essentially, the biopsychosocial model outlines the direct interaction between the mind, body, and one's environment. It considers how pain-related cognitions (thoughts) influence the pain experience, often assessed by intensity and unpleasantness. Below is an outline of common topics reviewed in the biopsychosocial conceptualization of pain. For a more thorough explanation of these topics, please refer to the recent Lancet Child & Adolescent Health Commission on Pediatric Pain [20].

Biological

- Sex and age
- Disease-specific and any additional somatic and physical symptoms (includes details related to onset, frequency of symptoms, duration, symptom triggers and exacerbating factors, and related functional impairment)
- Lifestyle factors (i.e., sleep, nutrition, engagement in exercise, general level of physical activity)
- History of previous injuries, surgeries, and other medical interventions
- Genetic predisposition (i.e., family history of chronic pain)

Psychological

- Changes in mood related to pain
  - Either precipitating pain or as a result of experiencing pain
- Cognitive factors
  - Pain-specific beliefs, fear of pain, pain catastrophizing

- Developmental considerations (e.g., autism spectrum disorder)
- Emotional factors

  – E.g., depression, anxiety, anger, history of trauma, psychosis

- Presence of executive functioning difficulties (e.g., ADHD) or learning disabilities
- Recent stressful events

  – Disruptions to family systems, world events, and peer, family, or school-related stress

- Coping style

  – Approach vs. avoidant, active vs. passive

- Personality characteristics (e.g., perfectionism)

Social (sociocultural)

- Socioeconomic status
- Race and ethnicity
- Cultural and community interactions

  – Including religious and/or spiritual beliefs and cultural understanding or interpretation of pain

- Peer relationships and responses to pain

  – Bullying or acceptance by peers and friends, level of support provided by peers, any changes in the amount of time spent with friends due to pain, etc.

- Family relationships and responses to pain

  – Parenting styles, level of support, and role of siblings and extended family members

- School functioning

  – Changes in attendance, grades, and amount of support—or lack thereof—that school provides with pain management

- Recreational, sport, and leisure activities

  – Engagement in extracurricular activities, hobbies, and any athletic endeavors

By identifying biopsychosocial factors that influence pain, providers are also able to identify important treatment targets that ultimately will aid with pain management and a return to functioning. We began this chapter by presenting the case of Taylor, an adolescent female who sustained a serious ankle injury during her soccer practice. Below, we outline a biopsychosocial conceptualization using the above framework.

Taylor completed a comprehensive evaluation by the Pain Service that revealed several biopsychosocial factors that likely influenced the development and maintenance of her pain:

Biological: *Taylor described her ankle pain as "sharp" and "aching." Her pain was constant, but fluctuated in intensity throughout the day. Identified pain triggers included prolonged walking, standing, any intense physical activity, changes in weather and/or temperature, and school- and family-related stress. Taylor reported a high level of functional impairment, as she could not participate in soccer or any other sport, and struggled to participate in school-related (i.e., extracurricular), social, and recreational/leisure activities. Sleep became significantly disrupted due to ongoing pain, as she noted that pain interfered with both sleep onset and sleep maintenance. As a result, she was reporting less than 6 h of sleep per night and noted taking at least one 2 h nap per day.*

She reported a history of frequent headaches, which began prior to her injury but worsened after her surgery, and a history of several prior sports-related injuries, including multiple concussions and sprains. Prior treatment interventions included over-the-counter medications, physical therapy, and massage. Taylor's family medical history was significant for arthritis, back pain, and migraines.

Psychological: *Taylor endorsed significant changes in her mood related to her pain. Following her injury and subsequent surgery, she reported overall low mood and significant anxious (i.e., excessive worry surrounding return to sport and school-related activities) and depressive (i.e., feelings of sadness, hopelessness, passive suicidal ideation without plan or intent) symptomatology. She noted a significant history of longstanding Generalized Anxiety Disorder, diagnosed in middle school. Taylor also reported that she believed pain was indicative of a more serious injury that her team was misdiagnosing. She described catastrophic thinking related to pain, as indicated by thoughts related to pain magnification, feeling helpless in her ability to manage her pain, and rumination over her pain symptoms. Taylor also described difficulties with sustaining attention and processing speed, which reportedly worsened after sustaining several concussions. She endorsed increased frustration stemming from feeling a lack of motivation to engage in social activities, increased school- and sport-related anxiety, and not meeting her own expectations (of note, she described herself as being "very perfectionistic").*

In terms of coping with pain, Taylor shared that she felt she had limited strategies and described taking a more passive (i.e., resting, avoiding activity) approach to pain management. In addition to her injury and ongoing struggles with pain, recent stressors included thinking about college and maintaining her ability to be competitive for a soccer scholarship, changes in her family system (parents recently separated), and school-related stress (due to declining grades and an increasingly unmanageable workload).

Social: Taylor is a White cisgender adolescent female from a middle-class family living in an affluent county. She attended a competitive high school, where she described significant pressure to "be the best in everything." Taylor's social life changed dramatically after her injury, as her primary social contact and source of social support came through participation in soccer. At school, she stated that her friends and teachers were generally supportive, but often would not know how to respond during pain flares. She experienced some bullying from other student athletes, who reportedly made comments about her "making it up" or "not being able to handle a small injury." She felt invalidated when they told her to "get over it" and to "stop making it a big deal." Some relationships with her teammates became strained, as they reportedly expected her to be able to return and support the team's progress toward championships. Her coach was initially supportive, but over time, became frustrated with her lack of progress and inability to return to play.

Taylor detailed significant conflict and stress in her home, which she attributed to the recent separation of her parents. Further, her parents responded quite differently to her pain. Her father would become seemingly irritated when she reported pain, telling her to "push through and stop complaining" while her mother frequently attended to her (i.e., by frequently asking her about pain and accommodating reports of pain by allowing Taylor to stay home, avoid activity, and engage in passive pain management strategies). She described sadness related to her father's perceived lack of support and interest in her recovery and frustration related to her mother's overprotective nature. On the days that Taylor's mother allowed Taylor to stay home instead of going to school, she would watch movies on the couch, spend time on social media, and relax. She had one younger brother who was generally supportive at home; however, she described feeling guilty for not being able to spend as much time supporting him in his various sports-related activities as she used to.

In terms of school, Taylor stated that she missed at least one full day of school per week, in addition to being frequently late or leaving early. She found it difficult to ambulate around school, given how large it was, and would commonly spend part of her school day with the school nurse. Due to her absences, her work began to pile up. In class, she found it difficult to concentrate and her grades fell, as she was formerly earning straight As and now having difficulty maintaining a C average across her courses. Her school was initially supportive immediately after her ankle injury and surgery; however, as her pain has progressed and she has continued to struggle, supports at school waned. She did not have a formalized school plan in place (e.g., 504 plan or IEP) to provide her with accommodations.

The above information was obtained during a comprehensive, multidisciplinary pain treatment evaluation by a pain physician, physical therapist, and clinical psychologist. When the pain is as complex as Taylor's, it is best for the orthopedist or surgeon to refer to a pediatric pain service for a comprehensive evaluation. There is significant evidence to suggest that interdisciplinary pain treatment programs for patients suffering from chronic pain provide the best clinical treatment for pain and associated disability and in the long run are the most cost-effective option [21–23]. Below, we further highlight these biopsychosocial risk factors and treatment options.

Psychological Factors Impacting Pain

While internalizing mental health concerns, such as anxiety, depression, and post-traumatic stress symptomatology are highly co-morbid in youth with chronic pain [24–26], pain-specific constructs such as pain catastrophizing [27], fear of pain [28], and avoidance of activities [29] are also known to significantly contribute to pediatric pain and pain-related disability. The Fear Avoidance Model (FAM) of Chronic Pain, which describes how pain-specific psychological constructs predict avoidant behaviors and result in impaired functioning (as outlined in Fig. 8.2), originally stemmed from the adult pain literature [30]. However, evidence from the pediatric literature supports the applicability of this model to the pediatric pain population [31]. Pain catastrophizing, or a negative cognitive attributional style marked by the tendency to ruminate over and magnify the experience of pain, is a powerful predictor of poor pain-related outcomes in children, as it has been consistently linked with higher pain intensity ratings [32, 33] and poor functioning [27, 33]. Likewise, fear of pain has also been associated with significant functional impairment in both pediatric chronic pain patients and youth experiencing acute postsurgical pain [34–36].

Central to the FAM [30] are several key psychological factors, including negative affectivity, pain catastrophizing, fear of pain, and avoidance of behaviors and associated functional impairment. At the time of the injury, a child will experience acute

Fig. 8.2 The fear avoidance model of chronic pain. (Reprinted from Vlaeyen JWS, Linton SJ. Fear-avoidance model of chronic musculoskeletal pain: 12 years on. *Pain.* 2012;153(6):1144–1147. https://doi.org/10.1016/j.pain.2011.12.009)

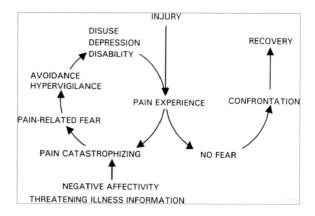

pain. Those youth who catastrophize (i.e., magnify, ruminate, or feel helpless in managing their pain [27]) typically report more fear of re-injury, movement, or of pain itself. These fears lead to avoidance of activity and instead, youth utilize more passive behaviors that guard or protect their body, such as not participating in usual activity and engaging in more sedentary behaviors. Ultimately, decreases in activity lead to physical deconditioning, greater functional impairment, and declines in mood. When applying the FAM to a pediatric pain population, it has been demonstrated that *direct* pathways also exist between depressive symptoms and pain catastrophizing and fear of pain, suggesting that psychological treatments focused on learning skills to modify catastrophic thought patterns and address fear of pain or movement may also improve depressive symptomatology [31].

Conversely, the right side of Fig. 8.2 outlines the pathway by which pain does not lead to high levels of disability or functional impairment and as such, serves as a potential treatment plan for chronic pain. In those with less fear of pain and/or movement, patients can more easily build confidence to gradually participate in activities that may cause or exacerbate pain. In the absence of avoidance, patients are able to gain mastery of pain management strategies, which puts them on the road to recovery. **Of note, it is important to recognize that recovery in the context of chronic pain does not mean complete remission of pain; rather, recovery is the ability to participate in everyday, normal activities while effectively managing their pain**. For patients who experience high fear of pain, behavioral treatment approaches will focus on graded exposures (i.e., gradually facing the feared activity) while engaging in active coping strategies (e.g., deep breathing; cognitive re-framing) with a focus on activity pacing and a return to the activity [37].

Taylor experienced an acutely painful ankle injury which ultimately led to surgical intervention. She continues to experience postsurgical pain beyond what she had been told to expect. She found it hard not to think about if something was really wrong. Thoughts such as "is this ever going to get better?," "did something go wrong with the surgery?," and "it's only getting worse ... there's nothing that makes it better" were an all-too-frequent occurrence. As a result, she became worried about re-injuring her ankle. She avoided situations and activities that she feared would stress or might reinjure her ankle, such as returning to soccer. Even navigating her large school was concerning to her, as she felt she had to walk too far and use too many stairs to get to each of her classes. Instead, she opted to minimize physical activity and movement and would frequently be found resting in bed, isolated from her family and peers.

Taylor's parents were becoming increasingly frustrated and distressed due to her lack of progress and continued decline in functioning, further contributing to Taylor's overall level of stress, low mood, and poor functioning.

Parent and caregiver factors, such as their emotional and behavioral responses to their child's pain as well as their own physical health, are well-known predictors of pediatric pain outcomes [38]. Emotional distress and catastrophic thinking about their child's pain have been associated with parental protective behaviors (i.e., activity restriction) and as a result, greater child functional impairment [39–41].

The Interpersonal Fear Avoidance Model of Pain (IFAM; Fig. 8.3 [42]) expands upon the Fear Avoidance Model of Chronic Pain (Fig. 8.2; outlined above) to include parent cognitive-affective and behavioral factors known to influence child pain outcomes. Essentially, parent interpretation of their child's pain is influenced by their own tendency to engage in catastrophic thinking or their own pain-related fears. Parent pain catastrophizing and fear of pain often lead to hypervigilance and maladaptive parenting behaviors such as overprotecting or minimizing their child's pain, which can reinforce their child engaging in avoidant behaviors and thus contribute to greater declines in functioning.

Ultimately, assessing and addressing caregiver factors is a key component of successful treatment for the child with chronic pain. Just as youth learn the skills they need to effectively manage pain during treatment, their caregivers must also develop skills to not only support their children's management of pain, but also address any of their own behaviors that could be helping to maintain their child's pain or poor functioning. Comprehensive, multi- and interdisciplinary pain treatment approaches are discussed in the next section.

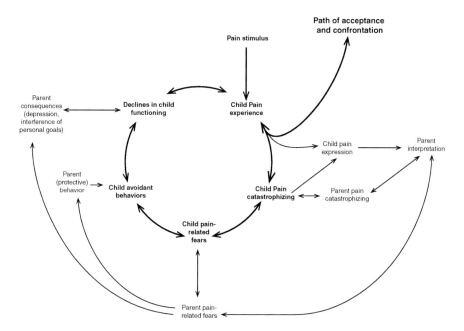

Fig. 8.3 The interpersonal fear-avoidance model of chronic pain. (Reprinted from Simons LE, Smith A, Kaczynski K, Basch M. Living in fear of your child's pain: the Parent Fear of Pain Questionnaire. *Pain*. 2015;156(4):694–702. https://doi.org/10.1097/j.pain.0000000000000100)

While there is a plethora of risk factors that contribute to the development and maintenance of chronic pain, it must be highlighted that there are many child and caregiver factors that confer resilience in the context of pediatric chronic pain. Individual, family, and social-environmental resilience resources (e.g., optimism, mindfulness, adaptive family functioning, social support) and resilience mechanisms (e.g., child and parent pain acceptance, pain-related self-efficacy, psychological flexibility, parent active coping) have all been identified as having protective effects, as outlined by the Ecological Resilience-Risk Model in Pediatric Chronic Pain [43].

Pain is threatening to anyone and particularly to young athletes for whom an injury usually is the trigger. It is quite stressful to endure limited functioning, be uncertain about length of recovery, and worry about whether recovery will ever be complete. While acute injury-related pain usually responds to a prescribed treatment program for the injury that triggered it, all pain is influenced by factors beyond the mechanical. Rather than simply focusing on the injury, it is helpful to use the biopsychosocial approach as a guiding therapeutic principle and as a way to understand the complex interactions between the mind and body.

Psychoneuroimmunology: Examining Mind-Body Interactions in the Context of Pain

Mind-body interactions are best encapsulated by the field of psychoneuroimmunology, which is the study of the complex relationships between psychological factors (e.g., behavior, depression, anxiety, coping, stress, and optimism, among others), the brain, and the immune and endocrine systems [44]. From acute conditions to chronic diseases, a vast literature has demonstrated that the relation between psychological and biological factors is bi-directional, as illness onset and progression, pain, and healing are all known to influence (and be influenced by) psychological processes [45–50]. Awareness of mind-body relationships in the context of pain is key. Numerous studies demonstrate the adverse impact of stress and challenging emotions on the immune, endocrine, and nervous systems (i.e., poor cytokine production, increased cortisol, chronic activation of the "fight-or-flight" response), which have been subsequently linked to poor wound healing [51, 52].

A considerable amount of research in the field of psychoneuroimmunology has been conducted with adult populations. Studies examining these relationships in youth—and young athletes in particular—are extremely limited. In the most recent reviews examining psychoneuroimmunology in pediatric populations [53, 54], only a handful of studies were identified. These studies examined the influence of psychological intervention (e.g., relaxation strategies, hypnosis, conditioning) on immune function in pediatric populations [55–59]. Of note, none of these studies examined the relation between psychological and biological factors relating to the experience or effects of acute or chronic pain.

Recently, some research examining the neuroendocrine mechanisms related to the development and maintenance of pediatric chronic pain has emerged. In a study examining the biomarkers of allostatic load (i.e., "wear and tear" on the nervous system due to significant, repeated, or prolonged exposure to stress) and functional disability in youth with various chronic pain conditions, results demonstrated significant associations between glucocorticoids (cortisol, dehydroepiandrosterone [DHEA]) and measures of pain and pain-related functional disability [60]. Youth with chronic pain evidenced a flattened morning cortisol response that was associated with higher functional disability, suggesting HPA axis dysregulation. Further, youth with higher DHEA levels reported better "best pain" scores (i.e., the lowest level of pain experienced over the last 2 weeks), which is consistent with research demonstrating the "neuroprotective" effects of DHEA [61]. How these results translate in the athlete population is currently unknown; however, these initial neuroprotective findings are promising.

Integrating Mind-Body Approaches into Clinical Practice

Pain Assessment

A comprehensive pain assessment in children typically involves several developmentally appropriate and well-established measures, including self-report (via a numerical pain rating scale, visual analog scale, or faces scales), parent report of their own observations of their child's pain behaviors, and clinician observations of patient pain behaviors (e.g., grimacing, guarding behaviors). For a full evidence-based summary of pediatric pain measures, please see the comprehensive review by Cohen et al. [62]. As outlined by the biopsychosocial model, obtaining relevant information about cognitive, social, emotional, cultural, and additional biological factors provides the most holistic and dynamic understanding of a child's pain experience [63].

Pain Neuroscience Education

The multi- or interdisciplinary pain evaluation can become an intervention in and of itself via psychoeducation about pain and the brain, a model that can also be incorporated into orthopedic clinics. Providing basic pain neuroscience education [64] (also frequently referred to as "pain education" or "psychoeducation") to patients and their families is the first—and perhaps most simple intervention—for clinicians, especially as it can be used as a stand-alone intervention [65].

The primary goal of pain neuroscience education is to explain the biopsychosocial processes involved in the pain experience and address misconceptions associated with pain. While pain neuroscience education can be delivered as its own intervention, it is also frequently combined with other therapeutic approaches such as pain-focused cognitive-behavioral therapy (CBT) or as part of physical therapy [66].

Pain can be easily explained through the use of analogies, many of which have been published and are available to providers through resources such as *Explain Pain* (a well-known book explaining pain biology to patients and providers alike [67]) and a comprehensive list of pain analogies by Coakley and Schechter [68]. For example, one such analogy that describes the phenomenon of chronic pain is as follows:

Technology glitch

Everyone has had the experience of technology that has not worked as planned. This analogy works well when discussing that persistent pain itself can be like a technology failure or glitch.

- Persistent pain is like a software failure. When your computer freezes or crashes, it's almost always a software error. If you looked inside the computer you wouldn't find anything wrong with the hardware. You don't run out to a computer store and replace the hard drive or internal modem, because the problem is the software, not the hardware. Chronic pain is a problem with the software. There is nothing wrong with the hardware in the body (e.g. bones, muscles, organs), but the software that sends messages throughout your system has a glitch (N. Schechter).

Reprinted with permission from the Pediatric Pain Letter Source: Coakley, R, Schechter, N, 2013. Chronic pain is like … The clinical use of analogy and metaphor in the treatment of chronic pain in children. *Pediatric Pain Letter*. 2013;*15*(1): 1–8

Loeser's onion model (Fig. 8.4) offers a clear visual of the components of the pain experience, including nociception, pain, suffering, and pain behavior [69]. When it comes to pain, what is observed by those on the outside are the pain behaviors (e.g., verbalizations of pain, body language, facial expression, avoidance of activity) while the remaining layers of suffering, pain, and nociception are experienced internally by the child with chronic pain. By describing each layer of the onion, a clinician provides both pain psychoeducation and validation by acknowledging and validating the suffering and loss endured by youth who experience chronic pain.

Beyond explaining chronic pain with the use of analogies or models, it is often useful to describe the approach to treatment in a similar fashion given that treatment has multiple components which—under ideal circumstances—should be engaged in concurrently by the patient. The following example outlines two variations of an analogy that provides the rationale for the recommended treatment approach:

Fig. 8.4 Loeser's onion model visually representing the four components of pain phenomena. (Reprinted from Loeser, J.D., 2006. Pain as a disease. *Handbook of clinical neurology*, *81*, pp. 11–20)

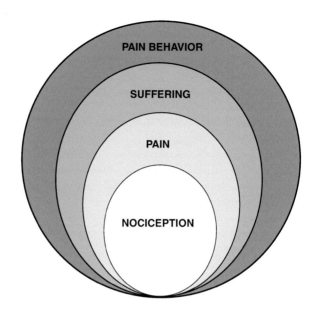

Car with flat tires / Legs on a stool

• The recovery from chronic pain is like trying to get a car with four flat tires moving again. You can fill one tire with medication, but you still won't go anywhere unless you fill the other three tires. You might fill one tire with cognitive behavioral skills, one with physical therapy, and one with acupuncture (The American Chronic Pain Association, 2013). A similar analogy is that a stool requires all four legs to stand. Each treatment modality can be conceptualized as a leg on the stool and without all four legs; the stool won't stand (B. Dick, personal communication, 2013).

Reprinted with permission from the Pediatric Pain Letter Source: Coakley, R, Schechter, N, 2013. Chronic pain is like … The clinical use of analogy and metaphor in the treatment of chronic pain in children. *Pediatric Pain Letter*. 2013;*15*(1): 1–8

Pain Treatment

Chronic pain is a complex phenomenon which naturally requires a comprehensive treatment approach that addresses the intricate interactions between identified biological, sociocultural, and psychological factors influencing the pain experience. As such, pediatric pain treatment typically takes a highly collaborative team- and family-based approach.

Multidisciplinary Clinics Grounded in the biopsychosocial approach, multidisciplinary pediatric pain clinics have gained increasing support in offering effective, comprehensive treatment for chronic pain. Teams often include providers from various disciplines including medicine (most commonly anesthesiologists), nursing, clinical psychology, physical and occupational therapy, and psychiatry [70], among others. Some clinics also offer services such as acupuncture or massage therapy. Treatment guidelines available from the International Association for the Study of Pain (IASP) recommend a multidisciplinary approach in order to thoroughly assess the biological, psychological, sociocultural, and environmental contributors to pain [71]. Further, treatment calls for providers to work in close collaboration to not only improve pain, but also improve overall physical and psychosocial functioning.

Intensive Interdisciplinary Pain Treatment (IIPT) Programs When it comes to pain treatment interventions, the IIPT programs are the highest level of care available—and gold standard of treatment—when a patient is significantly functionally impaired by chronic pain [72]. The central goal of intensive, interdisciplinary pediatric pain rehabilitation programs is not pain reduction nor elimination, but rather, learning and practicing pain management skills to support a return to functioning and valued activities. In an IIPT, teams are typically comprised of several members, including physicians and nurse practitioners, physical therapists, occupational therapists, psychologists, recreational therapists, music therapists, and social workers. Team members take a coordinated treatment approach and work with their patients to develop shared treatment goals and engage in an intensive (i.e., full days on weekdays for several weeks), family-based approach to treatment. Treatment also typically includes meetings with the patient's school and athletics team (e.g., coaches, athletic trainers, etc.) to help with school integration, return to sports, and to provide ongoing recommendations to maximize support for the patient following discharge.

We must highlight the key role that mental health providers play in the treatment of pediatric chronic pain. In addition to collecting data from standardized measures of anxiety and depression (among other factors that influence pain, such as pain catastrophizing), a pediatric pain psychologist conducts a thorough clinical interview to develop the biopsychosocial case conceptualization and help guide treatment goals.

Through individual and family-based treatment, psychologists collaboratively work with youth and their caregivers to teach a broad array of evidence-based pain treatment strategies, typically taking a cognitive-behavioral, biobehavioral, or acceptance and commitment therapeutic (ACT)-based approach. In addition to learning pain neuroscience education, as previously described earlier in this chapter, those who work with a clinical psychologist will receive emotional support and validation while also learning and practicing a host of pain management skills, including [73]:

- **Cognitive skills**, such as cognitive reframing (the process of learning how to modify and challenge maladaptive or unhelpful thoughts in order to reduce associated difficult emotional responses to such thoughts) or positive self-statements (generating helpful coping statements in an effort to increase one's pain-related self-efficacy)
- **Systematic desensitization**, a process by which a patient gradually increases their exposure to a feared situation or stimulus (i.e., movement of an affected limb) over time while learning how to manage associated fear and anxiety
- **Activity pacing**, or implementing breaks at timed intervals during activity, with the goal of increasing their level of activity gradually over time with fewer and shorter breaks required
- **Relaxation techniques**, such as diaphragmatic breathing, progressive muscle relaxation, guided imageries or meditations (note: *biofeedback* is often used when practicing relaxation strategies, as it provides children with a visual representation of physiological changes related to the relaxation response)
- **ACT-based strategies** [74], such as acceptance (acknowledging pain and suffering without attempting to control it), cognitive defusion (noticing thoughts or "watching your thinking"), increasing psychological flexibility, practicing mindfulness (taking a nonjudgmental stance while being in the present moment), and taking committed action towards values-based goals
- **Sleep hygiene strategies**, which may include cognitive skills in addition to practicing good sleep hygiene (i.e., eliminating screen time 1 hr before bed, eliminating naps, developing a consistent bedtime routine, gradually moving bedtime to an appropriate hour)
- **Parent training and support**, including helping parents and caregivers scaffold behaviors, respond to pain appropriately, support their child's return to activity, and manage their own distress surrounding their child's pain

Whether through individual treatment or group-based programs, such as The Comfort Ability pain management workshop (a manualized intervention designed to provide brief, cognitive-behavioral intervention to youth with chronic pain in addition to working with parents to provide parent training [75]), psychological intervention is an essential component of treatment.

Taylor was evaluated by a multidisciplinary team of providers (e.g., anesthesiologist, pain psychologist, and physical therapist) through a pediatric pain clinic.
Treatment recommendations:

1. Acknowledgment and validation of her experience with pain. *Pain is* ***always*** *real.*
2. Provide basic pain neuroscience education. Providers described the biopsychosocial factors that influence and maintain pain to Taylor and her family using clear, concise language and a pain analogy. Further, providers similarly explained the gold standard treatment approach to chronic pain, which includes a multidisciplinary team of providers (e.g., physicians, psychologists, OTs, and PTs) and various supports (e.g., massage, acupuncture, engagement in brief, group-based pain-focused interventions such as The Comfort Ability or other pain management support groups led by mental health professionals).
3. Collaboratively develop a treatment plan with Taylor and her family that includes the multidisciplinary supports outlined above. Other, more intensive, treatment options (such as engaging in an intensive interdisciplinary pain treatment rehabilitation program) were outlined as next steps should Taylor continue to struggle with pain and functioning over time.
4. The team also provided several resources and made school-based recommendations to Taylor and her family. Taylor was given a list of phone applications that help support adaptive pain coping. Further, she and her family were provided with handouts that outlined additional resources (e.g., books, websites, and online videos) the family could reference to learn more about the neuroscience behind pain. The team also prepared a letter to give to Taylor's school that advocated for additional accommodations and supports to help her manage pain in the school setting.
5. The team helped Taylor and her family establish a plan for follow-up. This included scheduling sessions with a pain psychologist, physical therapist, and follow-ups with her medical providers.

Ultimately, Taylor and her family worked closely with her medical team to follow all of the recommendations. She began a prescription medication, engaged in consistent physical therapy with a provider who specialized in pediatric chronic pain, started working with a pediatric pain psychologist on a weekly basis, and began acupuncture. Within weeks, Taylor started to experience significant improvements in her mood and functioning. She and her family learned new skills in physical therapy and in pain-focused psychotherapy that allowed her to gradually participate in more activities over time. She felt more supported by her family and school, more hopeful about her future, and more confident in her ability to independently manage her pain.

Summary

While all athletes will experience acute pain, a significant subset of youth develop chronic pain or chronic postsurgical pain. As a complex phenomenon, pain is best understood through the lens of the biopsychosocial model, an approach that examines the physical, emotional, cognitive, behavioral, and sociocultural factors influencing the experience, development, and maintenance of pain. Mind-body interactions examine the intricate relationships between psychological factors (e.g., behavior, mood, coping strategies, and risk and resilience factors), the brain, and the immune and endocrine systems. The relation between mind and body is bidirectional and given that chronic pain is a disorder of the nervous system, effective treatment approaches target relevant biopsychosocial factors.

In terms of treatment, providers can begin by providing basic pain neuroscience education to patients and families. If possible, integrating providers from other specialties such as psychology and physical therapy into orthopedic clinics will allow teams to take a multidisciplinary approach to pain management. Utilizing established multidisciplinary pain clinics and intensive interdisciplinary pain treatment programs ultimately allows for patients to engage in *actively* managing their pain, with the support of their caregivers and care team.

The world of pediatric pain research is rapidly growing, with the identification of novel pain mechanisms and the examination of treatment approaches and targets that continue to be developed, studied, and refined. However, there remains ample opportunity to examine pain more thoroughly within the pediatric athlete population. Despite this gap in the literature, several key points will always remain true to any patient experiencing pain: pain is *always* real, pain is most comprehensively understood and approached using the biopsychosocial model, and the most effective interventions are multi- or interdisciplinary in nature.

References

1. Maffulli N, Longo UG, Gougoulias N, Loppini M, Denaro V. Long-term health outcomes of youth sports injuries. Br J Sports Med. 2010;44(1):21–5. https://doi.org/10.1136/bjsm.2009.069526.
2. Hsu C, Loecher N, Park AL, Simons LE. Chronic pain in young athletes: the impact of athletic identity on pain-related distress and functioning. Clin J Pain. 2021;37(3):219–25. https://doi.org/10.1097/AJP.0000000000000917.
3. Becker AJ, Heathcote LC, Timmers I, Simons LE. Precipitating events in child and adolescent chronic musculoskeletal pain. Pain Rep. 2018;3(Suppl 1):e665. https://doi.org/10.1097/PR9.0000000000000665.
4. King S, Chambers CT, Huguet A, et al. The epidemiology of chronic pain in children and adolescents revisited: a systematic review. Pain. 2011;152(12):2729–38. https://doi.org/10.1016/j.pain.2011.07.016.
5. Perquin CW, Hazebroek-Kampschreur AAJM, Hunfeld JAM, et al. Pain in children and adolescents: a common experience. Pain. 2000;87(1):51–8. https://doi.org/10.1016/S0304-3959(00)00269-4.

6. Manzione M, Pizzutillo PD, Peoples AB, Schweizer PA. Meniscectomy in children: a long-term follow-up study. Am J Sports Med. 1983;11(3):111–5. https://doi.org/10.1177/036354658301100301.
7. Medlar RC, Mandiberg JJ, Lyne ED. Meniscectomies in children. Report of long-term results (mean, 8.3 years) of 26 children. Am J Sports Med. 1980;8(2):87–92. https://doi.org/10.1177/036354658000800205.
8. Wroble RR, Henderson RC, Campion ER, el-Khoury GY, Albright JP. Meniscectomy in children and adolescents. A long-term follow-up study. Clin Orthop Relat Res. 1992;(279):180–9.
9. Rabbitts JA, Fisher E, Rosenbloom BN, Palermo TM. Prevalence and predictors of chronic postsurgical pain in children: a systematic review and meta-analysis. J Pain. 2017;18(6):605–14. https://doi.org/10.1016/j.jpain.2017.03.007.
10. Werner MU, Kongsgaard UE. I. Defining persistent post-surgical pain: is an update required? Br J Anaesth. 2014;113(1):1–4. https://doi.org/10.1093/bja/aeu012.
11. Woolf CJ. Central sensitization: implications for the diagnosis and treatment of pain. Pain. 2011;152(3 Suppl):S2–S15. https://doi.org/10.1016/j.pain.2010.09.030.
12. Graven-Nielsen T, Arendt-Nielsen L. Peripheral and central sensitization in musculoskeletal pain disorders: an experimental approach. Curr Rheumatol Rep. 2002;4(4):313–21. https://doi.org/10.1007/s11926-002-0040-y.
13. Raja SN, Carr DB, Cohen M, et al. The revised International Association for the Study of Pain definition of pain: concepts, challenges, and compromises. Pain. 2020;161(9):1976–82. https://doi.org/10.1097/j.pain.0000000000001939.
14. Duncan G. Mind-body dualism and the biopsychosocial model of pain: what did Descartes really say? J Med Philos. 2000;25(4):485–513. https://doi.org/10.1076/0360-5310(200008)25:4;1-A;FT485.
15. Chorney JM, Crofton K, McClain BC. Theories on common adolescent pain syndromes. In: McClain BC, Suresh S, editors. Handbook of pediatric chronic pain. New York, NY: Springer; 2011. p. 27–44.
16. Melzack R, Wall PD. Pain mechanisms: a new theory. Science. 1965;150(3699):971–9. https://doi.org/10.1126/science.150.3699.971.
17. Melzack R. Pain: past, present and future. Can J Exp Psychol. 1993;47(4):615–29. https://doi.org/10.1037/h0078871.
18. Moayedi M, Davis KD. Theories of pain: from specificity to gate control. J Neurophysiol. 2013;109(1):5–12. https://doi.org/10.1152/jn.00457.2012.
19. Basch MC, Chow ET, Logan DE, Schechter NL, Simons LE. Perspectives on the clinical significance of functional pain syndromes in children. J Pain Res. 2015;8:675–86. https://doi.org/10.2147/JPR.S55586.
20. Eccleston C, Fisher E, Howard RF, et al. Delivering transformative action in paediatric pain: a Lancet Child & Adolescent Health Commission. Lancet Child Adolesc Health. 2021;5(1):47–87. https://doi.org/10.1016/S2352-4642(20)30277-7.
21. Danilov A, Danilov A, Barulin A, Kurushina O, Latysheva N. Interdisciplinary approach to chronic pain management. Postgrad Med. 2020;132(Suppl 3):5–9. https://doi.org/10.1080/00325481.2020.1757305.
22. Simons LE, Sieberg CB, Pielech M, Conroy C, Logan DE. What does it take? Comparing intensive rehabilitation to outpatient treatment for children with significant pain-related disability. J Pediatr Psychol. 2013;38(2):213–23. https://doi.org/10.1093/jpepsy/jss109.
23. Simons LE, Logan DE, Chastain L, Cerullo M. Engagement in multidisciplinary interventions for pediatric chronic pain: parental expectations, barriers, and child outcomes. Clin J Pain. 2010;26(4):291–9. https://doi.org/10.1097/AJP.0b013e3181cf59fb.
24. Soltani S, Kopala-Sibley DC, Noel M. The co-occurrence of pediatric chronic pain and depression: a narrative review and conceptualization of mutual maintenance. Clin J Pain. 2019;35(7):633–43. https://doi.org/10.1097/AJP.0000000000000723.
25. Asmundson GJ, Katz J. Understanding the co-occurrence of anxiety disorders and chronic pain: state-of-the-art. Depress Anxiety. 2009;26(10):888–901. https://doi.org/10.1002/da.20600.

26. Asmundson GJ, Coons MJ, Taylor S, Katz J. PTSD and the experience of pain: research and clinical implications of shared vulnerability and mutual maintenance models. Can J Psychiatr. 2002;47(10):930–7. https://doi.org/10.1177/070674370204701004.
27. Vervoort T, Goubert L, Eccleston C, Bijttebier P, Crombez G. Catastrophic thinking about pain is independently associated with pain severity, disability, and somatic complaints in school children and children with chronic pain. J Pediatr Psychol. 2006;31(7):674–83. https://doi.org/10.1093/jpepsy/jsj059.
28. Fisher E, Heathcote LC, Eccleston C, Simons LE, Palermo TM. Assessment of pain anxiety, pain catastrophizing, and fear of pain in children and adolescents with chronic pain: a systematic review and meta-analysis. J Pediatr Psychol. 2018;43(3):314–25. https://doi.org/10.1093/jpepsy/jsx103.
29. Beeckman M, Simons LE, Hughes S, Loeys T, Goubert L. A network analysis of potential antecedents and consequences of pain-related activity avoidance and activity engagement in adolescents. Pain Med. 2020;21(2):e89–e101. https://doi.org/10.1093/pm/pnz211.
30. Vlaeyen JWS, Linton SJ. Fear-avoidance model of chronic musculoskeletal pain: 12 years on. Pain. 2012;153(6):1144–7. https://doi.org/10.1016/j.pain.2011.12.009.
31. Simons LE, Kaczynski KJ. The Fear Avoidance model of chronic pain: examination for pediatric application. J Pain. 2012;13(9):827–35. https://doi.org/10.1016/j.jpain.2012.05.002.
32. Hermann C, Hohmeister J, Zohsel K, Ebinger F, Flor H. The assessment of pain coping and pain-related cognitions in children and adolescents: current methods and further development. J Pain. 2007;8(10):802–13. https://doi.org/10.1016/j.jpain.2007.05.010.
33. Vervoort T, Eccleston C, Goubert L, Buysse A, Crombez G. Children's catastrophic thinking about their pain predicts pain and disability 6 months later. Eur J Pain. 2010;14(1):90–6. https://doi.org/10.1016/j.ejpain.2009.03.001.
34. Simons LE, Sieberg CB, Carpino E, Logan D, Berde C. The Fear of Pain Questionnaire (FOPQ): assessment of pain-related fear among children and adolescents with chronic pain. J Pain. 2011;12(6):677–86. https://doi.org/10.1016/j.jpain.2010.12.008.
35. Wilson AC, Lewandowski AS, Palermo TM. Fear-avoidance beliefs and parental responses to pain in adolescents with chronic pain. Pain Res Manag. 2011;16(3):178–82. https://doi.org/10.1155/2011/296298.
36. Pagé GM, Campbell F, Isaac L, Stinson J, Martin-Pichora AL, Katz J. Reliability and validity of the Child Pain Anxiety Symptoms Scale (CPASS) in a clinical sample of children and adolescents with acute postsurgical pain. Pain. 2011;152(9):1958–65. https://doi.org/10.1016/j.pain.2011.02.053.
37. Simons LE, Vlaeyen JWS, Declercq L, et al. Avoid or engage? Outcomes of graded exposure in youth with chronic pain using a sequential replicated single-case randomized design. Pain. 2020;161(3):520–31. https://doi.org/10.1097/j.pain.0000000000001735.
38. Palermo TM, Valrie CR, Karlson CW. Family and parent influences on pediatric chronic pain: a developmental perspective. Am Psychol. 2014;69(2):142–52. https://doi.org/10.1037/a0035216.
39. Caes L, Vervoort T, Eccleston C, Vandenhende M, Goubert L. Parental catastrophizing about child's pain and its relationship with activity restriction: the mediating role of parental distress. Pain. 2011;152(1):212–22. https://doi.org/10.1016/j.pain.2010.10.037.
40. Goubert L, Eccleston C, Vervoort T, Jordan A, Crombez G. Parental catastrophizing about their child's pain. The parent version of the Pain Catastrophizing Scale (PCS-P): a preliminary validation. Pain. 2006;123(3):254–63. https://doi.org/10.1016/j.pain.2006.02.035.
41. Lynch-Jordan AM, Kashikar-Zuck S, Szabova A, Goldschneider KR. The interplay of parent and adolescent catastrophizing and its impact on adolescents' pain, functioning, and pain behavior. Clin J Pain. 2013;29(8):681–8. https://doi.org/10.1097/AJP.0b013e3182757720.
42. Simons LE, Smith A, Kaczynski K, Basch M. Living in fear of your child's pain: the Parent Fear of Pain Questionnaire. Pain. 2015;156(4):694–702. https://doi.org/10.1097/j.pain.0000000000000100.

43. Cousins LA, Kalapurakkel S, Cohen LL, Simons LE. Topical review: resilience resources and mechanisms in pediatric chronic pain. J Pediatr Psychol. 2015;40(9):840–5. https://doi.org/10.1093/jpepsy/jsv037.
44. Ader R, Cohen N. Psychoneuroimmunology: conditioning and stress. Annu Rev Psychol. 1993;44:53–85. https://doi.org/10.1146/annurev.ps.44.020193.000413.
45. Lovallo WR. Stress and health: biological and psychological interactions. 2nd ed. London: Sage; 2005.
46. Segerstrom SC, Miller GE. Psychological stress and the human immune system: a meta-analytic study of 30 years of inquiry. Psychol Bull. 2004;130(4):601–30. https://doi.org/10.1037/0033-2909.130.4.601.
47. Lutgendorf SK, Costanzo ES. Psychoneuroimmunology and health psychology: an integrative model. Brain Behav Immun. 2003;17(4):225–32. https://doi.org/10.1016/s0889-1591(03)00033-3.
48. Kiecolt-Glaser JK, McGuire L, Robles TF, Glaser R. Psychoneuroimmunology: psychological influences on immune function and health. J Consult Clin Psychol. 2002;70(3):537–47. https://doi.org/10.1037//0022-006x.70.3.537.
49. Kiecolt-Glaser JK. Psychoneuroimmunology: psychology's gateway to the biomedical future. Perspect Psychol Sci. 2009;4(4):367–9. https://doi.org/10.1111/j.1745-6924.2009.01139.x.
50. Kiecolt-Glaser JK, Marucha PT, Malarkey WB, Mercado AM, Glaser R. Slowing of wound healing by psychological stress. Lancet. 1995;346(8984):1194–6. https://doi.org/10.1016/s0140-6736(95)92899-5.
51. Marucha PT, Kiecolt-Glaser JK, Favagehi M. Mucosal wound healing is impaired by examination stress. Psychosom Med. 1998;60(3):362–5. https://doi.org/10.1097/00006842-199805000-00025.
52. McGuire L, Heffner K, Glaser R, et al. Pain and wound healing in surgical patients. Ann Behav Med. 2006;31(2):165–72. https://doi.org/10.1207/s15324796abm3102_8.
53. Nassau JH, Tien K, Fritz GK. Review of the literature: integrating psychoneuroimmunology into pediatric chronic illness interventions. J Pediatr Psychol. 2008;33(2):195–207. https://doi.org/10.1093/jpepsy/jsm076.
54. Tagge EP, Natali EL, Lima E, Leek D, Neece CL, Randall KF. Psychoneuroimmunology and the pediatric surgeon. Semin Pediatr Surg. 2013;22(3):144–8. https://doi.org/10.1053/j.sempedsurg.2013.05.002.
55. Kern-Buell CL, McGrady AV, Conran PB, Nelson LA. Asthma severity, psychophysiological indicators of arousal, and immune function in asthma patients undergoing biofeedback-assisted relaxation. Appl Psychophysiol Biofeedback. 2000;25(2):79–91. https://doi.org/10.1023/a:1009562708112.
56. Olness K, Ader R. Conditioning as an adjunct in the pharmacotherapy of lupus erythematosus. J Dev Behav Pediatr. 1992;13(2):124–5. https://doi.org/10.1097/00004703-199204000-00008.
57. Olness K, Culbert T, Uden D. Self-regulation of salivary immunoglobulin A by children. Pediatrics. 1989;83(1):66–71.
58. Hewson-Bower B, Drummond PD. Secretory immunoglobulin A increases during relaxation in children with and without recurrent upper respiratory tract infections. J Dev Behav Pediatr. 1996;17(5):311–6. https://doi.org/10.1097/00004703-199610000-00004.
59. Hewson-Bower B, Drummond PD. Psychological treatment for recurrent symptoms of colds and flu in children. J Psychosom Res. 2001;51(1):369–77. https://doi.org/10.1016/s0022-3999(01)00212-4.
60. Nelson S, Bento S, Enlow MB. Biomarkers of allostatic load as correlates of impairment in youth with chronic pain: an initial investigation. Children. 2021;8(8):709. https://doi.org/10.3390/children8080709.
61. Farooqi NAI, Scotti M, Lew JM, et al. Role of DHEA and cortisol in prefrontal-amygdalar development and working memory. Psychoneuroendocrinology. 2018;98:86–94. https://doi.org/10.1016/j.psyneuen.2018.08.010.

62. Cohen LL, Lemanek K, Blount RL, et al. Evidence-based assessment of pediatric pain. J Pediatr Psychol. 2008;33(9):939–57. https://doi.org/10.1093/jpepsy/jsm103.
63. Adams LM, Turk DC. Central sensitization and the biopsychosocial approach to understanding pain. J Appl Biobehav Res. 2018;23(2):e12125.
64. Louw A, Puentedura EL, Zimney K. Teaching patients about pain: it works, but what should we call it? Physiother Theory Pract. 2016;32(5):328–31. https://doi.org/10.1080/0959398 5.2016.1194669.
65. Robins H, Perron V, Heathcote LC, Simons LE. Pain neuroscience education: state of the art and application in pediatrics. Children. 2016;3(4):43. https://doi.org/10.3390/children3040043.
66. Louw A, Puentedura EJ, Zimney K, Schmidt S. Know pain, know gain? A perspective on pain neuroscience education in physical therapy. J Orthop Sports Phys Ther. 2016;46(3):131–4. https://doi.org/10.2519/jospt.2016.0602.
67. Butler DS, Moseley G. Explain pain. Adelaide, SA: Noigroup Publications; 2013.
68. Coakley R, Schechter N. Chronic pain is like… The clinical use of analogy and metaphor in the treatment of chronic pain in children. Pediatr Pain Lett. 2013;15(1):1–8.
69. Loeser JD. Pain as a disease. Handb Clin Neurol. 2006;81:11–20.
70. Odell S, Logan DE. Pediatric pain management: the multidisciplinary approach. J Pain Res. 2013;6:785–90. https://doi.org/10.2147/JPR.S37434.
71. International Association for the Study of Pain. Pain treatment services. 2021. https://www.iasp-pain.org/resources/guidelines/pain-treatment-services/. Accessed 20 May 2022.
72. Hechler T, Kanstrup M, Holley AL, et al. Systematic review on intensive interdisciplinary pain treatment of children with chronic pain. Pediatrics. 2015;136(1):115–27. https://doi.org/10.1542/peds.2014-3319.
73. Coakley R, Wihak T. Evidence-based psychological interventions for the management of pediatric chronic pain: new directions in research and clinical practice. Children. 2017;4(2):9. https://doi.org/10.3390/children4020009.
74. Pielech M, Vowles KE, Wicksell R. Acceptance and commitment therapy for pediatric chronic pain: theory and application. Children. 2017;4(2):10. https://doi.org/10.3390/children4020010.
75. Coakley R, Wihak T, Kossowsky J, Iversen C, Donado C. The comfort ability pain management workshop: a preliminary, nonrandomized investigation of a brief, cognitive, biobehavioral, and parent training intervention for pediatric chronic pain. J Pediatr Psychol. 2018;43(3):252–65. https://doi.org/10.1093/jpepsy/jsx112.

Chapter 9
Youth Sport Specialization: Risks, Benefits, and Mental Health Considerations

Kristin E. Whitney, Pierre A. d'Hemecourt, and Andrea Stracciolini

Key Points
- Sport specialization is becoming increasingly common among youth athletes, and at younger ages.
- Youth athletes who specialize in sport are at increased risk for injuries compared to their multisport athlete peers.
- Sport specialization is associated with adverse outcomes including reduced sleep, poorer quality of life outcomes, and increased risk for anxiety and depression.

K. E. Whitney (✉)
Division of Sports Medicine, Department of Orthopedic Surgery, Boston Children's Hospital, Boston, MA, USA

The Micheli Center for Sports Injury Prevention, Waltham, MA, USA

Harvard Medical School, Boston, MA, USA
e-mail: Kristin.Whitney@childrens.harvard.edu

P. A. d'Hemecourt · A. Stracciolini
Division of Sports Medicine, Department of Orthopaedics, Boston Children's Hospital, Boston, MA, USA

The Micheli Center for Sports Injury Prevention, Waltham, MA, USA

Harvard Medical School, Boston, MA, USA
e-mail: Pierre.DHemecourt@childrens.harvard.edu;
Andrea.Stracciolini@childrens.harvard.edu

© The Author(s), under exclusive license to Springer Nature   179
Switzerland AG 2023
M. A. Christino et al. (eds.), *Psychological Considerations in the Young Athlete*,
Contemporary Pediatric and Adolescent Sports Medicine,
https://doi.org/10.1007/978-3-031-25126-9_9

Introduction

Sport specialization has received much attention in the pediatric sports medicine arena over the last decade. The main goal of health care providers for young athletes is to "keep kids in the game". With this, we must continue to strive to understand risk factors for injury, keeping in mind the impact of injury on both physical and mental well-being. The current paradigm shift in youth sports participation is toward participation with greater intensity, at higher competitive levels, with a single sport focus and toward "elite" participation. This may lead to time away from family and friends, sleep, academics, and free play. The result may be an adverse effect on physical health (increased risk for physical injuries) and mental health, including anxiety, depression, and burnout.

Sport Specialization: Definition

As youth sport participation continues to rise, so has the trend toward specialization. Historically, sport specialization was born from the 10,000-Hour Rule whereby *"outstanding"* violinists practiced 10,000 h versus 8000 h for *"good"* and 4000 h for *"normal", and* started early with at least 10 years of experience. This led to high volumes of *deliberate practice* (i.e., specific, focused, skill-based practice) at a very young age, and was expanded by some to include sports training [1]. Perhaps Malcolm Gladwell drew major attention to the concept with his examination of the factors that contribute to high levels of success. To support his thesis, he examined why the majority of Canadian ice hockey players are born in the first few months of the calendar year, and placed emphasis on the "10,000-Hour Rule", claiming that the key to achieving world-class expertise in any skill, is, to a large extent, a matter of practicing the correct way, for a total of around 10,000 hours.

In the medical arena, Jayanthi et al. brought this phenomenon to light, and operationalized the definition of "specialized" as any two of the following three criteria; single sport training, playing greater than 8 months of the year, and playing one sport at the exclusion of other sports [2, 3]. The definition was expanded to allow for a *spectrum of sport specialization*. More specifically, a highly specialized athlete may be able to (1) choose a main sport, (2) participate for greater than 8 months per year in 1 main sport, and (3) quit all other sports to focus on 1 sport [3, 4]. With this, the degree of sport specialization was further defined as low, moderate, or high based on the number of definition components to which a young athlete may respond in a positive way [4].

Concerns surrounding the process by which this definition came to pass and the rapid widespread use of the definition in a variety of ways throughout research has made the understanding of the true effects of sport specialization on physical and mental health difficult to ascertain [5]. The most common method of operationalizing the definition is the 3-point specialization scale, which has been linked with injury [4, 6–8]. To this end, Bell et al. [5] recently conducted a Delphi Study to develop a consensus definition of youth sport specialization, and identify elements that support the construct of specialization. In four Delphi consensus rounds, 17 experts reviewed the umbrella definition and six elements, before consensus was reached. The umbrella definition and three of the initial six elements achieved greater than 80% agreement for importance, relevance, and clarity after the fourth round of review. The remaining three components did not reach greater than 80% agreement. The process resulted in a final consensus definition: Sport specialization is intentional and focused participation in a single sport for a majority of the year that restricts opportunities for engagement in other sports and activities.

Sport Specialization and Overuse Injuries

One of the early studies on sport specialization investigated a cohort of 519 youth tennis players and reported "tennis specialized" versus multiple sport athletes, who played competitive tennis, were more likely (OR 1.5 ($P < 0.05$) for withdrawal from a match due to any injury in the previous year compared to athletes who were specialized in tennis only [9]. A case-control study of 1190 athletes, 7–18 years, which explored the relationship between specialization and incidence of overuse injury, while controlling for age and hours of participation, showed that specialized athletes were more likely (OR 1.36 ($P < 0.01$)) to sustain a serious overuse injury (e.g., spondylolysis, stress fracture) compared to non-specialized athletes [4]. This landmark study was followed by another important study by McGuine et al. [7] which investigated the association of sport specialization with risk of lower extremity injuries in 1544 high school athletes over 2843 athletic seasons. In this study, sport specialization was classified as low, moderate, or high. The results showed that the incidence of lower extremity injuries for moderate participants was higher than for low participants ([95% CI, 1.04–2.20]; $P = 0.03$), and the incidence of lower extremity injuries for high participants was greater than for low participants ([95% CI, 1.12–3.06]; $P = 0.02$). Taking this one step further, Post et al. [10] from Wisconsin reported on the ability of several of these "rules of thumb" to determine the likelihood of injury, in a cohort of 2011 male and female athletes aged 12–18 years. Participants were recruited from athletic competitions around the Badger State, rather than from hospital injury clinics. Using a historical questionnaire, the authors evaluated three common recommendations: Don't specialize in 1 sport; limit participation to 8 months per year; and limit participation to fewer hours per week than your age in years. The researchers found that all three guidelines were meaningful. Highly specialized athletes were more likely to report injuries in general and overuse injuries in particular than those in the low specialization category. Young athletes whose weekly participation exceeded more hours than their age in years also were more likely to recall an injury of any type than those who adhered to this guideline. Finally, youth who played their primary sport 8 months per year were more likely to report overuse injuries in both upper and lower limbs. As the research on youth sport specialization and overuse injury continue to evolve Bell et al. [6] conducted a systematic review and meta-analysis of the literature to determine if sport specialization was associated with overuse musculoskeletal injuries. Studies were included if their population was ≤18 years of age, if they compared athletes with high or single-sport specialization with athletes with low or multisport specialization, and focused on overuse injuries. Five studies were included (1 prospective and 4 retrospective). Pooled estimates and data analysis of greater than 3000 athletes showed that highly specialized athletes had a greater risk of overuse injury versus moderately specialized (RR: 1.18 [95% CI: 1.05–1.33]) and low specialized participants. Moderate specialized participants had a higher risk of overuse injury versus low specialized athletes (RR: 1.39 [95% CI: 1.04–1.87]).

Sport specialization in unique populations has also been studied. Sugimoto et al. [11] focused their research on female athletes and the effect of single-sport participation on lower extremity overuse injuries. This study found an independent association between increased weekly hours of training for a sport, and greater likelihood of history of lower extremity overuse injuries (OR = 1.091, 95% CIs: 1.007–1.183, $p = 0.034$). Notably in this study, increased training volume was an independent contributing factor for lower extremity overuse injury, and single-sport athletes were found to have trained nearly twice as many hours per week compared to multisport athletes. The authors comment on volume being a major factor underlying the risk for injury of sport specialization.

Shephard et al. [12] conducted a retrospective study that examined the effects of high, moderate, and low levels of sport specialization on subjective hip and groin dysfunction in collegiate ice hockey athletes. The study reported that the high-specialization group of ice hockey athletes had lower scores compared to the low-specialized ice hockey athletes in symptoms, pain, activities of daily living, sport/recreation, and quality of life measures, and the moderate-specialization group had lower scores than the low-specialization group in symptoms and activities of daily living subscales.

Survey data among little league baseball players showed that just about 10% of those surveyed met criteria for high specialization. Notably, behaviors associated with specialization such as year-round play and receiving of private coaching were more common among highly specialized little leaguers, and the highly specialized little league players demonstrated worse throwing arm health compared with low-specialization players [13]. Survey data among 102 middle and high school long-distance runners showed that highly specialized male and female long-distance runners reported more months of competition per year, higher weekly run distance, more runs per week, higher average distance per run, and greater running enjoyment. Unexpectedly, no differences among sport specialization levels were found for running-related injuries, quality of life, sleep quality, or sleep duration among male or female middle school and high school runners [14].

More studies continue to emerge that seek to dissect risk-benefit profile for injury under sport specialization. Carder et al. [15] conducted a systematic review and meta-analysis which sought to determine if *sport sampling* was associated with a lower sports injury rate in youths compared with youths who specialize in one sport. From the six studies that met inclusion criteria, the total participant number was 5736. Of those, 2451 (42.7%) were classified as "sport samplers," and 1628 (28.4%) were classified as "sport specializers," and 1657 (28.9%) were considered "others" (i.e., could not be classified as true samplers or true specializers). *Sport specializers* had a higher injury risk than the *sport samplers* (RR, 1.37; 95% CI, 1.19–1.57;

$P < 0.0001$). There also was a higher risk of injury found in the "others" group when compared with the "sport sampler" group (RR, 1.21; 95% CI, 1.14–1.29; $P < 0.0001$). Lastly, the study reported a higher risk of injury in the "sport specializer" group over the "others" group (RR, 1.09; 95% CI, 1.04–1.14; $P < 0.005$). The authors concluded from this study that sport sampling was associated with a decreased risk of sports injury in youth athletes when compared with those who specialize in one sport.

Early Vs. Late Sport Specialization

Early sports specialization is most often defined as the pre-adolescent athlete limitation to a single sport for at least 8 months of a year, excluding other sports participation [2, 4]. This involves the pre-pubertal years when sport specialization is undertaken by children under the age of 12. Notably, this group often includes young school-age children. As previously mentioned, there has been an association with injuries when specialization initiates in the pre-adolescent years. With increased risk for injury at an early age, special consideration must be made for the pathogenesis of injury and the socio-emotional implications of early-life exposure to injury in sport in this uniquely vulnerable population of athletes in early development.

It is well established that a significant disparity of skeletal maturation occurs in this early development [16]. It has also been established that dynamic neuromuscular skills at the prepubertal stage are developed with a combination of genetic predisposition as well as the environment of neuromuscular training incorporating both general and specific skills [17, 18]. This neuromuscular training incorporates a combination of resistance, dynamic stability, plyometrics, and core stability. Neuromuscular adaptations are responsible for most of the adaptations in the pre-adolescent, not muscular hypertrophy. These skills must be instructed by individuals knowledgeable about pediatric science. Pubertal athletes that participated in lower extremity strengthening in the pre-pubertal ages have been shown to have a significant increase in strength than control groups [19]. Furthermore, it has been established that early neuromuscular integrative programs help prevent injury in youth sports [20]. Meeuwisse and Emery demonstrated this in youth soccer [21]. These integrative neuromuscular skills should be kept fun and out of the competitive range in the early youth training [22].

Following this thought process, Balyi proposed the long-term athletic development program [23]. The first stage is the FUNdamental phase (ages 6–10). This phase emphasizes the ABCs (agility, balance, coordination, and speed). The second stage is the training to train (males 10–14 years old/females 10–13 years old). This phase emphasizes the specific sport skills along with emphasis on appropriate nutrition and stretching, where athletes mostly focus on training with the initiation of some competition. Stage 3 is train to compete (males 14–18 years old/females 13–17 years old). This involves high-intensity and sport-specific training. Competition is increased to 50% of the sport-specific time. Stage 4 is the train to win phase (males 18 years/females 17 years and older). Competition is as much as 75%. All of the athlete's physical, tactical, and mental capacities are fully established.

The United States Olympic Committee formed the American Development Model (ADM) to address this long-term development from pre-pubertal to adult athletics. The five key elements are:

1. Universal access for all athletes.
2. Activities that develop fundamental skills and motor development in the early phases.
3. Multisport activities in early development.
4. Progressive challenging activities that are fun and engaging.
5. Quality coaching specific to the age group.

These principles reflect the appropriate progressive stages of sport participation over the lifespan during athlete development [24, 25].

There are some sports that have traditionally embraced sport specialization at an early age. These include artistic and rhythmic gymnastics as well as diving and dance [26]. Typical Olympic-level gymnastics peaks at an earlier age than other sports. The youngest champion gymnast was 15 and a number appears at the age of 16. For gymnastics, the anthropomorphic requirement is a key factor including body size. Kaur and Koley performed a systematic review and showed that body size was a significant factor in the success of the gymnast [27]. This may also be involved with dancers and divers but needs further study. Nonetheless, gymnasts and dancers experience high levels of stress fractures and other injuries. Consequently, they need close monitoring. In this group of early sports specialization, there are some strong recommendations to prevent injury and burnout. Recommendations for those participating in early sports training include:

1. Limiting hours of participation to less than chronologic age.
2. Monitor training and coaching.
3. Monitor overscheduling.
4. Have at least 3 months off per year and 1–2 days off per week.
5. Monitor physiologic and psychologic development [28].

Injury Risk in the Developing Athlete: Physical and Mental Health Considerations

Injury risk is an important consideration for all athletes, as sports-related injuries can have substantial impact on athletes' physical and mental health. It is likely that the repetitive nature of sport-specific athletic activity is a substantial driver of over-use injuries among young athletes—particularly in light of youth-specific risk factors in skeletally immature athletes with developing skeletal growth cartilage, musculotendinous development, and immature neuromuscular patterning. Recent research has suggested that sport specialization in youth athletes may be associated with increased risk for certain types of injuries, including serious overuse injuries [4, 9]. Although some have suggested that this may be due to overall training volume among specialized athletes, McGuine et al. demonstrated increased risk of lower-extremity injuries among specialized athletes from multiple sports, even when controlling for competition volume [4]. In a large cohort study conducted by Hall et al., including female athletes participating in basketball, soccer, or volleyball, among sport-specialized athletes compared to multisport athletes, the relative risk of anterior knee pain (diagnoses including patellofemoral pain, Osgood-Schlatter disease, and Sinding-Larsen-Johansson syndrome) was 1.5 times that of multisport athletes [29]. Notably, the anterior knee pain diagnoses included in this study all have pathophysiologic links to factors related to skeletal immaturity and skeletal growth, along with repetitive mechanical strain. Thus, sport specialization and repetitive loading in the developing athlete is of particular concern.

Injuries to the growth cartilage represent a significant portion of injuries to the young athlete population. This includes apophyseal as well as physeal injuries. In the growing athlete, growth cartilage is the weak link of the musculoskeletal chain [30]. It is less resistant to repetitive tensile, compressive, and shear forces. As such, the gymnast repetitively loads the distal radial physis and may cause premature closure of this physis resulting in positive ulnar variance [31]. For the lower extremities, athletic compressive forces may affect the distal femoral physis with resultant angular developmental abnormalities [32]. Finally, physeal stress at the femoral head may affect the development of a CAM impingement so frequently seen in the hockey player [33]. As such, young athletes, particularly those who are sport-specialized, need to be monitored for the development of these sport-specific injuries, along with the mental health implications of these types of injuries when they do occur in the developing athlete. Injury risk among specialized athletes warrants special consideration in the context of mental health in light of injuries' potential impact on an athlete's normal social contexts and routines.

Sleep

Sleep is a crucial part of recovery, and is closely linked to physical and mental health. Poor sleep has been associated with an increased risk of injury in youth athletes, and youth athletes are at an increased risk of sleep problems compared with nonathletes, potentially due to competing demands of academics, social, and athletics participation [34, 35]. Watson et al., prospectively evaluated the independent relationships between sport specialization, sleep, and subjective well-being in female youth soccer players, while adjusting for the influence of training load and age [36]. Specialized athletes reported significantly worse sleep quality during the season, although there was not a significant difference in total hours of sleep duration between specialized soccer players and multisport athletes [37]. Poor sleep quality has been demonstrated to be an independent predictor of decreased competitive success in athletes, and is associated with worse subjective well-being [38].

Well-Being and Quality of Life

Quality of life (QOL) has been increasingly recognized as an important primary health endpoint by clinicians, researchers, and the Department of Health and Human Services [39]. While athletes in general have higher health-related QOL compared to non-athletes, there are important risk factors which can be detrimental to an athletes' QOL [40, 41]. Athletic identity is higher in those athletes who are more specialized, and although sport specialization may confer some advantages in terms of coping skills in young athletes, these athletes may be at heightened risk for worry compared to less specialized athletes [42]. Studies have shown that injuries can negatively impact QOL in athletes, and some injuries can even ultimately result in symptoms consistent with features of posttraumatic stress disorder [43]. Sport specialization has been associated not only with overuse injuries as previously mentioned, but also with increased risk of burnout [44]. Highly sport-specialized athletes have demonstrated worse subjective well-being in terms of overall fatigue, mood, and soreness compared to multisport athletes, even after controlling for confounding factors including age, sleep, and training load [36]. Watson et al. evaluated QOL among high school female volleyball players and determined that highly sport-specialized athletes were more likely to report increased daytime sleepiness, and decreased QOL, when compared to athletes with low sport specialization. Decreased QOL scoring among specialized athletes was primarily driven by lower ratings on physical QOL. In this study population, highly specialized athletes were more likely to report an injury, and when both injury history and sport specialization was incorporated into multivariable model analysis, specialization was no longer significantly associated with QOL—suggesting that the negative association between sport specialization and QOL was due to higher rates of injuries as a mediator [45]. Of note, even those specialized athletes who had fully physically recovered from certain recent injuries reported continued lower QOL, consistent with prior studies that have shown that injuries' impact on QOL persists long after physical recovery [46]. This persistent negative impact on athlete quality of life may potentially be due to certain residual and long-lasting effects on athletes' social environment and athletic identity that may be slow to return to pre-injury baseline.

Anxiety and Depression

Sport specialization often requires increased training hours and may predispose young athletes to social isolation, increased stress and anxiety, inadequate sleep, and burnout [46, 47].

Research assessing anxiety and depression in the North American youth athlete population has been somewhat limited to date. One study by Pluhar et al. included a survey of 756 athletes ages 6–18 years, and found that a higher proportion of individual sport athletes reported anxiety or depression than team sport athletes (13% vs. 7%, $p < 0.01$) [48]. A mental health assessment instrument called the Hospital Anxiety and Depression Scale was administered to 326 elite German athletes between 12 and 18 years old, most of whom were enrolled at German elite sport schools. Of those surveyed, 7% met the criteria for "possible anxiety," 3% with "probable anxiety," 10% with "possible depression," and 4% with "probable depression." These findings did not differ by sex or age, and the study did not include a control group [49]. In a Norwegian study, rates of psychological distress were compared between participants in elite sport high schools ($n = 611$, representing 50 sports) and a control population of general high school students ($n = 355$). Symptom checklists demonstrated higher levels of psychological distress among the control group (18.9%) compared to the elite athletes (7.1%). Sex differences were identified, with higher rates of distress in female athletes (13.2%) as compared with male athletes (3.6%), and these rates were 11% higher in both male and female control participants compared to their elite-athlete counterparts [50]. Perfectionistic traits were the greatest predictors of psychological distress in this population, and have been associated with burnout in other studies as well [51].

Specialized athletes tend to have higher training volumes [11, 52]. A number of studies have illuminated the relationship between training volume and mental health. To some extent, exercise can be beneficial for mental health. In a cross-sectional study of 481 adolescents, those who reported more than 60 min of physical activity per day, 5–7 days per week, had 56% reduced odds of depression and 47% reduced odds of trait anxiety compared with adolescents who reported physical activity only 0–2 days per week [53]. A Swiss survey distributed to 1245 16–20 year-old participants (or athletes) showed that peak mental well-being was evident at a mean of 14 h of sports per week, whereas athletes at the extremes of exercise patterns, either high or low (over 17.5 h per week, or less than 3.5 h per week), had greater odds of poorer mental well-being (OR = 2.29 and OR = 2.33 respectively) [54].

Athletes with higher training volumes are at risk for less total sleep duration, and the interaction between sleep duration and mental health in adolescents is significant, with insufficient sleep and daytime sleepiness having a very close relationship with mood disorders [35, 55].

Sport environment and interpersonal dynamics between athletes and coaches can have a substantial impact on athlete mental health, with supportive environments helping to bolster resilience and mental toughness [56, 57]. Conversely, abusive environments can compromise mental health, and unfortunately, specialized athletes can oftentimes be in intensive training environments that place them at risk for abuse [57].

Athletic Success and Lifelong Participation

The motivation for many young athletes who are becoming sport-specialized is oftentimes the misconception that year-round intensive training, and specialization in a single sport from an early age will lead to better opportunities for future athletic success. However, studies have demonstrated that early sport specialization leads to increased risk of injuries, burnout, and lower lifelong sports participation without increasing the likelihood of elite achievement [58]. In the United States, Collegiate-level NCAA Division I athletes have a propensity to play multiple sports during high school, rather than just one [47]. At the 2015 National Football League Scouting Combine, 87% of the 322 participants played multiple sports during their youth, compared with only 13% who exclusively played football throughout their upbringing [47].

Not only do athletes with more diversified athletic backgrounds seem to reach higher echelons of sport, they tend to have more competitive success, as well. A longitudinal evaluation of 1558 elite athletes compared athletes who ranked in the top 10 of international competitions (Olympics or World Championships) to athletes who had not yet achieved international rankings, but placed in the top 10 in national-level competitions. The internationally ranked athletes showed significantly more variety in their sports backgrounds, having spent more time training and competing in sports other than their dominant sport from a young age, and their onset of sport specialization was much later in life [59]. Gullich et al. compared sport histories between medalists and non-medalists in international competitions with similar findings. This study found that athletes with greater success had less specialized sport backgrounds [60].

The underlying mechanism for sport diversification as a favorable predictor of sport success may be that playing multiple sports during childhood and throughout one's athletic career, exposes athletes to various neuromuscular-activation and neuromuscular-control patterns to enhance general athleticism and physical fitness [3]. Although specialized practice may enhance some sport-specific skills, training various muscle groups through different sports during childhood may facilitate greater overall athletic development while avoiding certain repetitive injury risks that may come along with highly specialized sport practice [3].

Conclusion

Sport specialization represents a widely prevalent paradigm shift in youth sports participation toward participation with greater intensity, at higher competitive levels, with a single sport focus and toward "elite" participation. This may lead to time away from family and friends, sleep, academics, and free play. The result may be an adverse effect on physical health and mental health, including anxiety, depression, and burnout. Heightened awareness among young athletes, parents, coaches, primary care physicians, mental health professionals, and orthopedics-sports medicine specialists is needed in order to support athletes, mitigate risks, and optimize youth athlete health and developments.

References

1. Ericsson KA. Towards a science of the acquisition of expert performance in sports: clarifying the differences between deliberate practice and other types of practice. J Sports Sci. 2020;38(2):159–76.
2. Jayanthi N, Pinkham C, Dugas L, Patrick B, Labella C. Sports specialization in young athletes: evidence-based recommendations. Sports Health. 2013;5(3):251–7.
3. Myer GD, Jayanthi N, Difiori JP, et al. Sport specialization, part I: does early sports specialization increase negative outcomes and reduce the opportunity for success in young athletes? Sports Health. 2015;7(5):437–42.
4. Jayanthi NA, LaBella CR, Fischer D, Pasulka J, Dugas LR. Sports-specialized intensive training and the risk of injury in young athletes: a clinical case-control study. Am J Sports Med. 2015;43(4):794–801.
5. Bell DR, Snedden T, Biese K, et al. Consensus definition of sport specialization in youth athletes using a Delphi approach. J Athl Train. 2021;56:1239.
6. Bell DR, Post EG, Biese K, Bay C, Valovich MLT. Sport specialization and risk of overuse injuries: a systematic review with meta-analysis. Pediatrics. 2018;142(3):e20180657.
7. McGuine TA, Post EG, Hetzel SJ, Brooks MA, Trigsted S, Bell DR. A prospective study on the effect of sport specialization on lower extremity injury rates in high school athletes. Am J Sports Med. 2017;45(12):2706–12.
8. Bell DR, Post EG, Trigsted SM, et al. Sport specialization characteristics between rural and suburban high school athletes. Orthop J Sports Med. 2018;6(1):2325967117751386.
9. Jayanthi N, Durazo R, Luke A. Training and specialization risks in junior elite tennis players. J Med Sci Tennis. 2011;16(1):14–20.
10. Post EG, Trigsted SM, Riekena JW, et al. The association of sport specialization and training volume with injury history in youth athletes. Am J Sports Med. 2017;45(6):1405–12.
11. Sugimoto D, Jackson SS, Howell DR, Meehan WP 3rd, Stracciolini A. Association between training volume and lower extremity overuse injuries in young female athletes: implications for early sports specialization. Phys Sportsmed. 2019;47(2):199–204.
12. Sheppard M, Nicknair J, Goetschius J. Early sport specialization and subjective hip and groin dysfunction in collegiate ice hockey athletes. J Athl Train. 2020;55(3):232–7.
13. Post EG, Rosenthal MD, Pennock AT, Rauh MJ. Prevalence and consequences of sport specialization among little league baseball players. Sports Health. 2021;13(3):223–9.
14. Garcia MC, Taylor-Haas JA, Rauh MJ, Toland MD, Bazett-Jones DM. Sport specialization in middle—and high-school long-distance runners. J Athl Train. 2021;56:1003.
15. Carder SL, Giusti NE, Vopat LM, et al. The concept of sport sampling versus sport specialization: preventing youth athlete injury: a systematic review and meta-analysis. Am J Sports Med. 2020;48(11):2850–7.
16. Malina RM, Cumming SP, Morano PJ, Barron M, Miller SJ. Maturity status of youth football players: a noninvasive estimate. Med Sci Sports Exerc. 2005;37:1044–52.
17. Davids K, Baker J. Genes, environment and sport performance: why the nature-nurture dualism is no longer relevant. Sports Med. 2007;37:961–80.
18. Faigenbaum AD, McFarland J. Make time for less intense training. Strength Cond J. 2006;28:77–9.

19. Ford KR, Myer GD, Hewett TE. Longitudinally decreased knee abduction and increased hamstrings strength in females with self-reported resistance training. Med Sci Sports Exerc. 2011;43:77.
20. Faigenbaum AD, Myer GD. Resistance training among young athletes: safety, efficacy and injury prevention effects. Br J Sports Med. 2010;44:56–63.
21. Emery CA, Meeuwisse WH. The effectiveness of a neuromuscular prevention strategy to reduce injuries in youth soccer: a cluster-randomised controlled trial. Br J Sports Med. 2010;44:555–62.
22. Myer GD, Faigenbaum AD, Ford KR, Best TM, Bergeron MF, Hewett TE. When to initiate integrative neuromuscular training to reduce sports-related injuries and enhance health in youth? Curr Sports Med Rep. 2011;10(3):155–66.
23. Balyi I, Way R, Higgs C. Long-term athlete development. Champaign, IL: Human Kinetics; 2013.
24. American Development Model. United States Olympic Committee Web site. https://www.teamusa.org/About-the-USOC/Athlete-Development/Coaching-Education/American-Development-Model. Accessed 27 Jun 2018.
25. Hainline B. Early sport specialization: shifting societal norms. J Athl Train. 2019;54(10):1011–2. https://doi.org/10.4085/1062-6050-251-18.
26. Hume PA, Hopkins WG, Robinson DM, Robinson SM, Hollings SC. Predictors of attainment in rhythmic sportive gymnastics. J Sports Med Phys Fitness. 1993;33(4):367–77.
27. Kaur K, Koley S. Anthropometric determinants of competitive performance in gymnastics: a systematic review. Int J Health Sci Res. 2019;9(7):249–56.
28. LaPrade RF, Agel J, Baker J, Brenner JS, Cordasco FA, Côté J, Provencher MT. AOSSM early sport specialization consensus statement. Orthop J Sports Med. 2016;4(4):2325967116644241.
29. Hall R, Barber Foss K, Hewett TE, Myer GD. Sport specialization's association with an increased risk of developing anterior knee pain in adolescent female athletes. J Sport Rehabil. 2015;24(1):31–5. https://doi.org/10.1123/jsr.2013-0101.
30. Flachsmann R, Broom ND, Hardy AE, Moltschaniwskyj G. Why is the adolescent joint particularly susceptible to osteochondral shear fracture? Clin Orthop Relat Res. 2000;381:212–21.
31. Difiori JP. Overuse injury of the physis: a "growing" problem. Clin J Sport Med. 2010;20(5):336–7.
32. Laor T, Wall EJ, Vu LP. Physeal widening in the knee due to stress injury in child athletes. AJR Am J Roentgenol. 2006;186(5):1260–4.
33. Novais EN, Maranho DA, Kim YJ, Kiapour A. Age- and sex-specific morphologic variations of capital femoral epiphysis growth in children and adolescents without hip disorders. Orthop J Sports Med. 2018;6(6):232596711878157.
34. Copenhaver EA, Diamond AB. The value of sleep on athletic performance, injury, and recovery in the young athlete. Pediatr Ann. 2017;46:e106–11.
35. Milewski MD, Skaggs DL, Bishop GA, et al. Chronic lack of sleep is associated with increased sports injuries in adolescent athletes. J Pediatr Orthop. 2014;34:129–33.
36. Watson A, Brickson S. Relationships between sport specialization, sleep, and subjective well-being in female adolescent athletes. Clin J Sport Med. 2019;29(5):384–90. https://doi.org/10.1097/JSM.0000000000000631.
37. Brandt R, Bevilacqua GG, Andrade A. Perceived sleep quality, mood states, and their relationship with performance among Brazilian elite athletes during a competitive period. J Strength Cond Res. 2017;31:1033–9.
38. Juliff LE, Halson SL, Hebert JJ, et al. Longer sleep durations are positively associated with finishing place during a national multiday netball competition. J Strength Cond Res. 2018;32:189–94.
39. U.S. Department of Health & Human Services. Healthy People 2020. Washington, DC: U.S. Department of Health and Human Services, Office of Disease Prevention and Health Promotion; 2020. Accessed 3 Dec 2022.
40. Snyder AR, Martinez JC, Bay RC, Parsons JT, Sauers EL, Valovich McLeod TC. Health-related quality of life differs between adolescent athletes and adolescent nonathletes. J Sport Rehabil. 2010;19:237–48.

41. Valovich McLeod TC, Bay RC, Parsons JT, Sauers EL, Snyder AR. Recent injury and health-related quality of life in adolescent athletes. J Athl Train. 2009;44:603–10.
42. Christino MA, Coene R, O'Neil M, Daley M, Williams KA, Ackerman KE, Kramer DE, Stracciolini A. Sport specialization, athletic identity, and coping strategies in young athletes. Abstract presented at: Pediatric Research in Sports Medicine (PRISM) National Conference, Houston TX; 2022.
43. Padaki AS, Noticewala MS, Levine WN, Ahmad CS, Popkin MK, Popkin CA. Prevalence of posttraumatic stress disorder symptoms among young athletes after anterior cruciate ligament rupture. Orthop J Sports Med. 2018;6:2325967118787159.
44. Brenner JS. Overuse injuries, overtraining, and burnout in child and adolescent athletes. Pediatrics. 2007;119:1242–5.
45. Watson A, McGuine T, Lang P, et al. The relationships between sport specialization, sleep, and quality of life in female youth volleyball athletes. Sports Health. 2022;14(2):237–45. https://doi.org/10.1177/19417381211014867.
46. Brenner JS. American Academy of Pediatrics Council on sports medicine and fitness. Overuse injuries, overtraining, and burnout in child and adolescent athletes. Pediatrics. 2007;119(6):1242–5.
47. Brenner JS, Council on Sports Medicine and Fitness. Sports specialization and intensive training in young athletes. Pediatrics. 2016;138(3):e20162148.
48. Pluhar E, McCracken C, Griffith KL, Christino MA, Sugimoto D, Meehan WP 3rd. Team sport athletes may be less likely to suffer anxiety or depression than individual sport athletes. J Sports Sci Med. 2019;18(3):490–6. PMID: 31427871; PMCID: PMC6683619.
49. Weber S, Puta C, Lesinski M, et al. Symptoms of anxiety and depression in young athletes using the hospital anxiety and depression scale. Front Physiol. 2018;9:182.
50. Rosenvinge JH, Sundgot-Borgen J, Pettersen G, Martinsen M, Stornaes AV, Pensgaard AM. Are adolescent elite athletes less psychologically distressed than controls? A cross-sectional study of 966 Norwegian adolescents. Open Access J Sports Med. 2018;9:115–23.
51. Gustafsson H, Hill AP, Stenling A, Wagnsson S. Profiles of perfectionism, parental climate, and burnout among competitive junior athletes. Scand J Med Sci Sports. 2016;26(10):1256–64.
52. Field AE, Tepolt FA, Yang DS, Kocher MS. Injury risk associated with sports specialization and activity volume in youth. Orthop J Sports Med. 2019;7(9):2325967119870124–232596711987012.
53. McDowell CP, MacDonncha C, Herring MP. Brief report: associations of physical activity with anxiety and depression symptoms and status among adolescents. J Adolesc. 2017;55:1–4.
54. Merglen A, Flatz A, Belanger RE, Michaud PA, Suris JC. Weekly sport practice and adolescent well-being. Arch Dis Child. 2014;99(3):208–10.
55. Stracciolini A, McCracken CM, Meehan WP III, Milewski MD. Lack of sleep among adolescent athletes is associated with a higher prevalence of self-reported history of anxiety and depression. J Clin Sport Psychol. Published online 2021. https://doi.org/10.1123/jcsp.2021-0004.
56. Gerber M, Best S, Meerstetter F, et al. Effects of stress and mental toughness on burnout and depressive symptoms: a prospective study with young elite athletes. J Sci Med Sport. 2018;21(12):1200–5.
57. Mountjoy M, Sundgot-Borgen J, Burke L, et al. The IOC consensus statement: beyond the female athlete triad. Relative energy deficiency in sport (RED-S). Br J Sports Med. 2014;48(7):491–7.
58. Anderson FL, Knudsen ML, Ahmad CS, Popkin CA. Current trends and impact of early sports specialization in the throwing athlete. Orthop Clin North Am. 2020;51(4):517–25.
59. Gullich A, Emrich E. Considering long-term sustainability in the development of world class success. Eur J Sport Sci. 2014;14(suppl1):S383–97.
60. Gullich A, Kovar P, Zart S, Reimann A. Sport activities differentiating match-play improvement in elite youth footballers: a 2-year longitudinal study. J Sports Sci. 2017;35(3):207–15.

Chapter 10
How Parents and Coaches Can Support Positive Development

Julie McCleery and Monique S. Burton

Key Points
- The quality of the youth sports experiences for children and adolescents depends on the behaviors and approaches of their parents and coaches.
- Understanding youth physiological and psychological growth and development is critical to creating an optimal youth sports environment.
- Research-based approaches, including creating a mastery climate and focusing on relationship building, help coaches achieve positive outcomes for youth.
- Parents navigate many roles in the youth sports sphere and their supportive engagement is crucial for positive outcomes.
- Parents and coaches need to work together and center youth in their own sports experiences in order to protect them from potentially damaging or abusive practices.

J. McCleery (✉)
Center for Leadership in Athletics, University of Washington, Seattle, WA, USA
e-mail: juliem4@uw.edu

M. S. Burton
Department of Pediatrics, Seattle Children's Hospital, University of Washington, Seattle, WA, USA

Department of Orthopedics and Sports Medicine, Seattle Children's Hospital, University of Washington, Seattle, WA, USA
e-mail: monique.burton@seattlechildrens.org

© The Author(s), under exclusive license to Springer Nature Switzerland AG 2023
M. A. Christino et al. (eds.), *Psychological Considerations in the Young Athlete*, Contemporary Pediatric and Adolescent Sports Medicine, https://doi.org/10.1007/978-3-031-25126-9_10

Introduction

Youth sport offers a space with so much potential for positive youth outcomes. The positive impacts are well documented and reach across social, emotional, physical, cognitive, and psychological domains [1, 2]. Physical activity, accessed through youth sport, also offers substantial physical and psychological benefits that are well-studied including facilitating healing, promoting resiliency, and mitigating the effects of trauma [3–5]. Particularly during this time of increased stress on youth and community health and well-being due to COVID-19, the ability to move and play is essential for physical and mental health.

However, the youth sports landscape is also fraught with practices that can undermine positive youth development. As Fraser-Thomas and Cote [2] note, "there appears to be a void between the potential positive outcomes, and some of the negative realities of youth sport programs". For example "sport participation" has been linked to increases in anxiety, decreases in motivation, and increases in negative affect (see [1, 6]) and youth who play sports may be more prone to some risky behaviors including substance abuse and aggression [1, 2, 7]. For both coaches and parents, understanding the ways sports can best support positive outcomes, and the necessary role parents and coaches play in mediating those outcomes, is essential for youth to thrive in a sports setting [1, 2, 7].

The majority of parents say their main reason for youth to play sports is for the development of life skills [8, 9]. The top reason children participate in sports is "to have fun" [10, 11]. Other top reasons for playing sports include "to learn/improve my skills" and "to be with friends/be part of a team" [12]. The youth sport "skills and excellence" system [13]—with its travel teams, tournaments, and focus on competitions—is not always geared for these outcomes or toward the developmental needs of youth. For both coaches and parents navigating a youth sports system that is not oriented toward long-term athlete development can be a challenge. In this chapter, we review the concept of long-term athlete development, highlight physiological and psychological developmental processes, and discuss the specific ways parents and coaches can keep these in mind, and help youth thrive, as they navigate the youth sports landscape.

Sport Contexts

Youth sports take place in a variety of contexts, from schools to camps to clubs, each offering unique constraints and facilitators for positive youth experiences. The role of parents in a high school sports setting may be quite different from the role of parent in an under-12 travel team. In this chapter, we consider all of the contexts in which 6–18 year olds play sports with an eye toward the common considerations for parents and coaches across the contexts. The vast majority of the 60 million [14] of kids who play sports from ages 6–18 are doing so to reap the participatory benefits. Only 6.3% of male high school athletes and 8.2% of female high school athletes go on to become college athletes (NCAA). Of those collegiate athletes, the majority—as the NCAA tag line reminds us—"will go pro in something other than sports." Despite the small odds of high-performance participation in sports past high school, "it is estimated that between 10% and 30% of youth athletes in the United States specialize in a single sport at a mean age of approximately 12–14 years'' [15] ostensibly to achieve elite levels of performance and participation. While there may be some individual sports, especially those like gymnastics and figure skating where achieving elite status can happen before puberty, our primary aim is to identify concepts and frameworks that support the 93% of kids playing participatory sports recognizing that these concepts are also important in a performance context.

We also note that some structural elements of youth sports, especially those outside of school, present substantial challenges for many families including cost, transportation, travel, and equipment. Sports sociologist Jay Coakley refers to this prevailing model of youth sports, characterized by "achievement at progressively higher levels of competition," the "skills and excellence model" [13]. Coakley notes that the pay-to-play approach that is "built into the skills and excellence model in the United States....reproduces the patterns of income and wealth inequality in the society as a whole" [13]. A 2021 Aspen Institute study found that "Travel is now the costliest feature in youth sports. On average across all sports, parents spent more annually on travel ($196 per sport, per child) than equipment ($144), private lessons ($134), registration fees ($125), and camps ($81)" [16]. This chapter does not specifically address those structural elements but acknowledges that parents and coaches participating in youth sports may bump up against financial and other constraints to varying degrees and those elements will impact the experience of those in the youth sports system and also prevent many families from participating at all.

Long-Term Athlete Development

Over the last decade, researchers have tried to establish a framework to guide youth sport practitioners that accounts for child and adolescent physiological and psychological growth and readiness for sport [13]. While a number of different models exist, and there is some debate about their empirical base [17], the underlying ideology at play is a good one: children are not mini adults and their youth sports experience, training, and competition should not be modeled on pro teams. According to Zwick & Kocher, "Age-appropriate training and conditioning of junior athletes is one of the biggest challenges for trainers, coaches, and administrators today" [18].

A number of factors need to be taken into account by coaches and parents alike. Some key guidelines relative to physiological growth and maturation:

- "Children's skeletal, muscular and nervous systems develop at different rates throughout childhood, and the variance associated with these different rates has significant implications for each child's physical development, and consequently, their sporting performance and improvement" [19].
- Growth plates and growth centers are open during childhood and through adolescence making youth more injury prone and vulnerable to physical load and stressors [20, 21].
- During adolescence, in particular, the body is under physiological stress related to growth [20].
- At a time when coaches and parents think youth can handle more load because they are physically maturing, youth might actually be at their most vulnerable [18].

Because of the current youth sports model's orientation to competitive success, growth and maturation plays an oversized role in many youth sports contexts: early developing youth are often afforded more competitive opportunities than late developers [22]. What is referred to as relative age effect (RAE) is a by-product of grouping kids by chronological age; whereby those born in the first quartile of a year have a physiological growth advantage over those born in the later half of the year and tend to be over-represented on sports teams [11]. Looking at professional leagues and national teams in a variety of sports—from Brazilian U14 volleyball players to American youth soccer players—reveals those born in the first quartile of a year continue to be over-represented all the way up the sports chain [11].

Case
- Parents and coaches should be on the lookout for the pattern of differential treatment for early and late developing youth and recognize that early physiological development and talent are not necessarily the same thing.
- An early developing girl, Hannah, is the tallest on her sixth grade basketball team and in the whole sixth grade league. Hannah's coach has her play the post position and draws up an offense that calls for lobbing Hannah the ball for easy layups over her smaller opponents. The team wins most games, struggling only when Hannah is out. Despite the excitement of winning, this type of approach is, in the long term, detrimental not just for Hannah but for all the girls on the team. As Hannah gets older many peers will likely catch—and maybe even pass—her in height. Hannah will not have learned the ball handling and passing skills she needs by being pigeonholed as a post player so early on in her basketball life. Other girls on the team also might have missed opportunities to develop their offensive skills due to the over-reliance on Hannah's height and the coach's choice to focus on winning over skill development and mastery.

Psychological Readiness

While children's bodies are growing so are their brains: children and adolescents are developing self-regulatory and meta-cognitive skills necessary for learning through sport until adulthood [19]. The "skills and excellence model" [13] has children engaged in competition-focused sport as early as 6 years old. However, most children do not develop the capacity for understanding competition and utilizing it to build skills and learn from until much later: "It is only at about the age of 12 or 13 that children are able to fully understand the differing effects that effort, practice, and ability have on their performances" [2]. For example, due to their not yet developed abstract thinking, youth under 12 might not "understand that their ability to hit a pitched ball during a baseball game is related to how much time they spend practicing hitting a ball between games" [23].

Other skills that assist with competitive engagement include causal attribution, delayed gratification, language use, abstract thinking, self-awareness, and emotional regulation [11, 19, 23]. Many of these skills are being built well into adulthood. Sports may, in fact, be a space where youth can build these skills, but only if the adults around them are intentional and explicit about building them [1, 11]. Further, coaches and parents need to be aware that these psycho-social skills are not built in a linear fashion, and youth may make gains and also regress as they experience new types of stressors and challenges.

Children may also be coming into sports spaces having experienced psychological stressors that are impacting their social, emotional, and cognitive development. While we know sport can, potentially, provide opportunities for mitigating the impacts of stress and trauma [24, 25], coaches and parents need to be aware of the ways trauma and stress can present in behavior. Trauma-informed approaches to teaching and coaching are becoming more common [26], and some organizations are offering training specifically focused on using sport to help kids regulate and recover after experiencing trauma. Coaches and parents should be aware that the social isolation and disruptions of COVID have impacted a generation of young people [27], and some behavioral consequences of this may appear on the playing field. Further, youth who are participating in sports and also dealing with chronic stressors like racism and poverty deserve a sporting experience that is attuned to and supportive of their needs.

The primary goal of adopting a long-term athlete development approach, and keeping youth physical and psychological growth in mind, are to sustain youth engagement in physical activity and sport for the long haul. The longer youth sustain participation in a positive youth sport setting, the more of its benefits they can reap. Further, physically active youth go on to become physically active adults. Additionally, youth who move through sports in developmentally appropriate ways are gaining the fundamental knowledge and physical literacy skills to pursue performance-oriented sports when they are ready. While reliable data is hard to come by on this front, estimates suggest that 70% of youth drop out of sports by age 13 [28]. Parent and coach familiarity with these ideas could help shift the sports landscape from one of a pyramid approach—where over time fewer and fewer youth participate to a model where youth are encouraged and supported to participate into adulthood (Figs 10.1 and 10.2).

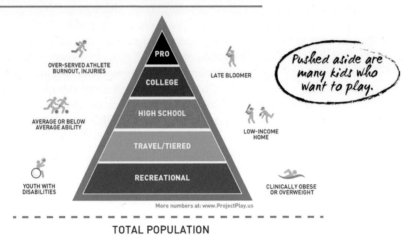

Fig. 10.1 Credit: Aspen Institute Project Play initiative [29]. Current Youth Sports Model

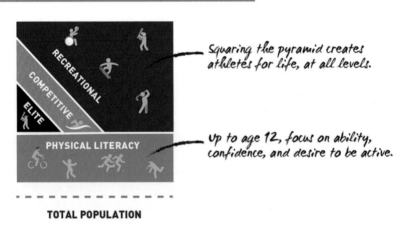

Fig. 10.2 Credit: Aspen Institute Project Play initiative. A more inclusive Youth Sports Model [29]

Coaches

Coaches are essential to creating this climate in which youth can thrive and experience positive outcomes physically, psychologically, and socially [30–33]: "The goal priorities they promote, the attitudes and values they transmit, and the nature of their interactions with athletes can markedly influence the effects of sport participation on children and youth" [34]. In the United States, however, the majority of youth sport coaches are not required to be trained prior to working with children and adolescents [35, 36]. While first aid/CPR and concussion protocol training are now legally required in many states [37], training on youth development and basic pedagogical approaches appropriate for children are not typically required for school or recreational sports [35, 38]:

> Many, if not the vast majority of coaches in youth sport lack specified training in the science of coaching [39]. This phenomenon is only magnified in the volunteer coach [40], who is the least resourced, yet represents the largest percentage of youth coaches in the United States [35].

While one chapter in a book cannot replace the need for a comprehensive coach education and certification process in youth sports, this chapter spells out some of the foundational elements of coaching that can keep youth athletes safe and healthy and retain them in sport. At their core, all of the frameworks below—psychological safety, mastery climate, social-emotional skill building, and quality coach-athlete relationships—take an orientation toward coaching that is holistic in nature. That is, good coaching is recognized as that which attends, simultaneously, to both performance and social-emotional growth and well-being [41].

Psychological Safety

Foundational to youth being able to experience positive outcomes in sport is that they have a sense of both physical and psychological safety:

Psychological safety is defined as a 'shared belief held by members of a team that the team is safe for interpersonal risk taking' [42] without the fear of being ridiculed, punished, or rejected when engaging in interpersonally risky behaviours [43].

Attending to physical safety is something coaches do routinely by doing warm-up and cool-down routines, monitoring the field of play for potential hazards, teaching proper technique, being trained in First Aid/CPR and concussion protocols, and helping players return to play post injury. However, emotional safety may be something with which coaches are less familiar as it is a relatively new concept in the coaching education realm—being translated from the organizational leadership literature. Recent research has found that coaches have just as important a role to play in attending to psychological safety [43, 44] as to physical safety. Similar to monitoring for physical safety, monitoring for psychological safety may include being attuned to bullying, recognizing signs of emotional distress, facilitating interpersonal problem solving, and creating a welcoming and inclusive culture for athletes of minoritized identities. Coaches who attend to these issues will create higher quality coach-athlete relationships and athlete flourishing [43].

Another, more heavily researched, and similarly important concept for coaches to understand is mastery climate.

Mastery Climate

Achievement goal theory categorizes achievement motivation into an ego orientation (performance) and mastery orientation (task) [31, 45]. An ego-involving climate is created in sport when coaches place value on winning and outperforming others as the primary measures of success. A mastery climate, on the other hand, is created when coaches focus on learning, effort, self-improvement, task mastery, having fun, and achieving personal goals [32]. Youth sports settings that create a mastery environment produce tremendous gains for young people including:

- "Greater well-being and adaptive achievement-related thoughts, emotions and behaviours" [46].
- Increased enjoyment of sport [31].
- Higher regard for their coach [31].
- Increased intention to continue to play for their coach in the future [31].
- Decreased anxiety [34].
- Increased self-esteem and intrinsic motivation [34].
- Greater life-skill gains [47].

The adoption of an ego-evolving motivational climate is, on the other hand, associated with a number of negative sport participation outcomes for the athletes such as practicing "winning at all costs" philosophy, inconsistent effort, lower self-esteem, fear of failure, decreased intrinsic motivation, and anxiety [31].

To create a mastery climate coaches should focus on rewarding and emphasizing effort and process over outcome, setting personalized learning goals for improvement, and encouraging mistakes and risk-taking which are essential for learning [31, 32]. The Positive Coaching Alliance (PCA) (see Box 10.1) is a national coach training organization, founded by Jim Thompson that helps coaches learn how to, among other things, create a mastery climate. PCA uses the acronym the E.L.M. tree of mastery where E is for effort, L is for learning, and M is for mistakes to help coaches understand the concept. The excerpt from Thompson's book The Power of Double Goal Coaching provides a good example of the way this training gives coaches specific tools to help create and maintain this environment [48].

Box 10.1 Parent and Coach Free Resources
Positive Coaching Alliance
National Council for Youth Sports: How to Coach Kids
Center for Healing and Justice Through Sports
SafeSportParent Toolkit
Aspen Institute Project Play Parent Checklist
National Federation of State High School Associations Coach Resources
National Alliance for Youth Sports Coach & Parent Free Trainings
ICOACHKIDS
Parent Values: 100 Point Exercise

This excerpt from Jim Thompson's book *Power of Double Goal Coaching* (2010) describes creating a "mistake ritual" to help young athletes recover and learn from mistakes, an important component of a mastery climate.
Mistakes are what youth athletes worry about most. Once a player makes a mistake in public (and the playing field, even with few spectators, is very public for youth athletes), they are no longer in the moment. Negative self-talk kicks in, they berate themselves silently for making a mistake, and are usually not ready for the next play. A mistake ritual is a gesture and statement that coaches and players use to transform the fear of mistakes so they don't play timidly. A mistake ritual allows athletes to quickly "reset" for the next play without beating themselves up for having made a mistake. Here are a few examples Double-Goal Coaches have used successfully:

- *The Flush: Motion like you're flushing a toilet. "It's okay, Omar. Flush it. Next play."*
- *No Sweat: Wipe two fingers across your forehead as if flicking sweat from your brow. "No sweat. Forget it. Get ready for the next play!"*
- *Brush It Off: Motion as if brushing dirt off your shoulder while yelling, "Brush it off."*
- *Encourage your team to not fear mistakes and discuss what mistake ritual they'd like to use. Urge players to use it with each other whenever a mistake is made [48].*

Intentional Social Emotional Skill Building

As noted earlier, parents see sports as a space for building important life skills. If sports are to meet that aim, then coaches are the ones who will need to do that work. Practicing skills like empathy, emotional regulation, teamwork, and respect for others needs to have the same place in the training plan as defensive footwork and flip turns. In order to successfully facilitate positive youth development outcomes through sport, coaches must engage athletes in activities that define, develop and transfer life skills. Expert coaches intentionally designate time to collect athletes' input on transferable life skills, integrate discussions that explicitly define life skills, discuss their importance, and list specific behaviors associated with them in the sport context [49]. Through discussing life skills, coaches will accomplish two goals: (1) increase their ability to use life skills as "keywords" to activate behavioral change in athletes during practice and competition (e.g., What does a coach mean by saying "patience" in the middle of the practice? What exactly am I supposed to do?) and (2) enhance confidence for life skills development among athletes through encouragement and reinforcement [50]. Further, research shows that for athletes to draw meaningful connections between the discussion of life skills and practical application, they must engage in opportunities to practice life skills outside of the sports setting and reflect on the success or failure of the application process [49].

A 2021 scoping review of explicit practices coaches use to support life skills transfer includes:

- Discussing and teaching life skills
- Creating opportunities to practice life skills in sport
- Supplying direct feedback related to using life skills
- Debriefing sport experiences to enhance life skill transfer
- Providing opportunities to transfer outside of sport [51].

Making time to practice life skills and their transfer outside of sports can be challenging for coaches, especially those who see athletes only a few hours a week. However, this type of "practice" is imperative to the holistic approach to coaching and to meeting the stated aims of the majority of sport parents—life skills development.

Coach: Athlete Relationship

At the heart of any of these approaches is a strong, caring coach-athlete relationship. Jowett and Shanmugam [52] suggest three elements essential to a high-quality coach-athlete relationship: closeness, commitment, and complementarity. Closeness is defined by trust, respect, and appreciation; commitment by loyalty and stability, and complementarity by cooperation and receptiveness—essentially that both coach and athlete are oriented toward helping the athlete meet their goals [43].

Quality relationships have been shown to contribute to team cohesion [44] and create environments where youth feel comfortable taking risks [42], which—as noted above—is an important element of a mastery climate. "In contrast, lack of quality relationships is likely to weaken interpersonal psychological safety and augment exploitation, intimidation and humiliation in the coach–athlete interactions affecting athletes' well-being (see [43, 53])".

For coaches, creating quality relationships can begin with simple approaches like learning all athletes' names and using them routinely. Expert coaches use relationship-building routines, like pre and post practice celebratory huddles and differentiated individual feedback, to support both performance gains and social-emotional development [41].

Being a youth sports coach is something many parents and adults do to support their child and their community; volunteer coaches drive the majority of introductory and recreation sports in the United States. This can make widespread and consistent coach education challenging, but adults working with youth owe it to those young athletes and their families to understand the basic principles supportive of a positive youth sports experience. There are a number of good coach education resources available to support coach training and development. Box 10.1 contains a list and links to those resources.

Parents

While coaches are the most direct mediators of young athletes' experiences while they are in the pool or on the court, parents and guardians play an essential role in their child having a positive youth sport experience. Parents are tasked with navigating and balancing numerous roles and responsibilities to support their child's sport participation: time, finances, transportation, emotions and most importantly child satisfaction. Parents may also bring experience from their past sports participation that includes both positive and negative experiences and outcomes that can influence their attitudes and behaviors toward their child's participation. As youth become increasingly involved in the "skills and excellence" model of youth sports—including select, travel, and professional development teams—parents are often confronted with balancing youth athlete desire and enjoyment, external pressures, and youth emotional and physical well-being.

Given these, sometimes competing interests and external influences, it can be challenging for parents to balance the various roles and provide an ideal parent-child support relationship. As noted earlier in this chapter, the number one reason children enjoy sports is fun. Sports also provide an opportunity for growth through experiences of navigating success, disappointments, friendships, teamwork, and mentorship. Youth athlete success can bring tremendous joy, confidence, sense of accomplishment and pride for youth that can be carried into other skills throughout their life. Likewise, negative experiences and pressures can impact confidence and self-worth in detrimental ways. Finding the most beneficial way to support the youth athlete, in both the short and long term, presents challenges each caregiver must navigate to help provide an ideal experience.

Parent Roles

Literature on parental roles in youth sports includes everything from cheering on the sidelines, providing financial support, transportation, organizing schedules, coaching a team fundraising, or acting as a team manager [54]. Hoyle and Leff [55] categorize these roles in three overarching descriptors: motivator, facilitator, and coach. More recently Vealey and Chase [11] describe the three main parental role categories as manager, model, and meaning maker.

In the role of manager, parents provide financial support, which not only includes supporting the expenses of the sport but also contributing to team expenses through other mechanisms including volunteering, fundraising, celebrations, etc. [11]. Costs associated with "sport and excellence model" of pay to play sports and its related expenses may be prohibitive for some families, placing parents in situations of personal sacrifice to support their children, seeking additional sources of income, balancing choices of most affordable team options or having to make the difficult decision to choose other options for their child. As managers, parents are tasked with managing their child's schedule including transportation coordination either through their own means or in partnership with other families through carpooling. Parents also must constantly assess the sport environment to ensure safe and ideal settings for their child's growth and development [11, 56]. The American Academy of Pediatrics (AAP) [57] recommends early sports sampling as beneficial to the development of motor skills and long-term athlete development. To accomplish this, parents must also seek opportunities for exposure to various sports to help assess physical abilities and what sports may best suit them from both a physical and personal satisfaction perspective. While acting as manager for their child may be challenging and somewhat stressful, most parents enjoy the opportunity to play an active supportive role in their child's youth sport journey.

The role of model includes helping set standards and showing an example for their child [11]. This role provides opportunities for growth and development of the child's life skills. Parental and family values are an integral part of how parents navigate youth sports participation in a way that fosters and supports meaningful experiences and contributes to their moral compass. Parents can model behavior in their actions through sports that are consistent with their beliefs including, sideline reactions and interactions with other parents and coaches that youth observe [56]. Parents also can utilize sports experience to provide examples of work ethic and support of others/teammates and cultivation of important life skills.

Finally, as meaning makers, parents have the opportunity to provide guidance and framework for youth athletes to understand their participation in sports [11].

They can support their child in finding enjoyment, motivate them, and build self-esteem and feelings of competence. In this role, parents can do the most to stay oriented toward the dual aims of performance and life skills development. While coaches have to work hard to help youth apply life skills learned in sport off the field, parents have the perfect vantage point to "make meaning" of sports experiences in everyday life. Parental support through challenges that arise in sports participation, including performance disappointments, helps children navigate emotions and learn from the experience [56]. This role also provides an opportunity for parents to demonstrate and reinforce unconditional love and acceptance regardless of performance and provide stability without conditions in line with their values as a family.

Parent Support, Pressure, and "Push"

Across all of these roles, parents will need to determine an optimal level of engagement and "push," [11] which means distinguishing between *supporting* a child in sports and *pressuring* a child. Parental support is associated with greater enjoyment of sport, more positive performance outcomes, and more positive appraisals [55]. Support influences motivation and enjoyment by youth and as a result supports long-term development [58]. Parental pressure, on other hand, is associated with discontent with the sport, stress, negative, and uncertain appraisal of self-worth [55].

Youth athletes often seek parental support and guidance in navigating their experiences in sports. Parents may influence sport enjoyment, experience, and desire to continue in sports through their direct and indirect or observable interactions, including parental facial expressions and body language or comments directly to them, or overhead to other parents and coaches. Support helps establish confidence to participate, competence in their sports, and self-esteem to continue. Youth athletes seek and desire parent validation and approval without conditions or contingent upon their performance. This allows a space to make mistakes, learn and grow from them, and be supported for effort and behaviors that support family values (such as cheering and supporting teammates).

Even when parents believe they are providing support, certain "parent backfires" [11] can come across to a child as pressure. This includes statements such as "I'm proud of you," "you should win this," and unintentional nonverbal communication which are most often well intended but provide limited context and can result in the athlete creating their own story and attaching meaning of these phrases and behaviors. For example, a young child may think a parent is proud only because they won a swim meet. For parents, as for coaches, providing specific feedback about behaviors or—more importantly—about effort, attitude, process, and preparation are great ways to show support and encouragement. Finding a delicate balance between genuine engagement and pressure is both crucial and challenging. The term "optimal push" has been used by researchers to describe the ways parents can support and execute their roles in the youth sports realm without tipping over into pressure [11, 56]. The push needs to be delivered in a supportive manner with ideal timing, not directly linked to competition, practice, and performance to help avoid perception of judgment and pressure from the child as well. Optimal push accompanied with listening and showing unconditional support helps facilitate growth and accomplishment for the youth athlete. However, as Lauer and colleagues note:

> It is hard to find the fine line between motivating and challenging a child and pressuring them. This fine line is based on the player's perceptions of his or her parents' behaviors and attitudes. Thus, one athlete's optimal push is another athlete's controlling parental behavior [56].

Therefore, it is important for parents to keep open lines of communication with their child and continually check-in with their child. This is discussed in more detail below.

Parental experience and familiarity with the sport their child is participating in is common and brings the possibility of both benefits and challenges [54]. Parents' sports familiarity may help provide a deeper understanding of the details of the sport including not only logistics, but also experiences. It may also present challenges in separating personal goals, beliefs, and experiences they had from those of their child, including the pitfall of *living dreams through the child*. Participation goals should rather be framed around the child's enjoyment, skill level, experience, and development. Parents with positive sports experience are eager to support their children to share the same benefits they gained [54, 58]. However, parents with negative experiences are motivated to prevent similar experiences. As a result, they may demonstrate more empathy for various circumstances the youth may experience [54, 58]. Although empathy may be beneficial to help navigate youth sports, it can also lead to inappropriate reactive parent responses, blurring past parental experiences with those of the child's current circumstance [54]. Parents with less sports familiarity rely on others, such as other parents and coaches, to guide their reactions and behavior in the sports. Likewise, this can have both positive and negative implications from relying on the reactions of those they are deferring behavior to [54].

Approach to Supporting the Youth Athlete

We know that enjoyment of sports comes from having fun, sharing experiences with others, and finding "success." We also know that youth desire unlimited unconditional support from their parents, with very limited to no pressure. Keeping all of this in mind we look at ways parents can, logistically, support a positive youth sports experience and make good decisions throughout the process.

Parent Values

First, parents need to identify and stay true to their reasons for enrolling their child in youth sports. If the familial motivation for youth sports is friendship, fun, exercise, and life skills development, as it is for many parents, those values should drive choices and decisions. Aligning parent and family values from the beginning when selecting a sport, team, program, and environment is essential to provide a foundation on which to build. As youth navigate their sport journey at different levels of play and teams, connecting back to the original values may help guide decision-making to ensure the focus continues to be on that foundation. These values can be demonstrated in the form of conversations and reactions with the youth athlete related to navigating success and disappointment, demonstrating a culture of support modeled to the child through peer parent and coach interactions witnessed by the child.

Sport and Team/Program/Environment Selection

Selecting a sport, team, and program environment that supports positive growth and development is essential. It is important to find an environment with not only a positive culture, but also one that limits negative exposures, including a mismatch in competitive goals, negative peer or parent culture, and poor and excessively pressuring coaches. Use of a checklist such as the one developed by The Aspen Institute can help serve as a resource to ensure an environment that is safe and supports growth mindset culture and positive sport participation experience (See the Resource Section). Parents can use this as a starting point to build their own list of goals and expectations for a positive youth sports experience and make sure they align with their core values.

Sideline Behavior

Parents watching their child participate in sports can experience a range of emotional responses. Given we know children look to their parents' reactions for feedback on how they should feel and validation for their performance, parents should be mindful of body language and reactions that can be observed by youth from afar and may impact their perception of parental approval. Behavior should be respectful with positive body language and provide encouragement for both the child and team in a respectful manner that doesn't draw unnecessary attention and distraction to the child. Parents should avoid being overly loud, sideline coaching, and negative comments [11]. It is also important to be mindful of ongoing parent-peer, parent-coach, and parent-official reactions to model a supportive environment that provides an opportunity for learning.

Parent Check-In and Monitoring

Successful youth sports parents are active listeners, curious, and open to what the child is thinking and feeling. Checking in with the youth athlete on a regular basis allows opportunity to ensure the sport is still providing the desired outcomes of fun and growth and assess their enjoyment of the sport as well as feedback about parental involvement. It establishes a behavior pattern the youth can rely upon as an invitation for discussion when desired. In addition to checking in with the child, parents should periodically assess the environment of participation to make sure it continues to be a safe supportive experience.

Many sports come with some financial investment. In most circumstances, services requiring a fee also come with an expectation for the service being purchased. Parents can apply this concept to sports and make sure the fee they are paying for is resulting in the service they expect their child to receive including all the components previously discussed. If the experience and conditions of the sports are not meeting these expectations it is reasonable to provide feedback, engage in discussion, and advocate to work toward a more desirable situation. Offerings of parent coach conferences for youth athlete progress, open dialogue between the coaches when questions and concerns arise should be welcomed and appropriate updates on staffing or other changes are ideal. Finally, parents should check in with themselves to help ensure their values are being maintained and the child's experience is still the foremost goal. Using a tool such as the 100-point exercise may help parents gain clarity on their child's youth sports goals to best support them and make sure parental experiences are not influencing the child's participation. It is also reasonable to explore other options if the service provided is not meeting expectations, has undesirable consequences or inadequate results.

Parent Education

Looking for opportunities to learn more about positive parental support will help provide a foundation and allow growth as a parent. As youth sports evolve, parent education courses and classes increase as well. The resource section provides some suggestions of courses that provide tools to help navigate parental support. Youth sports organizations may offer learning opportunities to investigate as well.

Youth sports can bring incredible joy, growth, memories, and foundation for future life skills and goals. As a parent it can be a remarkable honor and pleasure to help support and facilitate the experience. Ideal youth sport-parent relationships are emotionally supportive with an optimal push, supportive of the coach without interfering with their job, and making sure participation is about the child's goals and desires, not the parents [11]. Providing an atmosphere with a foundation of fun, growth, and emotional support and encouragement will help provide the most ideal outcome for the youth athlete.

Communication Between Parent and Coach in Support of Athlete

In this chapter, we have primarily focused on the parental and coach role as distinct; however, the relationship between the family and the coach is also an important consideration. Research suggests that "organizational redundancy" is essential if sport is going to be supportive of positive youth development [59]. This means that "all agents that are part of a sport organization share a common PYD (positive youth development) philosophy" [59]. For parents, youth, and coaches to achieve positive aims of youth sports, they all have to be oriented toward those positive aims.

While the tenor and centrality of the parent-coach relationship will shift from childhood into adolescence, with the athlete having more autonomy and direct interaction with the coach as they get older, keeping the safety and needs of the athlete at the center of the parent-coach relationship is paramount. Parents and coaches each have specific roles to play in ensuring the physical and psychological safety of the athlete. Challenges may arise when either coach or parent feels the other has stepped into their domain regarding the athlete's experience. For example, coaches may want to prevent parents from talking to them about playing time and playing positions since that is largely a coaching domain. However, when the developmental needs of an athlete are being egregiously compromised by playing time and positional decisions (i.e., an 8 year old rides the bench for three games in a row or an 11 year old is considered a "pitcher only") parents have a right and responsibility to communicate directly with the coach. As noted above, parents should regularly check-in with the child and continually monitor whether the programming continues to align with the family's values, interests, and well-being. One of the challenges of youth sports is that the lines between parent and coach are often blurry and shift over the athlete's lifespan. Using the frameworks and concepts set forth in this chapter may offer some clarity as would training for both coaches and parents in youth sports setting.

One essential resource for all engaged in youth sports is SafeSport. Parents' and coaches' highest duty is to protect youth from harm. Unfortunately, due, in part, to blurry lines around roles and responsibilities and limited education and training for coaches, sexual, physical, and emotional abuse are all too prevalent in youth sport [60]. The SafeSport Parent Toolkit offers important definitions and guidelines for protecting youth from abuse in sports (see Resources). Abuse can often stem from a lack of understanding of many of the issues described in this chapter, including the specific physical, social, emotional, cognitive, and psychological needs of youth and developmentally appropriate ways to meet them. Because of the predominance of a skills and excellence model, which is often not aligned with youth developmental needs, some youth sports systems are built around practices that are potentially abusive. This means that coaches and parents might be cognizant of appropriate, supportive practices, but the program, league, or team itself has an infrastructure or system that is not safe for youth. According to Mountjoy et al. [60], these include systems which "promote over-training, the endorsement of abusive hazing rituals, the use of selection procedures which promote competing with an injury, and age cheating". For this reason, an integrated approach to safeguarding that involves all stakeholders agreeing on and identifying best practices in support of youth is the most effective.

Physical Activity

Youth sport is not the only way for children and adolescents to be physically active. In fact, since many youth drop out of sports as they move into and through adolescence, it is important for parents to keep in mind that encouraging free play, unstructured physical activity, and family movement-based activities are just as important as sports. About 75% of youth are not meeting physical activity standards set by the Centers for Disease Control and Prevention [61]. This lack of physical activity can cause a whole host of other mental and physical health problems [61]. Due to the cost of youth sports, as well as many of the challenges named above, parents should also encourage lifetime participation in physical activity by modeling it and supporting family-oriented activity time like walking in the neighborhood, biking, dance parties, and stretching and yoga.

Conclusion

A myriad of factors play a role in how children and adolescents experience sports. Parents and coaches are primary among those in mediating the sports programming and landscape so youth can experience the positive benefits. By recognizing the importance of their roles, educating themselves on the developmental needs of youth in sport and remembering children are not mini-adults, parents and coaches can have a profound impact at the individual level but also at the structural and organization level. Demanding programs that are developmentally appropriate, train coaches, and safeguard kids is the right and responsibility of all adults in the youth sports system.

References

1. Anderson-Butcher D, Riley A, Wade-Mdivanian R, Davis J, Reynolds J. Sports and youth development. In: Levesque RJR, editor. Encyclopedia of adolescence. New York: Springer; 2016. https://doi.org/10.1007/978-3-319-32132-5_372-2.

2. Fraser-Thomas J, Côté J. Youth sports: implementing findings and moving forward with research. Athl Insight. 2006;3(3):12–27.
3. Bell CC. Cultivating resiliency in youth. J Adolesc Health. 2001;29(5):375–81. https://doi.org/10.1016/S1054-139X(01)00306-8.
4. Hlavinka E. Sports a win for those with childhood trauma. 2019. https://www.medpagetoday.com/pediatrics/generalpediatrics/80105.
5. Savina E, Garrity K, Kenny P, Doerr C. The benefits of movement for youth: a whole child approach. Contemp Sch Psychol. 2016;20(3):282–92. https://doi.org/10.1007/s40688-016-0084-z.
6. Brustad RJ, Babkes ML, Smith AL. Youth in sport: psychological considerations. In: Handbook of sport psychology, vol. 2. Wiley: New York; 2001. p. 604–35.
7. Coakley J. Youth sports: what counts as "positive development?". J Sport Soc Issues. 2011;35(3):306–24. https://doi.org/10.1177/0193723511417311.
8. Neely KC, Holt NL. Parents' perspectives on the benefits of sport participation for young children. Sport Psychol. 2014;28(3):255–68.
9. Pracht DW, Houghton V, Fogarty K, Sagas M. Parents' motivations for enrolling their children in recreational sports. J Amat Sport. 2020;6(1):81–99. https://doi.org/10.17161/jas.v6i1.8250.
10. Murphy S. The cheers and the tears. San Francisco: Jossey-Bass; 1999.
11. Vealey RS, Chase MA. Best practice for youth sport. Champaign: Human Kinetics; 2016. https://books.google.com/books?id=cvF6DwAAQBAJ.
12. Weiss MR, Williams L. The why of youth sport involvement: a developmental perspective on motivational processes. In: Weiss MR, editor. Developmental sport and exercise psychology: a lifespan perspective. Queensland: Fitness Information Technology; 2004. p. 223–68.
13. Coakley J. Sports in society: issues and controversies. 13th ed. New York: McGraw-Hill; 2021. https://www.mheducation.com/highered/product/sports-society-issues-controversies-coakley/M9781260240665.html.
14. National Council of Youth Sports About Us. 2022. https://www.ncys.org/about-us/. Accessed 19 May 2022.
15. Kliethermes SA, Marshall SW, LaBella CR, Watson AM, Brenner JS, Nagle KB, Jayanthi N, Brooks MA, Tenforde AS, Herman DC, DiFiori JP, Beutler AI. Defining a research agenda for youth sport specialization in the United States: the AMSSM youth early sport specialization summit. Clin J Sport Med. 2021;31(2):103–12. https://doi.org/10.1097/JSM.0000000000000900.
16. Youth Sports Facts. Challenges. Project play. 2021. https://www.aspenprojectplay.org/youth-sports/facts/challenges#:~:text=Travel%20is%20now%20the%20costliest,%2C%20and%20camps%20(%2481. Accessed 19 May 2022.
17. Lloyd RS, Oliver JL, Faigenbaum AD, Howard R, De Ste Croix MBA, Williams CA, Best TM, Alvar BA, Micheli LJ, Thomas DP, Hatfield DL, Cronin JB, Myer GD. Long-term athletic development- part 1: a pathway for all youth. J Strength Cond Res. 2015;29(5):1439–50. https://doi.org/10.1519/JSC.0000000000000756.
18. Zwick EB, Kocher R. Growth dynamics in the context of pediatric sports injuries and overuse. Semin Musculoskelet Radiol. 2014;18(5):465–8. https://doi.org/10.1055/s-0034-1389263.
19. Muir B, Morgan G, Abraham A, Morley D. Developmentally appropriate approaches to coaching children. In: Stafford I, editor. Coaching children in sport. Abingdon: Routledge; 2011.
20. Caine D, Maffulli N, Caine C. Epidemiology of injury in child and adolescent sports: injury rates, risk factors, and prevention. Clin Sports Med. 2008;27(1):19–50. https://doi.org/10.1016/j.csm.2007.10.008.
21. Caine D. Physeal injuries in children's and youth sports: reasons for concern? Br J Sports Med. 2006;40(9):749–60. https://doi.org/10.1136/bjsm.2005.017822.
22. Malina RM, Cumming SP, Rogol AD, Coelho-e-Silva MJ, Figueiredo AJ, Konarski JM, Kozieł SM. Bio-banding in youth sports: background, concept, and application. Sports Med. 2019;49(11):1671–85. https://doi.org/10.1007/s40279-019-01166-x.

23. Patel DR, Pratt HD, Greydanus DE. Pediatric neurodevelopment and sports participation: when are children ready to play sports? Pediatr Clin. 2002;49(3):505–31. https://doi.org/10.1016/S0031-3955(02)00003-2.
24. Easterlin MC, Chung PJ, Leng M, Dudovitz R. Association of team sports participation with long-term mental health outcomes among individuals exposed to adverse childhood experiences. JAMA Pediatr. 2019;173(7):681–8. https://doi.org/10.1001/jamapediatrics.2019.1212.
25. Massey WV, Whitley MA. The role of sport for youth amidst trauma and chaos. Qual Res Sport Exerc Health. 2016;8(5):487–504. https://doi.org/10.1080/2159676X.2016.1204351.
26. Noel-London K, Ortiz K, BeLue R. Adverse childhood experiences (ACEs) & youth sports participation: does a gradient exist? Child Abuse Negl. 2021;113:104924. https://doi.org/10.1016/j.chiabu.2020.104924.
27. Chawla N, Tom A, Sen MS, Sagar R. Psychological impact of COVID-19 on children and adolescents: a systematic review. Indian J Psychol Med. 2021;43(4):294–9.
28. Miner J. Why 70% of kids quit sports by age 13. Washington post. 2016. https://www.washingtonpost.com/news/parenting/wp/2016/06/01/why-70-percent-of-kids-quit-sports-by-age-13/.
29. Youth Sports Playbook. Project play. https://www.aspenprojectplay.org/youth-sports/playbook.
30. Merkel DL. Youth sport: positive and negative impact on young athletes. Open Access J Sports Med. 2013;4:151–60. https://doi.org/10.2147/OAJSM.S33556.
31. Smoll FL, and Smith RE. Mastery approach to coaching manual—English PDF reinforcement motivation. Scr Theol. 2009. https://www.scribd.com/doc/296000407/Mastery-Approach-to-Coaching-Manual-English.
32. Vella S, Perlman D. Mastery, autonomy and transformational approaches to coaching: common features and applications. Int Sport Coach J. 2014;173–179:173. https://doi.org/10.1123/iscj.2013-0020.
33. Weiss MR, Wiese-Bjornstal DM. Promoting positive youth development through physical activity. Pres Counc Phys Fit Sports Res Dig. 2009;10:1–8.
34. Smith RE, Smoll FL, Cumming SP. Effects of a 2008 motivational climate intervention for coaches on young athletes' sport performance anxiety. J Sport Exerc Psychol. 2007;29(1):39–59. https://doi.org/10.1123/jsep.29.1.39.
35. Fawver B, Beatty GF, Roman JT, Kurtz K. The status of youth coach training in the United States: existing programs and room for improvement. Int Sport Coach J. 2020;7(2):239–51.
36. Vickers B, Schoenstedt L. Coaching development: methods for youth sport introduction. Strategies. 2011;24(4):14–9.
37. Kim S, Connaughton DP, Spengler J, Lee JH. Legislative efforts to reduce concussions in youth sports: an analysis of state concussion statutes. J Legal Asp Sport. 2017;27:162.
38. Project Play. State of play: trends and developments in youth sport. 2019. www.ProjectPlay.us.
39. Nelson LJ, Cushion CJ, Potrac P. Formal, nonformal and informal coach learning: A holistic conceptualisation. International journal of sports science & coaching. 2006;1(3):247–59.
40. Lemyre F, Trudel P, Durand-Bush N. How youth-sport coaches learn to coach. The sport psychologist. 2007;21(2):191–209.
41. McCleery J, Hoffman JL, Tereschenko I, Pauketat R. Ambitious coaching core practices: borrowing from teacher education to inform coach development pedagogy. Int Sport Coach J. 2021;1(aop):1–12.
42. Edmondson A. Psychological safety and learning behavior in work teams. Adm Sci Q. 1999;44:350–83. https://doi.org/10.2307/2666999.
43. Gosai J, Jowett S, Nascimento-Júnior JRAD. When leadership, relationships and psychological safety promote flourishing in sport and life. Sports Coach Rev. 2021;0(0):1–21. https://doi.org/10.1080/21640629.2021.1936960.
44. Edmondson AC, Harvey JF. Extreme teaming: lessons in complex, cross-sector leadership. New York: Emerald Group; 2017.
45. Nicholls JG. Achievement motivation: conceptions of ability, subjective experience, task choice, and performance. Psychol Rev. 1984;91(3):328. https://doi.org/10.1037/0033-295X.91.3.328.

46. Quested E, Duda J. Enhancing children's positive sport experiences and personal development: a motivational perspective. In: Stafford I, editor. Coaching children in sport. London: Routledge; 2011. p. 123–38.
47. Gould D, Flett R, Lauer L. The relationship between psychosocial developmental and the sports climate experienced by underserved youth. Psychol Sport Exerc. 2012;13(1):80–7.
48. Thompson J. The power of double-goal coaching: developing winners in sports and life. Portola Valley, CA: Balance Sports Publishing; 2010.
49. Bean C, Kramers S, Forneris T, Camiré M. The implicit/explicit continuum of life skills development and transfer. Quest. 2018;70(4):456–70. https://doi.org/10.1080/00336297.201 8.1451348.
50. Danish SJ, Petitpas AJ, Hale BD. Life development intervention for athletes: life skills through sports. Couns Psychol. 1993;21(3):352–85.
51. Newman T, Black S, Santos F, Jefka B, Brennan N. Coaching the development and transfer of life skills: a scoping review of facilitative coaching practices in youth sports. Int Rev Sport Exerc Psychol. 2021;1–38:1. https://doi.org/10.1080/1750984X.2021.1910977.
52. Jowett S, Shanmugam V. Relational coaching in sport: its psychological underpinnings and practical effectiveness. In: Schinke RJ, McGannon KR, Smith B, editors. Routledge International handbook of sport psychology. Abingdon: Routledge; 2016. p. 471–84.
53. Wachsmuth S, Jowett S. Conflict and communication in coach–athlete relationships. In The Routledge International Encyclopedia of Sport and Exercise Psychology. Routledge. 2020. p. 192–212.
54. Knight CJ, Dorsch TE, Osai KV, Haderlie KL, Sellars PA. Influences on parental involvement in youth sport. Sport Exerc Perform Psychol. 2016;5(2):161–78. https://doi.org/10.1037/ spy0000053.
55. Hoyle RH, Leff SS. The role of parental involvement in youth sport participation and performance. Adolescence. 1997;32(125):233.
56. Lauer L, Gould D, Roman N, Pierce M. Parental behaviors that affect junior tennis player development. Psychol Sport Exerc. 2010;11(6):487–96.
57. Brenner JS, Council on Sports Medicine and Fitness. Sports specialization and intensive training in young athletes. Pediatrics. 2016;138(3):e20162148. https://doi.org/10.1542/peds.2016-2148. PMID: 27573090
58. Knight CJ. Revealing findings in youth sport parenting research. Kinesiol Rev. 2019;8(3):252–9.
59. Santos F, Gould D, Strachan L. Research on positive youth development-focused coach education programs: future pathways and applications. Int Sport Coach J. 2019;6(1):132–8. https://doi.org/10.1123/iscj.2018-0013.
60. Mountjoy M, Rhind DJ, Tiivas A, Leglise M. Safeguarding the child athlete in sport: a review, a framework and recommendations for the IOC youth athlete development model. Br J Sports Med. 2015;49(13):883–6.
61. Centers for Disease Control and Prevention. Physical activity facts. https://www.cdc.gov/healthyschools/physicalactivity/facts.htm. Accessed 19 May 2022.

Chapter 11
Mental Skills Training and Treatment Interventions

Kelsey L. Griffith, Chelsea Butters Wooding, Erika D. Van Dyke, and Peter Kadushin

Key Points
- Mental skills training helps athletes strengthen their adaptability, confidence, and resilience to better navigate adversity and reach optimal performance in sport.
- While much of the research focuses on mental skills training with older, more elite athletes, these sorts of services are equally as valuable for youth athletes.
- In applied sport psychology, mental skills consultants combine the science of mental skills training with creativity and flexibility to best address and support the unique needs and circumstances of each client.
- Developing the athlete's mental skills toolbox requires an understanding that strategies are not hard-and-fast rules, but rather guides to building skills to better performance (i.e., stress management, imagery, self-talk, goal setting).

K. L. Griffith (✉)
Division of Sports Medicine, Boston Children's Hospital, Boston, MA, USA
e-mail: kelsey.griffith@childrens.harvard.edu

C. B. Wooding
Department of Exercise Science, North Park University, Chicago, IL, USA
e-mail: cwooding@northpark.edu

E. D. Van Dyke
Department of Psychology, Springfield College, Springfield, MA, USA
e-mail: evandyke@springfieldcollege.edu

P. Kadushin
Fifth Third Arena, Chicago, IL, USA
e-mail: pkadushin@blackhawks.com

Introduction

The aim of mental skills training (MST) is to help athletes achieve optimal performance [1]. MST educates athletes on cognitive behavioral strategies in a way that promotes sport- and non-sport successes [1]. Much like a strength and conditioning specialist, whose job is to aid an athlete's physical development, the role of a mental skills specialist is to enhance the athlete's mental game. Simply put, MST is another piece of the athlete puzzle. MST provides athletes with strategies and tools to promote a mindset that facilitates consistent performance. When athletes feel good (i.e., confident, focused, clear-headed), they are better able to effectively navigate adversity in sport. Mental skills programs emphasize the importance of adaptability, confidence, and resilience, [2] and provide athletes with a psychological edge that allows them to more efficiently pursue excellence [3].

For a number of decades, MST programs have provided athletes with strategies for improved performance, including education on goal setting, self-talk, imagery, relaxation, pre-competition routines, and arousal control [4–10]. There is a growing body of evidence that mindfulness- and psychological skills-based training promote mental toughness and optimize performance [11–14]. For instance, psychological skills training has been seen to improve strategies such as imagery, self-talk, goal setting, and arousal regulation [1, 15, 16]. Athletes trained in motivational self-talk demonstrate improved task performance, increased self-confidence, and decreased cognitive anxiety. Those trained in mindfulness-based stress reduction (MSBR) [12] and mindful sport performance [11] have shown improvement in areas such as psychological well-being, sleep quality, coping skills, performance, mental toughness, and emotional regulation.

Building upon past research and models, Vealey outlined a variety of mental skills essential to the success of athletes [1]. Separated into four categories, Vealey's model includes foundation skills, performance skills, personal development skills, and team skills. Within these categories exist skills such as drive, confidence, information processing, attentional focus, energy management, sense of relatedness, team cohesion, and communication. Vealey argues that MST is a multifaceted process wherein the consultant's individual approach, in combination with evidence-based techniques and strategies, combines to create a helpful, guiding framework for intervention [1].

Many people believe the myth that sport and performance psychology, and by extension MST, is a relatively new field. Actually, interest in the psychology of sport began in the late 1800s with experiments looking at a variety of topics, including reaction and movement time in athletes [17] and the effects of an audience on performance [18]. It is true that MST and consulting has gained in popularity in the last quarter century [19]; however, myths about the field still abound. Therefore, before diving into various strategies and skills that might be helpful, it is important to first understand the nature of MST.

It is often assumed that MST is most (if not only) beneficial when performers are experiencing a slump. Similarly, a common misperception is that MST is another form of clinical therapy. The goal of MST is to help performers of all types reach their potential through developing helpful mental strategies. In other words, the purpose of mental training is to "help people excel at the mental game for both

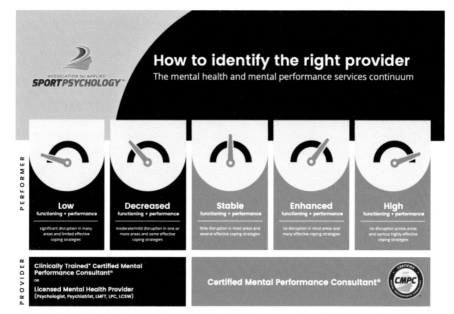

Fig. 11.1 The mental health and mental performance continuum is a guide to help athletes seeking support identify the appropriate provider based on circumstance. (Reprinted from The Association for Applied Sport Psychology. Accessed March 4th, 2022. https://appliedsportpsych.org/site/assets/files/33107/aasp_mental_health_services_continuum.pdf)

short- and long-term gains, which includes improved performance, health and happiness" [20]. Clinical therapy and counseling are crucial tools for performers, as research consistently shows that athletes do struggle with mental health concerns, [21] but clinical psychology and MST are unique disciplines. MST can be helpful when performance is suffering, but it can be just as helpful while performance is going well. In fact, MST and consulting is designed to benefit clients when performance is stable, enhanced, or high (see Fig. 11.1). By its nature, MST is educational, intended to teach skills, strategies, and information to athletes and performers interested in improving their mental approach to performance [22]. Just like an effective care team has both a Strength and Conditioning Coach (to build strength and prevent injury) along with an Athletic Trainer (to care for performers after injury has occurred), mental performance consulting allows performers to develop a strong foundation of tools and strategies to use in various performance domains, while clinical therapy and counseling are valuable when there are clinical mental health concerns that could also be impacting performance.

Crucially important to understand when working with mental skills is that, just like physical skills, mental skills take deliberate practice, patience, and time; it is *not* a "quick fix." Although language such as focus, confidence, and relaxation are common in most performance domains, the techniques behind developing skills to direct our focus, build our confidence, and manage our energy are complex.

Engaging in MST requires commitment from all involved [19, 20] along with time and self-discipline [23]. The greatest benefits from MST occur when mental skills can be rehearsed in practice on a day-to-day basis, offering performers opportunities to build their confidence in using mental skills appropriately when it matters most [23]. Reminding performers that they will get out of MST what they put into it, just like they do at practice or rehearsal, can be helpful to maintain realistic expectations of the process and hard work that will be involved.

Defining Mental Skills Training

What is it?	What is it not?
• Part of the athlete's toolbox in achieving optimal sport performance	• Something to engage in only when there's a problem
• Backed by evidential support and research	• The same as mental health
• A subset of training that requires intentional practice	• Training to eliminate all challenge in sport
	• Training that takes little time, dedication, or effort
• Training to develop strategies to navigate adversity in sport	• Something you have or you don't

Mental Skills Training with Youth Athletes

Much of the existing research on the efficacy of MST programs focuses on the performance of older, more elite athletes [24]. As a highly client-centered practice, the most effective MST will be geared toward the needs of the client at hand. Thus, while not necessary to "reinvent the wheel," it would benefit those working with youth athletes to take into consideration the developmental state of this subset of clients [25]. To look at youth athletes as identical to adult athletes would be a disservice. While the mental skills strategies employed with older athletes certainly have applicability with youth athletes, being sure to adapt these skills in a creative, age-appropriate way is essential [25]. Recent estimates report that, in the United States, close to 45 million children participate in sport [26]. Based on Wylleman and Lavallee's Long-Term Athlete Development Model, there are a number of changes that occur for the young athlete as they move through their athletic, psychological, and psychosocial development [27]. For those between ages 6 and 11, there starts to be improvement in language and communication, followed by the development of more abstract thought during adolescence [28]. Keeping in mind the physical, cognitive, emotional, and social growth that occurs during this time, one can assume that youth sport offers a unique opportunity for MST. Researchers have argued that during these formative years, youth athletes' understanding of achievement motivation and resultant definitions of success and failure are most likely to be influenced [29, 30]. If introduced to MST at a young, malleable age, youth athletes may develop more positive—and thus facilitative—perceptions of their athletic capabilities, which could increase their capacity for growth athletically and otherwise.

As proposed by Orlick and McCaffrey, the youth athlete population requires a different level of engagement in order to most positively benefit from MST [31]. They suggest that the best MST for kids keeps fun at the forefront. Approaching it from this lens, exercises should be simple, active, and creative [31]. For instance, an exercise on focus might involve developing patterns and tossing stuffed animals in those respective patterns, all the while increasing speed and complexity of task. To stop there, however, would be a disservice, as the young athlete's ability to transfer what's done in the exercise to its parallel in sport is likely far less innate than in an older population [28]. Thus, it is the responsibility of the consultant to engage in effective debriefing so those involved have the opportunity to process and collaborate with teammates, ask questions, and make connections between the exercises taught and their applicability to sport performance [25].

The better able mental skills consultants are to reach this particularly impressionable population, the greater the chance that such training may become a part of the game. As explained by Harwood and colleagues, with these sorts of services at their disposal, youth athletes have a choice as to what extent they invest in their mental skills [30]. They can decide whether to actively pursue MST with the same kind of vigor they do their physical training. They can decide whether to *trust* in MST when they encounter any one of the many difficulties so inherent in sport. Ultimately, these choices will impact the successes of the young athlete. [30] If consultants can attain buy-in at the youth sport level, the young athlete's chance for achievement—and enjoyment!—in sport will see far greater reach.

The Science and Art of Mental Skills Consulting

Sport and Performance Psychology is a scientific field rooted in the use of empirical evidence [32]. Relying on sound science provides a strong foundation for effective consulting work, and will be the crux of much of the evidence provided in this chapter. Of equal import, however, is the "art" of consulting, recognizing the unique contexts, settings, and individuals with whom we work. Preparation for any consultant is crucial, and that involves understanding the science guiding one's decisions. As the work begins and develops, however, flexibility becomes key. For instance, being able to recognize when a well-established plan requires changing (or completely abandoning) once in front of the client is an essential skill of the consultant [33]. Various situations inherently change the reality in which consultants must effectively work, and thus pre-packaged mental training programs become ineffective because they do not account for individual needs and circumstances [22]. Effective mental performance consultants will adjust their approach for what works with the athlete in front of them. In other words, there is no "right" or "wrong" approach to MST; instead, consultants understand the science behind various effective approaches and creatively select the approach that best fits this client in this moment in this context.

One variable that might impact a consultant's selection of various interventions is their theoretical orientation. As defined by Poznanski and McLennan, a theoretical orientation is "a conceptual framework used by a [practitioner] to understand client therapeutic needs" [34]. A theoretical orientation serves as a sort of "tool belt" that consultants can fill with various tools that serve various functions, including general skills like expressing empathy, confrontation skills, and asking open-ended questions, or more specific theoretical tools like cognitive modification (Cognitive-Behavioral), unconditional positive regard (Person-Centered), or meaning identification (Existential) [35]. While some consultants work from a single theoretical orientation, others use strategies and approaches of various orientations, creating an eclectic approach [36]. A thorough discussion of the various orientations popular in sport and performance psychology is beyond the scope of this chapter, however interested readers are encouraged to consider Halbur and Halbur, [35] Corey, [37] or Jarvis [36].

Rather than thinking of sport and performance psychology as either scientific or artistic, effective consultants understand the value and importance of both. As we discuss various skills and strategies that might be helpful with youth athletes, please note that these are not hard-and-fast rules that can be applied to all settings. As is true in so many professions, balancing sound empirical evidence with creative approaches to each client and situation leads to the best outcomes for all.

Mental Skills Consulting: A Case Study

To help readers understand mental skills that might be useful in work with youth athletes and the application of those skills, the following case study will be used to explore potential approaches in applied practice.

> **Exercise 1**
> *Kiara is a 12-year-old female soccer player. Recently, Kiara switched club teams in order to gain more experience playing at a higher competitive level. After her first few months with her new club, Kiara notices that she performs well in practice, but is not as consistent as she would like to be during games. She is playing well, but not necessarily up to her full potential. In noticing these newer – and somewhat unfamiliar – patterns in her performance, Kiara wants to learn some mental skills that might help her perform up to her potential, no matter the setting.*

Stress Management: The What and The Why

Sport presents both a demanding and rewarding environment in which athletes can learn physical, psychological, and social skills [38]. At the same time, positive growth and well-being are not guaranteed, and are contingent upon the environment created, the disposition and resources of the athlete, and the timing and type of stressors within the sport environment [38]. Youth sport, specifically, has a number of positive benefits for youth athletes, but can also impact participants negatively, such as physical (e.g., injuries) and psychological (e.g., pressure to improve and reach elite levels) risk [39].

According to Passer, the stress process involves four stages: (a) a demanding or opportunistic situation, (b) the person's appraisal of the situation based on the demand and available resources (e.g., either a threat or a challenge), (c) an emotional response occurring (in the instance of stress, this is an unpleasant or aversive emotional response), and (d) consequences occurring (e.g., behavioral, health-related, psychological, performance) [40]. The consequences of one situation can then start the four-step process over again, creating a stress cycle [40]. Understanding the relationship between the demands of a situation and the skills and resources to which the athlete has access to meet those demands allow for the prediction of whether a situation is appraised as a threat (i.e., demands > resources), or a challenge (i.e., resources > demands) [41].

Kellmann's work on burnout in sport highlights the nature of stress and recovery and how stress can shift from facilitative to detrimental [42]. Short-term stress (e.g., a practice session) where demand is balanced with athlete resources, followed by rest and recovery, allows for growth and consolidation. Kellmann's model shows that as the acute demand increases, the need for increased recovery arises [42]. Eventually, stress may outpace an individual's capacity for recovery, at which point an unsustainable cycle of distress takes hold, which is associated with overtraining, burnout, and significant negative physical and psychological consequences [43]. Understanding the factors associated with stress appraisal is critical, as stress is a necessary ingredient for both growth and peak performance, and can be detrimental when applied without a clear purpose or when the demand outpaces an athlete's resources and capacity to recover.

For many youth athletes, sport can become quite stressful. Therefore, learning effective coping strategies through various stress management approaches can help athletes both in and out of sport [44]. Generally, research has shown that youth athletes do not experience more significant stress when participating in sport than in other performance domains [45]. Yet, sport can be highly demanding and filled with various stressors, and that stress seems to only increase as youth become more talented [46]. For instance, youth and adolescent athletes often navigate dual career experiences, balancing their roles as both athlete and student [47]. Also, certain sport cultures, such as football, emphasize the athlete role over other roles in the athletes' lives [48]. The types of stressors experienced by youth athletes can change over time, and negative consequences can arise when stressors are not coped with effectively [49].

Sources of stress in sport are numerous, but Thatcher and Day argue that understanding the underlying properties of sport that lead to stress might help consultants teach clients to reduce stressful appraisals [50]. Lazarus and Folkman listed eight properties of stress that can impact a person's appraisal: novelty, predictability, event uncertainty, imminence, duration, temporal uncertainty, ambiguity, and timing of events in relation to the life cycle [51]. Thatcher and Day showed applicability of those properties to a sporting context, and added two others relevant to sport: self and other comparison, and preparation [50]. Stressors in sport can also be related to performance (i.e., preparation, injury, expectations, self-presentation, and rivalry) or the organization (i.e., factors intrinsic to the sport, organizational structure and climate of the sport, athletic career and performance development issues, sport relationships and interpersonal demands, and roles in the sport organization) [52].

There are significant individual differences in youth athletes' experiences of stress, and stakeholders in sport would benefit from teaching youth athletes stress management strategies that could help them manage stress in all areas of their lives, sport included [45]. Inside classrooms, various stress management programs have shown positive outcomes such as increasing coping skills and minimizing the symptoms of stress [53]. Trainings as short as 10 min a day were effective in decreasing anxiety symptoms, providing students skills they could use to better cope with stressors [54]. Stress management programs using a train-the-trainer approach (i.e., training teachers how to teach stress management to their students) also improved academic achievement and classroom social climate [55]. Similar positive outcomes are seen in sporting environments, like enhancing performance through helping athletes modify or control elements of the stress process [56].

Stress Management: The How

Changing Appraisal

There are times when it is appropriate and effective to help an athlete adjust their appraisal of a stressful situation to change their perception of the balance between demands and resources. It is important to recognize that not all stressors are healthy or productive, and that facilitating a shift from threat to challenge is not appropriate in every case.

There are two entry points for shifting the appraisal of a stressful situation. An athlete can either change the way they are thinking about the demands of the situation, or they can shift the way they are feeling about their skills and resources. For either approach, it is important to keep the athlete grounded in reality, rather than magical thinking. The athlete is not changing either the demand or their resources, so much as they are shifting their attention and self-talk to frame the demands as more manageable or to recognize the skills and resources they have already developed.

Exercise 2
To shift her appraisal of the situational demands, Kiara could:

- shorten her timescale and give herself permission to only feel responsible for the present moment while she's playing, rather than feeling overwhelmed by the whole game;
- recognize explicitly that the pitch, ball, and rules of the game do not change between practice and a game, even if the experience of pressure or expectation might feel different between the two spaces;

- focus on her specific role within each game, allowing her to shift from an outcome focus (e.g., winning, getting the best stats) to a task focus (e.g., improving in a specific area, focusing on one element of her role or position).

To shift her appraisal of her skills and resources, Kiara could:

- reflect on the progress she has made throughout her soccer career and remember the tools she has successfully used in the past to continue improving;
- communicate with the coaches that she is interested in learning and growing, and ask them for clear strategies she might be able to practice and use in game settings;
- build awareness to the conscious or unconscious pressure she is putting on herself in game settings (e.g., "I have to," "I should," "I need to") and return to thoughts that are more helpful for her (e.g., "I want to").

NOTE: When working with youth athletes, using the analogy of movies can be helpful. When a hero meets a villain, they have a demand being asked of them (e.g. beat the "bad guy") and they have resources (e.g. their "super powers" and fellow superheroes) to meet that demand. In helping Kiara shift her appraisals, this analogy might help her identify both the specific demands and resources available to her to become the hero of her story.

Breathing Strategies

Deep breathing has been shown as an effective strategy in improving mood and decreasing stress [57]. When stressed, our breathing tends to become fast and irregular [58]. However, diaphragmatic breathing can improve both sustained attention and affect [59].

Athletes can be trained to simply bring awareness to where they are feeling their breath. Diaphragmatic breathing is a specific strategy that teaches athletes to contract their diaphragm, drawing air down into the body, increasing diaphragm length, and making breathing more efficient [60]. When working with youth athletes, instructing them to place their hands, one on top of the other, on top of their diaphragm, then to think of their diaphragm as a balloon, can help them start creating a mind-body connection. If they are comfortable, asking them to close their eyes, and to see the balloon filling up (inhale) and emptying (exhale) can give them a visual aid to help maintain their focus. Although consultants understand the diaphragm contracts and, in actuality, flattens on the inhale to create space for the air, following the cue of their belly rising and falling can help athletes understand how to connect to, and deliberately change (if needed), their breathing.

Exercise 3
There are a number of different ways to teach breathing strategies. Below is a description of BOX BREATHING: [61]
    BOX BREATHING—*the how to:*

    Inhale for a count of four
    Hold for a count of four
    Exhale for a count of four
    Hold for a count of four

    NOTE: The count can also change based on a person's comfort and ability (e.g., shorter or longer).

Self-Efficacy

In 1977, Albert Bandura outlined Self-Efficacy Theory as a new approach to behavior change [62]. According to Bandura, self-efficacy—our beliefs about our abilities to effectively perform specific tasks within specific domains [63]—is impacted through four major sources: performance accomplishments, vicarious experience, verbal persuasion, and emotional arousal [62]. Although Kiara has not specifically discussed concerns about her self-efficacy, not playing up to her potential in games could be causing her to question her abilities. Using Bandura's approach to help Kiara build her self-efficacy might also help minimize her stress.

To focus on performance accomplishments, Kiara could be asked to think back to a time when she was able to perform well. What were the skills and strategies that helped then? What would it look like to incorporate those now? Vicarious experience is the second strongest source of self-efficacy, which can be built through watching others being successful or visualizing (through imagery) one's own abilities and strengths. A consultant might ask Kiara about other players she looks up to, and what she might learn from them? [1] Imagery (to be discussed below) could also be used as a vicarious experience. Exploring the verbal persuasion in Kiara's life is the third source of self-efficacy. What are other people in her life telling her, and what is she telling herself? Though she cannot necessarily change others, building awareness of her own self-talk (to be discussed below) might help increase her self-efficacy, and thus decrease her stress. The fourth and final source of self-efficacy is emotional arousal, which can be helped through a variety of relaxation strategies, including those discussed above.

---

[1] It might be helpful here to teach Kiara about the "Iceberg Illusion" [123]. When learning from the accomplishments of others, it can be important to help athletes remember that we often only see the 10% of their best (the part of the iceberg outside of the water). Rarely do we get to see the blood, sweat, and tears the athlete poured in behind the scenes (the 90% of the iceberg under the water).

Imagery: The What and The Why

Imagery is a multi-sensory recreation of a past-lived experience, and is a commonly used technique in MST [64, 65]. Imagery helps improve sport performance through the mental practice of skill development, emotional regulation, and attention control [66, 67]. To best reap the benefits of this tool, athletes must not only be able to conjure the image of their performance, but also control what they're seeing [65]. Through practice and repetition, imagery use can assist athletes in re-patterning the ways they think about, engage with, and interpret challenging situations. Imagery targets parts of the brain that are active during motor planning and execution [68]. Imagery and motor performance possess similar neural mechanisms to the extent that training both systems have the potential to improve physical output [69, 70].

Imagery can benefit athletes in a number of ways. The idea is to create a mental movie in which the athlete is the sole director. To help better understand why athletes engage in imagery, Paivio developed a conceptual framework to explore two distinct functions of this skill [71]. He proposed that the function of cognitive imagery is to help athletes envision sport skills (cognitive-specific) and game strategy (cognitive-general). In this sense, imagery works to improve athletes' physical skill and performance output [72, 73]. The framework went on to say that motivational imagery helps athletes experience goal achievement (motivational-specific), arousal regulation (motivation-general arousal), and skill mastery (motivational-general mastery) [71, 74]. Just as cognitive-specific and cognitive-general imagery speaks to the athlete's physical game, motivational-specific, motivational-general arousal, and motivational-general-specific bolster facets of the athlete's mental game. Researchers have found that athletes who use this type of imagery see improvement in things such as confidence [75] and drive [76].

To help athletes in successful creation of their own mental movies, Holmes and Collins set forth the PETTLEP imagery model, a checklist to assist in the creation of effective imagery scripts, where the acronym stands for physical, environment, task, timing, learning, emotion, and perspective [77]. This model is meant to help the athlete "[match] closely the imagined and actual skill-learning environments" [78]. In essence, a process such as this speaks to a "been there, done that" mindset, wherein the athlete not only strengthens the neural priming of the skill and performance, but also gleans confidence in knowing they have successfully executed said skill and performance once (or many times!) before.

While much of the past research has focused on the benefits of imagery in older populations, there is evidence that imagery also serves youth athletes in terms of performance output, strategy, and motivation [79–82]. Important to keep in mind, however, is the development of imagery skill for this particular population. This is critical for the mental skills consultant looking to engage youth athletes in imagery work, given that imagery ability—or athletes' capability of creating clear, strong, effective images of performance—starts to fully take shape and evolves significantly between five and 17 years of age [83, 84].

Imagery: The How

Imagery Mad Libs®

Drafting an imagery script can be a helpful first step in creating the athlete's mental movie. Some athletes may find it challenging to conjure the sensory and emotional details essential in this process. A fun, interactive way for young athletes to develop their imagery-crafting skills is to format the script as a sort-of imagery Mad Libs®. With first time imagers, the consultant might choose to include the word bank to help generate ideas. As the exercise progresses, the aim would be for the athlete to elicit language that is more personal and connected to their own performance. Alternatively, for athletes with more experience in imagery, the Mad Libs® could be entirely self-generated. In this instance, the consultant and athlete would work collaboratively to fill in the blanks and adapt the language for specificity of sport before recording the script aloud or leading it live. Below is an example of how consultants might engage the athlete in this process.

Exercise 4

As you stand, getting ready for practice, notice your body feeling loose and ready. As you begin your stretches, look to your left and right and take in your surroundings. As you notice _____, you can feel yourself getting ____ for practice. Specifically, you're thinking about _____ and how you're going to work hard to get better at it today.

You notice some of your teammates nearby, and see them _____. You smile, _____ to see some of your friends and _____ to spend some time with them today.

As you continue to move and stretch your body and breathe, you notice your body feeling more _____. The ____ under your feet feels ____ and the air on your skin is ____. You can clearly hear ____, and know that it's almost time to start practice. Before you go, you decide today is going to be _____, and you pause to really let that feeling sink into your body. You feel it in your _____, and know that it's time to have fun and get better with your teammates.

Word Bank		
Happy	Excited	Relaxed
Loose	Calm	Energized
Tingly	Ready	Pumped
Soft	Firm	Springy
Gentle	Loud	Silly
Fun	Better	Laugh

Self-Talk: The What and The Why

Self-talk has been defined as "the syntactically recognizable articulation of an internal position that can be expressed either internally or out loud, where the sender of the message is also the intended receiver" [85]. Put simply, self-talk is what we say to ourselves about ourselves. In applied sport psychology, self-talk is so commonly used that it has been considered a key part of the "canon" of psychological skills [15]. Self-talk has been widely studied among athletes in a variety of sport settings, and endorsed as a strategy for self-regulation and performance [85–87].

Drawing from self-talk theory and research, a sport-specific model of self-talk [85] was developed to help guide research and practice in sport psychology (see Fig. 11.2) [85]. In the model, self-talk is situated among personal factors (e.g., athlete preferences), contextual factors (e.g., motivational climate; sport setting), cognitive mechanisms (e.g., deliberate, effortful processing vs. more automatic, effortless processing), and behavior (e.g., performance), and the dynamic interrelationships among these factors are shown. The sport-specific model of self-talk provides both a theoretical and practical framework for understanding the features of self-talk, and relationships to the individual athlete, sport and cultural context, cognition, and behavior [85].

Hardy suggested that self-talk may be considered in terms of several key factors, including valence, function, and overtness [88]. The valence dimension refers primarily to positive, negative, and neutral self-talk. Positive self-talk refers to statements that are positive and encouraging in tone, such as "I can do it" or "That's it, keep it up!" Negative self-talk refers to statements that are negative, discouraging, or that reflect frustration or anger, such as "I feel off" or "That was terrible!" Neutral self-talk may include statements related to instruction or performance cues such as

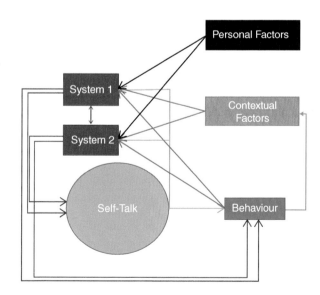

Fig. 11.2 The sport-specific model of self-talk diagrams both a theoretical and practical framework for understanding the features of self-talk, and relationships to the individual athlete, sport and cultural context, cognition, and behavior. (Reprinted from *Psychology of Sport and Exercise*, 22, Van Raalte, J. L., Vincent, A., & Brewer, B. W., Self-talk: Review and sport-specific model, 139–148, Copyright (2016), with permission from Elsevier)

"bend your knees" or other statements related to tactics or strategy such as "watch the defender." Positive self-talk has typically been shown to facilitate sport performance; [89] whereas, negative self-talk tends to be more complex. In some instances athletes may find that negative self-talk enhances motivation and performance, [90] but in general negative self-talk tends to be detrimental to sport performance [89]. Given the individual differences we see in self-talk preferences, using language such as "helpful" and "unhelpful" may be an appropriate way to discuss self-talk with athletes.

In terms of the function dimension, self-talk has often been described as serving instructional and motivational functions [86, 87]. A matching hypothesis has also been proposed, suggesting that self-talk may be most beneficial when the type of self-talk used is matched to the performance task [86]. For example, instructional self-talk may be best for fine motor tasks, whereas motivational self-talk may be best for gross motor tasks. This hypothesis has been met with mixed findings, [87] perhaps because many sports involve a blend of fine and gross performance tasks to be successful. Self-talk may also serve a variety of other self-regulatory functions, including directing attention, facilitating automatic skill execution, enhancing cognitive and emotional regulation, increasing confidence, and mobilizing effort, [91] as well as directing goal achievement [92]. Expressive and interpretive functions of self-talk have also been explored, as when athletes say something to themselves to express feelings and intuitions or to interpret performance and other sport experiences [89].

Another factor that may be considered is the overtness of self-talk [88]. For example, self-talk may be used completely internally, may be mouthed but inaudible, or may be spoken aloud. Interestingly, similarities between internal and overt self-talk have been noted through physiological research showing brain activation in areas involved in speech production [85]. Much of the self-talk science has used retrospective questionnaires to assess athletes' self-talk, although some research has explored observable self-talk [93, 94] and inner experience [95] in real-time performance. Self-talk by nature is directed toward the self, yet can influence contextual factors (i.e., coach or teammate perceptions and interactions) when articulated aloud. Learning about our athletes' preferences can help consultants be responsive to these different types of self-talk and what may resonate most with the individual.

Of primary interest to many athletes and coaches is the link between self-talk and performance. As outlined by Van Raalte and colleagues, self-talk has been found to facilitate performance in various sport settings including basketball, cycling, dressage, golf, gymnastics, running, skiing, soccer, swimming, tennis, volleyball, and water polo among others [85]. Some evidence suggests that self-talk is also beneficial for performing more consistently in sport [96–98]. Among youth athletes, self-talk has been supported as a helpful mental skill to facilitate performance [94, 99–101], as well as increase self-confidence and reduce anxiety [102, 103]. A key consideration regarding the effectiveness of using self-talk as a mental skill is believing the self-talk [93]. This may connect to notions of cognitive dissonance and consonance—when self-talk is compatible with impressions of self and abilities it tends to produce favorable experiences [85]. It is also helpful to note that just as self-talk influences performance, so too may performance influence self-talk. For instance, when an athlete performs well they may be more likely to experience positive or helpful self-talk, which may facilitate not only performance, but also well-being in sport.

Self-Talk: The How

Returning to the model of sport-specific self-talk, [85] we notice that personal and contextual factors are large influences on individual self-talk patterns. It is therefore important for consultants to keep in mind that there is often not a "one size fits all" approach. Working with athletes to tailor self-talk to their preferences is a key part of the "art" of consulting. As the science also supports self-talk as an effective mental skill for performance and performance consistency, self-talk may be quite useful in helping Kiara perform up to her potential. Equipped with the science and the art of self-talk, there are a variety of practical implications we might consider in working with Kiara.

Facilitating Awareness of Self-Talk

It is not uncommon for athletes to express the desire to rid themselves entirely of negative thoughts. The truth is that this sort of self-talk elimination is quite challenging and takes up a lot of mental space. Sometimes, the more athletes focus on *stopping* the negative thoughts, the louder they get. Think of it like playing whack-a-mole, where each time one thought gets shoved back in the hole, another unwanted one pops right up! Instead, it can be helpful to direct athletes toward thought acknowledgment and acceptance. The goal is to turn down the volume on the thoughts deemed unhelpful, and turn up the volume on those viewed as helpful or productive. Often, asking athletes to begin by noticing their typical self-talk can be a useful way to raise awareness of current patterns of internal dialogue. Depending on the helpfulness of these current self-talk patterns, consultants can work with athletes to develop intentional self-talk statements or to accept their inner experience. One approach to developing this awareness is the 3 A's of Self-Talk strategy.

Exercise 5
ACKNOWLEDGE where you're at
 ATTEMPT to make change (i.e., using established self-talk phrases)
 ACCEPT where you're at, change or not, and give your best focus to the task at hand

Further, Van Raalte and Vincent provide a collection of practical approaches to developing self-talk strategies with athletes [89]. In guiding Kiara to develop self-talk that matches her preferences, consultants might consider whether the self-talk matches the athlete's arousal level. When athletes tend to be highly activated during performance, self-talk such as "calm and confident" could be a nice fit. In contrast, when athletes tend to have lower levels of activation and need to increase their arousal or energy, self-talk such as "let's go!" could be more appropriate. Working with Kiara to develop self-talk that matches her preferences and fits the sport task can be an effective approach. This is an excellent way to encourage self-determined statements, and thus embed experiences of autonomy into athletes' MST. This has the added benefit of making self-talk feel familiar and comfortable to the athlete, and thus more easily used in sport performance.

A consultant might also consider how the self-talk Kiara uses fits with her beliefs. For example, when individuals who experience low self-esteem try to apply positive self-talk, performance decrements may follow as there is cognitive dissonance between the individual's beliefs and the self-talk used. Developing self-talk that feels true for the athlete, rather than self-talk that is overly positive or negative in tone, may be useful for facilitating performance. This links back to guiding athletes toward self-talk that is "helpful" for them.

Developing Self-Talk

When facilitating self-talk as a mental skill, it can be helpful for athletes to develop and practice their own self-talk statements. Tailoring self-talk to athletes' experiences and preferences can promote greater consonance between the chosen self-talk and the athletes' feelings, impressions, and abilities [85]. Practicing self-talk is one strategy to help make the mental skill become more natural or habitual, and thus require fewer cognitive demands while performing complex sport tasks. Given our relatively limited cognitive capacity, the more automatic we can make our mental skills through practice, the more cognitive space we have available for the task at hand.

Exercise 6

Step 1
Have the athlete free-write under the prompt, "I am my best when…"

[ex.]
I am clear-headed and calm. → breathe
I believe in my abilities. → trust
I feel ready, mentally and physically. → prepared
My teammates have my back. → supported
I realize I'm not alone on the field. ^
I play because I want to, not because I feel pressured. → "this is mine" / "own it"
I focus on one moment at a time and stay in the present moment.

STEP 2
Go through the free-write and identify if 1) any themes emerge, 2) there are certain words or phrases that stand out as important to you (see above -- highlighted in yellow) AND if these words lead to other more powerful words (see above -- highlighted in blue).

STEP 3
It can be helpful to combine *motivational self-talk* phrases (generated in STEPS 1 & 2) with *instructional self-talk* (i.e. skill specific, actionable / directional words or phrases -- "head up," "next play," "fast feet").

STEP 4
Creation of self-talk statement:
[ex.]
Want it. Trust it. Head up.

STEP 5
Self-talk is not a one-size-fits all situation, and development of phrasing is likely to morph over time in various circumstances. The aim of self-talk work is to develop statements in a way that best serves the athlete in performance and occupies as little mental space possible. Below are some tips athletes might use to help habituate their self-talk statements.
→ Write on your wrist pre-practice or pre-game.
→ Write it on a piece of paper pre-practice or pre-game and stick it in your shoe.
→ Incorporate self-talk statements into pre-performance training journals and goal setting.

Goal Setting: The What and The Why

Arnold Schwarzenegger said, "You must see it. You must believe it. And then you must never stop working to make it happen." This saying so eloquently and succinctly addresses two essential facets of goal setting, a commonly used tool within the world of MST and consulting [104, 105]. First, it is essential that athletes *dream big.* Sport is rife with challenge. The more athletes want it—whatever *it* may be— the easier it is to persist against adversity. Dreaming big and chasing after those goals is incredibly motivating; the *want* is so important. However, it can't stop there. The work athletes put in to reach those end goals—*the performance and process goals*—are the roadmap to their eventual success. When athletes overlook incremental progress and only seek out the end goal, they're likely to miss a whole lot of satisfaction along the way.

Locke and Latham proposed Goal Setting Theory (GST) as a framework to explain the purpose and function of goals [106–108]. They suggested that goal setting helps improve productivity and performance by focusing attention on a particular task, increasing invested effort and energy, encouraging greater persistence, and developing task-specific tools and strategies [107]. While the evidence stands that goals positively impact task performance, the *type* of goals and the *ways* in which goals are set are also of great import [106–110]. Things such as goal difficulty, specificity, proximity (i.e. short- versus long-term goals), and type impact goal function. Another contributor to the efficacy of goals is *how* and by *whom* goals are set.

In light of Locke and Latham's GST, it makes sense that goal setting became a go-to tool used within the sport setting [106–108]. With performance output a primary focus of sport, capitalizing on this strategy seemed a natural step in an arena where achievement sits atop the mountain of motivators. Interestingly, though, initial research regarding the value of goal setting in sport was a bit unclear. For instance, while Locke and Latham proposed that goal specificity was more effective in determining performance outcome, [111] other studies have been in opposition of this finding, stating that broader, more motivationally based goals can, too, enhance performance [112, 113]. Of interesting note, however, is the evolution of Locke & Latham's initial thoughts on goal type. Locke and Latham initially identified goal type as *learning* and *performance;* in sport, this has evolved into what many coaches and athletes are likely now familiar with—*process goals, performance goals,* and *outcome goals* [110]. As explained by Jeong and colleagues, this shift in labeling likely better accommodates the fact that while "the learning 'process' and individual 'performance' standards are dependent on one's goal commitment, … certain 'outcome' (e.g. winning a tournament) could be dependent on the opponents and external factors regardless of one's goal commitment" [114].

Harter argued that individuals have an innate drive to demonstrate competence [115, 116]. When presented with opportunities to demonstrate capability and skill proficiency, as is common in sport performance, athletes derive a sense of satisfaction in their work [115, 116]. Good breeds good. It has been shown that for most youth athletes, this drive for improvement and mastery, along with a sense of enjoyment, are at the forefront of sport participation [117, 118]. This is an important lens with which to approach goal setting with youth athletes. Amidst the many functions of goal setting should remain a strong sense of process over outcome. For youth athletes, the pursuit of success should encompass the "want tos" and the "how tos," rather than the "need tos" and the "shoulds." When athletes set regular goals for themselves—short-, medium- and long-term—they are better able to recognize the controllables and use these intermediary markers as stepping stones to success.

Goal Setting: The How

Training Journal

Using a daily training and performance journal helps athletes stay focused on the present and gives greater purpose to their training and competition. Below is a step-by-step guide for this tool. Before training and competition, athletes are instructed to set their mindset and process goals. This helps prime athletes for what's to come, providing them with an opportunity to seek out the controllables and find satisfaction in chasing their ultimate performance outcome.

Exercise 7
BEFORE TRAINING/COMPETITION:

1. The athlete is asked to set their **INTENTION.** This as an opportunity to identify their "mindset goals" for the day. The athlete is asked to take stock as to where they are, mentally, in that moment, and establish the mindset with which they want to step into training or performance.

KIARA'S **INTENTION**:

I will be patient with myself and allow myself space to make mistakes and move onto the next play.

2. The athlete is asked to set **3 FOCUS POINTS, or "baby goals."** This is their chance to reflect on past performances as a way to help guide their work in the present moment.

THINK: *how to?* ...and be specific!

KIARA'S **FOCUS POINTS**:

To *play my best, I will focus on:*

a quick first touch.

keeping my head up and looking for open space.

communicating with my teammates.

AFTER TRAINING/COMPETITION:

3. After practice/competition, it's important for the athlete to take a couple moments to **REFLECT** on their performance. *What went well? What do they want to work on tomorrow? ...the next day? How did their game plan lead them to "1% better?"*

4. To help strengthen the athlete's mental muscle of finding the positives, they are asked to finish off with **ONE WIN** from that day. *Remember: good breeds good!* The greater "collection" of wins the athlete has—big and small!—the easier it becomes to redirect focus when encountering challenge.

THE NEXT DAY OF TRAINING/COMPETITION:

...the athlete should reflect on their prior "entry" as a way to inform that day's performance.

SMART Goal Setting

While not fully grounded in empirical evidence, [119] SMART goals can be a helpful guide in terms of how to create goals that speak to process. Despite the fact that SMART goals veer off of the evidence track, the acronym's memorability [120] and practicality [119] make it a common tool across a number of performance arenas, including sport. The SMART goal template provided below is meant to help athletes identify their goals *and* create a roadmap to success.

Exercise 8

You want to get stronger?

HOW are you going to do it?

You want to improve your consistency from practice to performance?

WHAT STEPS do you need to take to get there?

Create a goal using the S.M.A.R.T guidelines. Use the below format to help create a pathway to success:

Specific

Measurable

Achievable

Realistic

Time sensitive

Kiara's *WORKING GOAL* is her S.M.A.R.T goal. What does she want to achieve?

Kiara's *PLAN OF ACTION* is the HOW. What steps does she need to take to work towards her goal?

Kiara's *ANTICIPATED BARRIERS* are the challenges she might encounter along the way. When athletes look ahead at what might be hard, they are far more prepared to navigate the challenge(s), rather than letting them stop them dead in their tracks.

Kiara's *STRATEGIES TO ADDRESS BARRIERS* are the detour. If she runs into one (or many!) of these challenges, how might she get around it?

Kiara's *SUPPORTS* are those who have her back. It's important for Kiara to remember she's not in this alone. For many, it can be helpful to create an environment wherein they feel supported and encouraged to actively pursue their goals.

Conclusion

Most athletes are quick to acknowledge the importance of the mental side of the game. And yet, many are equally as quick to acknowledge that they spend little to no time at all training their mental game. An athlete would never walk onto the field, court, ice, or stage without a proper physical warm-up. If the argument stands that a significant portion of the game is mental, why not address this facet of sport performance with equal weight? At the root of this question is the availability and accessibility of MST programs. Visek et al. argued the possibility that sport organizations, particularly those at the youth level, may be unaware that MST programs exist [25]. For those that do know about MST programs, they may be unsure of how to integrate such services into their existing sport training frameworks. Developing partnerships between mental skills consultants and local sport organizations is one way to increase program visibility and strengthen the relationships so that MST becomes a part of the game [25]. As the conversation around the athlete's mental game continues to grow, the hope is that MST and consultation at the individual and group level become more commonplace.

As the field of MST (ideally!) finds its way into the everyday practice of sport, it is important to emphasize the role of the consultant. The mental skills consultant is one who understands the science behind their work, and is able to creatively approach each client with tools and strategies to develop their mental performance [22]. This sort of work requires subject-specific training, be it from a master's or doctoral program. Hays proposed the question as to where the mental skills consultant fits within the framework of athlete well-being [121]. She asked, "as a performance consultant, are you a consultant, a coach, or a therapist" [121]? The answer is certainly complex, but Hays argues that clarification exists within "a mix of skill, focus, definition, legal regulation, clientele or setting, and common usage, as well as advertising and marketing" [121]. Regardless, those in search of a mental skills consultant want to be sure to explore the consultant's background, both educationally and experientially, to ensure the best possible outcome for the athlete [122].

For many, developing skills such as focus, confidence, and relaxation is key in achieving optimal, consistent performance. However, much like physical training, developing and strengthening mental skills tools does not happen overnight. Helping athletes understand that the work that goes into their mental game takes time is crucial in managing expectations for performance. The opportunity to work with youth athletes on the mental part of their performance is unique in that, developmentally, they are in a space to better develop constructive views of their successes and failures. Capitalizing on this mentality has the potential to positively shape the sport experience of young athletes, and set them up for growth and achievement in and outside of sport.

References

1. Vealey SR. Mental skills training in sport. In: Tenenbaum G, Eklund R, Singer R, editors. Handbook of sport psychology. Hoboken, NJ: Wiley; 2007.
2. Zinsser N, Bunker L, Williams JM. Cognitive techniques for building confidence and enhancing performance. In: Applied sport psychology: personal growth to peak performance. New York: McGraw-Hill; 2006. p. 349–81.
3. Jones G, Hanton S, Connaughton D. What is this thing called mental toughness? An investigation of elite sport performers. J Appl Sport Psychol. 2002;14(3):205–18.
4. Blakeslee ML, Goff DM. The effects of a mental skills training package on equestrians. Sport Psychol. 2007;21(3):288–301.
5. Brewer BW, Shillinglaw R. Evaluation of a psychological skills training workshop for male intercollegiate lacrosse players. Sport Psychol. 1992;6(2):139–47.
6. Gould D, Hodge K, Petlichkoff L, Simons J. Evaluating the effectiveness of a psychological skills educational workshop. Sport Psychol. 1990;4(3):249–60.
7. Greenspan MJ, Feltz DL. Psychological interventions with athletes in competitive situations: a review. Sport Psychol. 1989;3(3):219–36.
8. Martin GL, Vause T, Schwartzman L. Experimental studies of psychological interventions with athletes in competitions: why so few? Behav Modif. 2005;29(4):616–41.
9. Meyers M, Leunes A, Bourgeois A. Psychological skills assessment and athletic performance in collegiate rodeo athletes. J Sport Behav. 1996;19:132–46.
10. Weinberg RS, Comar W. The effectiveness of psychological interventions in competitive sport. Sports Med. 1994;18(6):406–18.
11. Ajilchi B, Amini HR, Ardakani ZP, Zadeh MM, Kisely S. Applying mindfulness training to enhance the mental toughness and emotional intelligence of amateur basketball players. Australas Psychiatry. 2019;27(3):291–6.
12. Jones BJ, Kaur S, Miller M, Spencer RMC. Mindfulness-based stress reduction benefits psychological well-being, sleep quality, and athletic performance in female collegiate rowers. Front Psychol. 2020;11:2373.
13. Röthlin P, Birrer D, Horvath S, Grosse HM. Psychological skills training and a mindfulness-based intervention to enhance functional athletic performance: design of a randomized controlled trial using ambulatory assessment. BMC Psychol. 2016;4(1):1–11.
14. Röthlin P, Horvath S, Trösch S, Holtforth MG, Birrer D. Differential and shared effects of psychological skills training and mindfulness training on performance-relevant psychological factors in sport: a randomized controlled trial. BMC Psychol. 2020;8(1):1–13.
15. Andersen MB. The "canon" of psychological skills training for enhancing performance. In: Performance psychology in action: a casebook for working with athletes, performing artists, business leaders, and professionals in high-risk occupations. Washington, DC: American Psychological Association; 2009. p. 11–34.
16. Hardy L, Jones GJ, Gould D. Understanding psychological preparation for sport: theory and practice of elite performers. Chichester: Wiley; 1996.
17. Scripture EW. Tests of mental ability as exhibited in fencing. Stud Yale Psychol Lab. 1894;2:122–4.
18. Triplett N. The dynamogenic factors in pacemaking and competition. Am J Psychol. 1898;9:507–53.
19. Fifer A, Henschen K, Gould D, Ravizza K. What works when working with athletes. Sport Psychol. 2008;22(3):356–77.
20. Halliwell W, Orlick T, Ravizza K, Rotella B. Consultants guide to excellence for sport and performance enhancement. Chelsea, PQ: Zone of Excellence; 2003.
21. Chang C, Putukian M, Aerni G, Diamond A, Hong G, Ingram Y, et al. Mental health issues and psychological factors in athletes: detection, management, effect on performance and prevention: American medical Society for Sports Medicine Position Statement-Executive Summary. Br J Sports Med. 2020;54(4):216–20.

22. Ravizza K. Sport psych consultation issues in professional baseball. Sport Psychol. 1990;4(4):330–40.
23. Ravizza K. Gaining entry with athletic personnel for season-long consulting. Sport Psychol. 1988;2(3):243–54.
24. Sharp LA, Woodcock C, Holland MJG, Cumming J, Duda JL. A qualitative evaluation of the effectiveness of a mental skills training program for youth athletes. Sport Psychol. 2013;27(3):219–32.
25. Visek AJ, Harris BS, Blom LC. Doing sport psychology: a youth sport consulting model for practitioners. Sport Psychol. 2009;23(2):271–91.
26. Swanson B. Youth sports participation by the numbers. ACTIVEkids. https://www.active-kids.com/football/articles/youth-sports-participation-by-the-numbers. Accessed 3 Mar 2022.
27. Wylleman P, Lavallee D. A developmental perspective on transitions faced by athletes. In: Weiss M, editor. Developmental sport and exercise psychology: a lifespan perspective. Queensland: Fitness Information Technology; 2004. p. 507–27.
28. Vernon A. Working with children, adolescents, and their parents: practical application of developmental theory. In: Vernon A, editor. Counseling children and adolescents. Denver, CO: Love Publishing; 2004. p. 163–87.
29. Harwood C, Swain A. The development and activation of achievement goals within tennis: II. A player, parent, and coach intervention. Sport Psychol. 2002;16(2):111–37.
30. Harwood C, Cumming J, Fletcher D. Motivational profiles and psychological skills use within elite youth sport. J Appl Sport Psychol. 2004;16(4):318–32.
31. Orlick T, McCaffrey N. Mental training with children for sport and life. Sport Psychol. 1991;5(4):322–34.
32. About sport & performance psychology association for applied sport psychology. https://appliedsportpsych.org/about-the-association-for-applied-sport-psychology/about-sport-and-performance-psychology/. Accessed 14 Feb 2022.
33. Ravizza K, Statler T. Lessons learned from sport psychology consulting. In: Morris T, Gordon S, Terry P, editors. Sport and exercise psychology: international perspectives. 1st ed. Queensland: Fitness Information Technology; 2007. p. 57–65.
34. Poznanski JJ, McLennan J. Conceptualizing and measuring counselors' theoretical orientation. J Couns Psychol. 1995;42(4):411–22.
35. Halbur DA, Halbur KV. Developing your theoretical orientation in counseling and psychotherapy. 2nd ed. Pearson, London; 2011.
36. Jarvis M. Sport psychology: a student's handbook. Routledge, New York; 2006.
37. Corey G. Theory and practice of counseling and psychotherapy. 9th ed. Boston, MA: Brooks/Cole Cengage Learning; 2013.
38. Ronkainen NJ, Aggerholm K, Ryba TV, Allen-Collinson J. Learning in sport: from life skills to existential learning. Sport Educ Soc. 2020;26(2):214–27.
39. Merkel DL. Youth sport: positive and negative impact on young athletes. Open Access J Sport Med. 2013;4:151.
40. Passer MW. Children in sport: participation motives and psychological stress. Quest. 1981;33(2):231–44.
41. Akinola M, Mendes WB. It's good to be the king: neurobiological benefits of higher social standing. Soc Psychol Personal Sci. 2014;5(1):43–51.
42. Kellmann M. Preventing overtraining in athletes in high-intensity sports and stress/recovery monitoring. Scand J Med Sci Sports. 2010;20(2):95–102.
43. Pelka M, Kellmann M. Relaxation and recovery in sport and performance. In: Oxford research encyclopedia of psychology. Oxford: Oxford University Press; 2017. p. 1–20.
44. Crocker PRE, Tamminen KA, Bennett EV. Stress, emotions, and coping in youth sport. In: Knight CJ, Harwood CG, Gould D, editors. Sport psychology for young athletes. London: Routledge; 2018. p. 164–73.
45. Gould D, Wilson CG, Tuffey S, Lochbaum M. Stress and the young athlete: the child's perspective. Pediatr Exerc Sci. 1993;5(3):286–97.

46. Elliott S, Drummond MJN, Knight C. The experiences of being a talented youth athlete: lessons for parents. J Appl Sport Psychol. 2017;30(4):437–55.
47. Stambulova NB, Engström C, Franck A, Linnér L, Lindahl K. Searching for an optimal balance: dual career experiences of Swedish adolescent athletes. Psychol Sport Exerc. 2015;21:4–14.
48. Christensen MK, Sørensen JK. Sport or school? Dreams and dilemmas for talented young Danish football players. Eur Phys Educ Rev. 2009;15(1):115–33.
49. Hayward FPI, Knight CJ, Mellalieu SD. A longitudinal examination of stressors, appraisals, and coping in youth swimming. Psychol Sport Exerc. 2017;29:56–68.
50. Thatcher J, Day MC. Re-appraising stress appraisals: the underlying properties of stress in sport. Psychol Sport Exerc. 2008;9(3):318–35.
51. Lazarus RS, Folkman S. Stress, appraisal, and coping. Cham: Springer; 1984.
52. Mellalieu SD, Neil R, Hanton S, Fletcher D. Competition stress in sport performers: stressors experienced in the competition environment. J Sports Sci. 2009;27(7):729–44.
53. Kraag G, Zeegers M, Kok G, Hosman C, Abu-Saad H. School programs targeting stress management in children and adolescents: a meta-analysis. J Sch Psychol. 2006;44:449–72.
54. Bothe DA, Grignon JB, Olness KN. The effects of a stress management intervention in elementary school children. J Dev Behav Pediatr. 2014;35(1):62–7.
55. Holen S, Waaktaar T, Lervåg A, Ystgaard M. Implementing a universal stress management program for young school children: are there classroom climate or academic effects? Scand J Educ Res. 2013;57(4):420–44.
56. Crocker PRE, Alderman RB, Murray F, Smith R. Cognitive-affective stress management training with high performance youth volleyball players: effects on affect, cognition, and performance. J Sport Exerc Psychol. 1988;10(4):448–60.
57. Perciavalle V, Blandini M, Fecarotta P, Buscemi A, Di Corrado D, Bertolo L, et al. The role of deep breathing on stress. Neurol Sci. 2017;38(3):451–8.
58. Conrad A, Müller A, Doberenz S, Kim S, Meuret AE, Wollburg E, et al. Psychophysiological effects of breathing instructions for stress management. Appl Psychophysiol Biofeedback. 2007;32(2):89–98.
59. Ma X, Yue ZQ, Gong ZQ, Zhang H, Duan NY, Shi YT, et al. The effect of diaphragmatic breathing on attention, negative affect and stress in healthy adults. Front Psychol. 2017;8:874.
60. Chen YF, Huang XY, Chien CH, Cheng JF. The effectiveness of diaphragmatic breathing relaxation training for reducing anxiety. Perspect Psychiatr Care. 2017;53(4):329–36.
61. Specht R. Examining the immediate effects of an online breathing meditation practice on working memory capacity. Arizona State University, Tempe; 2020.
62. Bandura A. Self-efficacy: toward a unifying theory of behavioral change. Adv Behav Res Ther. 1978;1(4):139–61.
63. Carr A. Positive psychology: the science of happiness and human strengths. 2nd ed. Routledge, London; 2011.
64. Cumming J, Ramsey R. Imagery interventions in sport. In: Mellalieu SD, Hanton S, editors. Advances in applied sport psychology. London: Routledge; 2009. p. 5–36.
65. Morris T, Spittle M, Watt AP. Imagery in sport. Human Kinetics, Champaign; 2005.
66. Cumming J, Williams SE. The role of imagery in performance. In: Murphy SM, editor. The Oxford handbook of sport and performance psychology. New York, NY: Oxford University Press; 2012. p. 213–32.
67. Martin KA, Moritz SE, Hall CR. Imagery use in sport: a literature review and applied model. Sport Psychol. 1999;13(3):245–68.
68. Jeannerod M. The representing brain: neural correlates of motor intention and imagery. Behav Brain Sci. 1994;17(2):187–202.
69. Finke RA. Levels of equivalence in imagery and perception. Psychol Rev. 1980;87(2):113–32.
70. Jeannerod M. The cognitive neuroscience of action. Hoboken: Wiley; 1997.
71. Paivio A. Cognitive and motivational functions of imagery in human performance. Can J Appl Sport Sci. 1985;10(4):22S–8S.

72. Driskell JE, Copper C, Moran A. Does mental practice enhance performance. J Appl Psychol. 1994;79(4):481–92.
73. Hall C, Schmidt D, Durand MC, Buckolz E. Imagery and motor skills acquisition. In: Shiekh AA, Korn ER, editors. Imagery in Sports and Physical Performance. New York: Baywood Publishing; 1994. p. 121–34.
74. Hall CR, Mack DE, Paivio A, Hausenblas HA. Imagery use by athletes: development of the sport imagery questionnaire. Int J Sport Psychol. 1998;29(1):73–89.
75. Callow N, Hardy L, Hall C. The effects of a motivational general-mastery imagery intervention on the sport confidence of high-level badminton players. Res Q Exerc Sport. 2001;72(4):389–400.
76. Callow N, Hardy L. Types of imagery associated with sport confidence in netball players of varying skill levels. J Appl Sport Psychol. 2001;13(1):1–17.
77. Holmes PS, Collins DJ. The PETTLEP approach to motor imagery: a functional equivalence model for sport psychologists. J Appl Sport Psychol. 2001;13(1):60–83.
78. Wakefield C, Smith D. Perfecting practice: applying the PETTLEP model of motor imagery. J Sport Psychol Action. 2012;3(1):1–11.
79. Li-Wei Z, Qi-Wei M, Orlick T, Zitzelsberger L. The effect of mental-imagery training on performance enhancement with 7-10-year-old children. Sport Psychol. 1992;6(3):230–41.
80. Munroe-Chandler KJ, Hall CR, Fishburne GJ, Murphy L, Hall ND. Effects of a cognitive specific imagery intervention on the soccer skill performance of young athletes: age group comparisons. Psychol Sport Exerc. 2012;13(3):324–31.
81. Munroe-Chandler KJ, Hall CR, Fishburne GJ, Shannon V. Using cognitive general imagery to improve soccer strategies. Eur J Sport Sci. 2006;5(1):41–9.
82. Munroe-Chandler KJ, Hall CR. Enhancing the collective efficacy of a soccer team through motivational general-mastery imagery. Imagin Cogn Pers. 2005;24(1):51–67.
83. Ashby AA. Developmental study of short-term memory characteristics for kinesthetic movement information. Percept Mot Skills. 1983;57(2):649–50.
84. Henderson A, Duncombe L. Development of kinesthetic judgments of angle and distance. Occup Ther J Res. 1982;2(3):131–44.
85. Van Raalte JL, Vincent A, Brewer BW. Self-talk: review and sport-specific model. Psychol Sport Exerc. 2016;22:139–48.
86. Hatzigeorgiadis A, Zourbanos N, Galanis E, Theodorakis Y. Self-talk and sports performance: a meta-analysis. Perspect Psychol Sci. 2011;6(4):348–56.
87. Tod D, Hardy J, Oliver E. Effects of self-talk: a systematic review. J Sport Exerc Psychol. 2011;33(5):666–87.
88. Hardy J. Speaking clearly: a critical review of the self-talk literature. Psychol Sport Exerc. 2006;7(1):81–97.
89. Van Raalte JL, Vincent A. Self-talk in sport and performance. In: Oxford research encyclopedia of psychology. Oxford: Oxford University Press; 2017. https://doi.org/10.1093/acrefore/9780190236557.001.0001/acrefore-9780190236557-e-157.
90. Hardy J, Hall CR, Alexander MR. Exploring self-talk and affective states in sport. J Sports Sci. 2001;19(7):469–75.
91. Theodorakis Y, Hatzigeorgiadis A, Chroni S. Self-talk: it works, but how? Development and preliminary validation of the functions of self-talk questionnaire. Meas Phys Educ Exerc Sci. 2008;12(1):10–30.
92. Latinjak AT, Zourbanos N, López-Ros V, Hatzigeorgiadis A. Goal-directed and undirected self-talk: exploring a new perspective for the study of athletes' self-talk. Psychol Sport Exerc. 2014;15(5):548–58.
93. Van Raalte JL, Brewer BW, Rivera PM, Petitpas AJ. The relationship between observable self-talk and competitive junior tennis players' match performances. J Sport Exerc Psychol. 1994;16(4):400–15.
94. Thibodeaux J, Winsler A. Careful what you say to yourself: exploring self-talk and youth tennis performance via hierarchical linear modeling. Psychol Sport Exerc. 2020;47:47.

95. Dickens YL, Van Raalte J, Hurlburt RT. On investigating self-talk: a descriptive experience sampling study of inner experience during golf performance. Sport Psychol. 2018;32(1):66–73.

96. Harvey DT, Van Raalte JL, Brewer BW. Relationship between self-talk and golf performance. Int Sport J. 2002;6(1):84–91.

97. Rogerson LJ, Hrycaiko DW. Enhancing competitive performance of ice hockey goaltenders using centering and self-talk. J Appl Sport Psychol. 2002;14(1):14–26.

98. Van Dyke ED, Van Raalte JL, Brewer BW, Mullin EM. Self-talk and competitive balance beam performance. Sport Psychol. 2018;32(1):33–41.

99. Hatzigeorgiadis A, Galanis E, Zourbanos N, Theodorakis Y. Self-talk and competitive sport performance. J Appl Sport Psychol. 2014;26(1):82–95.

100. Johnson JJM, Hrycaiko DW, Johnson GV, Halas JM. Self-talk and female youth soccer performance. Sport Psychol. 2004;18(1):44–59.

101. Meggs J, Chen MA. Competitive performance effects of psychological skill training for youth swimmers. Percept Mot Skills. 2019;126(5):886–903.

102. Hatzigeorgiadis A, Zourbanos N, Mpoumpaki S, Theodorakis Y. Mechanisms underlying the self-talk-performance relationship: the effects of motivational self-talk on self-confidence and anxiety. Psychol Sport Exerc. 2009;10(1):186–92.

103. Walter N, Nikoleizig L, Alfermann D. Effects of self-talk training on competitive anxiety, self-efficacy, volitional skills, and performance: an intervention study with junior sub-elite athletes. Sports (Basel). 2019;7(6):148.

104. Boyce BA. Effects of assigned versus participant-set goals on skill acquisition and retention of a selected shooting task. J Teach Phys Educ. 1992;11(3):220–34.

105. Ward P, Carnes M. Effects of posting self-set goals on collegiate football players' skill execution during practice and games. J Appl Behav Anal. 2002;35(1):1–12.

106. Locke EA, Latham GP. A theory of goal setting and task performance. New Delhi: Prentice-Hall; 1990.

107. Locke EA, Latham GP. Building a practically useful theory of goal setting and task motivation: a 35-year odyssey. Am Psychol. 2002;57(9):705–17.

108. Locke EA, Latham GP. The development of goal setting theory: a half century retrospective. Motiv Sci. 2019;5(2):93–105.

109. Latham G, Locke E. New developments in and directions for goal-setting research. Eur Psychol. 2007;12:290–300.

110. Locke EA, Latham GP. New developments in goal setting and task performance. Routledge, London; 2013.

111. Locke EA, Latham GP. The application of goal setting to sports. J Sport Psychol. 1985;7(3):205–22.

112. Burton D, Yukelson D, Weinberg R, Weigand D. The goal effectiveness paradox in sport: examining the goal practices of collegiate athletes. Sport Psychol. 1998;12(4):404–18.

113. Burton D, Weiss C. The fundamental goal concept: The path to process and performance success. In: Horn T, editor. Advances in sport psychology. 3rd ed. Champaign: Human Kinetics; 2008. p. 339–75, 470–4.

114. Jeong YH, Healy LC, McEwan D. The application of goal setting theory to goal setting interventions in sport: a systematic review. Int Rev Sport Exerc Psychol. 2021:1.

115. Harter S. Effectance motivation reconsidered: toward a developmental model. Hum Dev. 1978;21(1):34–64.

116. Harter S. The development of competence motivation in the mastery of cognitive and physical skills: is there still a place for joy? In: Nadeau CH, editor. Psychology of motor behavior and sport. Champaign, IL: Human Kinetics; 1981. p. 3–29.

117. McCarthy PJ, Jones MV. A qualitative study of sport enjoyment in the sampling years. Sport Psychol. 2007;21(4):400–16.

118. Weinberg RS, Burke KL, Jackson A. Coaches and players perceptions of goal setting in junior tennis: an exploratory investigation. Sport Psychol. 1997;11(4):426–39.

119. Swann C, Jackman PC, Lawrence A, Hawkins RM, Goddard SG, Williamson O, et al. The (over)use of SMART goals for physical activity promotion: a narrative review and critique. Health Psychol Rev. 2022:1–16.
120. McPherson KM, Kayes NM, Kersten P. MEANING as a smarter approach to goals in rehabilitation. Boca Raton, FL: CRC; 2014.
121. Hays KF. Being fit: the ethics of practice diversification in performance psychology. Prof Psychol Res Pract. 2006;37(3):223–32.
122. Hays KF, Brown CH. You're on! Consulting for peak performance. American Psychological Association, Washington, DC; 2004.
123. Ericsson KA, Simon HA. Protocol analysis: verbal reports as data. Cambridge: Bradford Books/MIT Press; 1984.

Chapter 12
Optimizing Mental Wellness Through Multidisciplinary Care

Mary M. Daley and Claudia L. Reardon

Key Points

- Psychological factors have tremendous influence on overall health, athletic performance, and recovery from illness or injuries.
- Multidisciplinary models allow providers to deliver comprehensive care that addresses the multifaceted needs of young athletes.
- While the expertise of mental health providers is instrumental, providers across all specialties and disciplines play a role in fostering mental and emotional wellbeing.

Introduction

Just as any successful sports team is comprised of players each bringing a specific skill set and working toward a common goal, optimal care of young athletes is best achieved with a multidisciplinary approach. The multidisciplinary model is not a

M. M. Daley (✉)
Division of Sports Medicine, Department of Orthopaedic Surgery, Children's Hospital of Philadelphia, Philadelphia, PA, USA

Pediatrics, Perelman School of Medicine, University of Pennsylvania, Philadelphia, PA, USA
e-mail: daleym2@chop.edu

C. L. Reardon
Department of Psychiatry, University Health Services, University of Wisconsin, Madison, WI, USA

Psychiatry, University of Wisconsin School of Medicine and Public Health, Madison, WI, USA
e-mail: claudia.reardon@wisc.edu

© The Author(s), under exclusive license to Springer Nature Switzerland AG 2023
M. A. Christino et al. (eds.), *Psychological Considerations in the Young Athlete*, Contemporary Pediatric and Adolescent Sports Medicine,
https://doi.org/10.1007/978-3-031-25126-9_12

243

new concept, but is arguably one that can vary widely in efficacy depending in part on its implementation. Young athletes inevitably encounter a variety of professionals who provide support, render treatment, and influence their wellbeing and development. Collaboration among these professionals can be invaluable not only when addressing physical manifestations of illness or injury, but just as importantly in fostering wellness in young athletes.

Prerequisites to implementing an effective multidisciplinary team include delineation of clear objectives, assembly of an appropriate group of professionals, establishment of a framework to meet the stated objectives, and identification and addressing of potential obstacles. Much of the early literature on multidisciplinary medical care was born from systems built to address the complex needs of patients with chronic medical conditions such as diabetes or cancer, many of which require treatment from multiple specialists [1, 2]. Given that athletes routinely interact with a wide spectrum of professionals across different settings, they represent a population that benefits from an organized multidisciplinary team approach that fosters collaboration and communication toward a common goal of optimizing outcomes for a variety of conditions—not just chronic medical ones.

Foundation for a Multidisciplinary Model

Broadly speaking, the primary aim of a multidisciplinary team is to provide comprehensive care designed with a patient-centered approach. In the case of children and adolescents, this concept is expanded to include emphasis on a *family*-centered approach, with attention to specific values, priorities, resources, and cultural beliefs and practices unique to each family. Common goals of providers involved in caring for athletes include supporting recovery and rehabilitation after injury and providing education and guidance around injury prevention. This typically involves some combination of physicians (e.g., pediatricians, sports medicine physicians, orthopedic surgeons), athletic trainers, and physical therapists. However, the establishment of a well-rounded multidisciplinary team allows for capabilities to provide specialized care that expands beyond the scope of many of these providers, including addressing the emotional and psychological needs of the young athlete.

Establishing a Framework

Though it is widely accepted that effective multidisciplinary teams are centered around the patient, in practice there are inevitably variations in the degree to which a hierarchal structure is adopted within the group. While some would argue that a purely collaborative approach without any designated principal leader is ideal, perhaps the more important point of emphasis is that the role of each team member is clearly stated and agreed upon, not only by team members but also, where relevant, by the patient and/or family. Regardless of the degree to which a hierarchical approach is employed, the contributions of every team member should be treated with due respect and consideration. Equally important is utilizing a shared language, and to that end in some cases a team leader who is well-versed in each of the contributing disciplines may be beneficial. Disagreements are to be expected and discussed in a constructive manner, and while ultimate responsibility may rest more heavily with one team member or another dependent on the scenario, the goal is to maintain a culture of collective decision-making that prioritizes the health and well-being of the patient [3, 4].

Thoughtful consideration of the details is paramount in designing a team-based model. This may involve determining the appropriate number of members (including the optimal number of professionals from each discipline), establishing guidelines and boundaries, and perhaps most importantly, ensuring a realistic plan for regular open communication, often in the form of recurring group meetings.

Addressing Mental Health

There are many psychological benefits of youth participation in sports, including higher levels of self-esteem, confidence, and social functioning, and decreased rates of depression, anxiety, and suicidality [5]. However, it is also clear that athletes are not immune to mental health challenges. Prior studies based largely on collegiate athletes are mixed, with some demonstrating lower rates of depression in athletes compared with non-athletes, and others suggesting that prevalence of depression in athletes is comparable to the general population [6–8]. Of course, there are also psychological challenges requiring unique consideration in athletes, including but not limited to performance anxiety, maladaptive weight management behaviors or disordered eating, psychological sequelae of concussion, and injury in sport, which can result in varying degrees of depression and/or fear of re-injury [9–14].

Given the myriad factors that can impact the mental health of young athletes, inclusion of appropriate professionals is essential in assembling a multidisciplinary team. Ideally this would include a sports psychiatrist and/or sports psychologist when possible, as familiarity with sports and the unique challenges that athletes face can be invaluable toward building a strong therapeutic alliance [15]. Unfortunately, the demand for mental health professionals with expertise in sports far exceeds the availability of such specialists, as sports psychiatry, in particular, is still an emerging field. Nonetheless, mental health providers can be invaluable in addressing the psychological needs of athletes even in the absence of specific expertise in sports. This is perhaps particularly true in the context of working within an interdisciplinary team, in which the quality of care offered by each provider is enhanced by the opportunity for professionals to learn from one another.

Multidisciplinary Team Members and Their Role in Addressing Mental Health

Sports Psychologists and Sports Psychiatrists

While there are certainly similarities between psychologists and psychiatrists, there are also important distinctions. Undergraduate training for sports psychologists is often in general psychology, potentially with a dual major in exercise physiology or related fields, but specialized training in sports psychology is achieved at the masters and doctoral levels. This specialized training incorporates topics not only in clinical psychology but also in exercise science and kinesiology. The role of the sports psychologist can vary, but generally involves efforts to optimize performance, including providing tools for coping with anxiety, developing mental skills to enhance confidence and focus, establishing healthy routines, and supporting return to sports after injury. Psychologists typically provide counseling and can offer various forms of therapy, which can be tailored to the needs of the individual and may include addressing mental health symptoms and disorders.

Psychiatrists obtain a medical degree before completing a residency in general psychiatry, which includes additional training in pharmacology and neurology, and can be followed by fellowship training in child and adolescent psychiatry or other areas. As sports psychiatry is an emerging field, a Certificate of Additional Training can be obtained through the International Society for Sports Psychiatry (ISSP) [16] or a Diploma of Additional Training from the International Olympic Committee [17], but at the time of this publication there are no accredited sports psychiatry fellowships in the United States. The first fellowship program dedicated to sports psychiatry training is set to begin in 2022, and with continually growing awareness of and interest in the mental health of athletes, this may be the first of many.

Sports psychiatrists are well-suited not only to diagnose and manage mental health conditions in athletes, but also to make recommendations around pharmacological interventions when indicated. Given that antidepressants and stimulants represent some of the most commonly prescribed medications in children and adolescents, [18] expertise in psychopharmacology can be extremely beneficial, particularly when considering that many pharmacological agents require unique considerations in athletes.

Neuropsychologists

Neuropsychology is a distinct field of study that encompasses neurology, psychology, and human behavior. Specialized training in neuropsychology begins at the doctoral level, after obtaining a bachelor's degree and often a master's degree in related fields. In the pediatric population, neuropsychologists can be instrumental in addressing cognitive problems such as those seen in concussion and other traumatic brain injuries, learning and attention deficit disorders, and complications of medical conditions including brain cancer and seizure disorders. Within the context of sports medicine, neuropsychologists are especially commonly involved in concussion management, for which their expertise is invaluable given the wide array of associated cognitive and psychological sequelae.

Mental Health Counselors, Clinical Social Workers, and Mental Skills Coaches

Mental health services can be provided by a variety of professionals with specialized training in counseling and psychotherapy, including mental health counselors and clinical social workers. Both of these professions require master's degrees in their respective fields, with the option to pursue further training at the doctoral level. Mental performance coaches, sometimes referred to as mental skills coaches, require training and certification by an accredited organization, and often aim to help athletes develop skills that can enhance sports performance. This can include goal setting, focus and motivation, and relaxation and stress management techniques. Importantly, mental performance coaches are commonly not licensed mental health professionals, and as such, while their role may be important in the care of the athlete, it is important to understand that mental health conditions are most appropriately managed by licensed mental health professionals.

Pediatricians, Sports Medicine Physicians, and Orthopedic Surgeons

Depending in part on the composition of the multidisciplinary team and availability of dedicated mental health professionals, the degree to which physicians are involved with addressing the psychological aspects of treatment can vary widely. Pediatricians, for example, including those who specialize in sports and/or adolescent medicine, might prescribe medications such as antidepressants or stimulants when access to psychiatrists is limited. Pediatricians also often have long-term relationships with patients and their families. This lends itself not only perhaps to an enhanced ability to identify when patients are struggling, but also positions them as trusted professionals upon whom families can rely for counsel and support. The specific roles of pediatricians and pediatric specialists can vary across settings and can be tailored to the individual needs of the patient.

Orthopedic surgeons can have enormous influence on the psychological wellbeing of athletes who sustain injuries requiring surgical intervention, particularly when recovery requires a prolonged time away from sports. Surgeons are in a unique position to provide detailed information regarding the rehabilitative process, to address specific questions and concerns, and to set realistic expectations from the outset. Further, given that psychological factors have been shown to impact surgical outcomes, mental health screening in the orthopedic office pre- and post-operatively might allow for early intervention and appropriate referrals when indicated [9, 19].

Physical Therapists and Athletic Trainers

Certified athletic trainers hold master's degrees with training in kinesiology, anatomy, and evaluation and management of musculoskeletal injuries. Particularly at the high school level and beyond, athletic trainers are often the medical professionals who not only are most familiar with the patient, but in many cases are present at the time of injury. As such, athletic trainers regularly perform the initial assessment, determine appropriate referrals, remain involved in the rehabilitation process, and ultimately participate in decisions around returning to sports.

Physical therapists are instrumental in facilitating recovery and rehabilitation from the full spectrum of overuse and acute injuries, including pre- and post-operatively. Their education is similar to athletic trainers in many ways, but physical therapists are increasingly encouraged to obtain a doctorate in physical therapy. Though they often meet athletes for the first time in the aftermath of an injury, physical therapists commonly spend about 2 to 3 h per week one on one with the patient throughout the recovery process. In many cases, physical therapists guide the activity progression based on their assessment of the patient's progress.

By virtue of the frequency of interactions that athletic trainers and physical therapists have with athletes, they are often in ideal position to provide encouragement and motivation, to address concerns that arise between appointments with other providers, and to identify athletes who may be struggling with the emotional and psychological impacts of the injury. Although physical therapists and athletic trainers may not have extensive training in mental health, they can have enormous impact by simply acknowledging the challenges associated with recovering from an injury and being away from sports, by allowing the patient to talk about their experience, and by coordinating referrals to specialized healthcare providers when needed.

Nutritionists

Nutritionists are often incorporated into the team of medical providers caring for athletes at the elite level including many collegiate teams. Although all young athletes would likely benefit from the opportunity to work with a registered dietician or other nutritionist, for most children and adolescents these professionals are more likely to be involved in caring for patients with concomitant nutritional deficits, gastrointestinal disorders, relative energy deficiency in sport (RED-S), or disordered eating/eating disorders. Patients with disordered eating or clinical eating disorders typically require regular visits with a nutritionist. Given the intricate relationship between psychological health and dietary practices, nutritionists inevitably must work through complex psychological barriers and undoubtedly provide a great deal of emotional support in their work with patients. This again underscores the essential role of every member of the multidisciplinary team in cultivating the emotional and psychological wellbeing of young athletes.

Special Populations

Concussion

Sport-related concussion is a form of mild traumatic brain injury affecting multiple systems and resulting in a broad range of clinical sequelae. Post-concussive syndrome consists of somatic symptoms such as headaches and nausea, vestibular symptoms such as dizziness and balance impairments, ocular symptoms including impairments in tracking and focus, cognitive symptoms such as difficulty with memory and concentration, dysfunction of the sleep-wake cycle, and psychological symptoms including depression, anxiety, and behavioral changes. Given the multidimensional nature of the injury, providing a multidisciplinary approach to treatment is imperative.

Naturally, multidisciplinary models will vary across settings. Large institutions may have the capability and structure to provide appropriate referrals and access to most if not all relevant specialists within the walls of the organization, while others may need to construct a model comprised of practitioners throughout the community. The initial referral to a concussion specialist often comes from emergency department providers, pediatricians, athletic trainers, or school nurses, the latter three of which remain involved to some extent throughout the recovery process. These providers are unique in that they generally have established relationships with patients and families and will continue to follow athletes even after they have fully recovered from concussion.

A comprehensive approach to concussion management can incorporate a wide range of specialties, including sports medicine, physical therapy, psychology and/or psychiatry, neuropsychology, ophthalmology, optometry, neurology and/or neurosurgery, and otolaryngology. Specific treatment plans and referrals can be catered to the needs of the individual. While we will focus on a subset of these specialties, it is important to recognize that, while depression has been linked to prolonged recovery, the association of psychological symptoms with concussion is very likely a reciprocal relationship. Persistent somatic, cognitive, vestibular, and ocular symptoms, for example, can certainly contribute to emotional and psychological distress. Therefore, addressing these symptoms with appropriate referrals and targeted treatment can have a substantial impact on the psychological wellbeing of the athlete, regardless of whether these providers are addressing mental health concerns directly.

Physical and Vestibular Therapists

Vestibular dysfunction is commonly seen after concussion, with dizziness affecting an estimated 50–90% of patients [20]. The initial approach to addressing post-concussion vestibular symptoms typically starts with referral to a physical therapist with training in vestibular rehabilitation. These referrals are generally made when symptom duration approaches or exceeds 4 weeks after the injury, but can be initiated sooner when indicated (e.g., in patients with a history of prior concussions with prolonged recovery and/or significant vestibular dysfunction). In addition to addressing vestibular function and balance, physical therapists can initiate basic ocular rehabilitation to address impairments in tracking and/or convergence, cervical stretching and strengthening, and sub-threshold aerobic activity.

The role of the physical therapist is multifaceted, and though not deliberately addressing psychological health per se, they can be instrumental in fostering emotional and psychological wellness in many ways. First, given the association between dizziness and psychological symptoms after concussion, it follows that addressing vestibular symptoms may help to alleviate psychological symptoms to some degree. Next, addressing sources of physical pain, often in the form of cervical stretching and strengthening, can mitigate both headaches and associated psychological distress. Finally, sub-symptom threshold aerobic activity is associated with faster recovery and reduced risk of persistent post-concussive syndrome [21, 22] as well as decreased anxiety, depression, and dizziness [23]. A gradual progression of activity as tolerated under the guidance of a physical therapist also provides a means by which the athlete is actively working toward a return to sport, thereby fostering motivation, encouraging a positive outlook, and in many cases restoring self-esteem.

Otolaryngologists

Visual and vestibular dysfunction can be predictive of prolonged recovery, and in some cases referrals to appropriate specialists are indicated [24]. Moderate to severe dizziness is associated not only with a greater symptom burden, but also with higher symptom scores specifically for depression and anxiety when compared with patients reporting mild to no dizziness [20]. At a single-center pediatric multidisciplinary concussion clinic, more than 95% of patients were seen by otolaryngology. They found that approximately one in four patients had abnormal dynamic visual acuity testing, approximately one in five had an abnormal Dix-Hallpike maneuver, and altogether one-third of patients had physical examination findings suggestive of peripheral vestibular dysfunction [25]. Although none of the patients had pre-existing vestibular diagnoses, nearly 40% required further follow-up with otolaryngology after the initial evaluation.

Neuropsychologists

Among the greatest challenges of caring for young athletes after concussion is attempting to distinguish whether symptoms are a direct result of concussion, as opposed to emergence or exacerbation of pre-existing conditions, including those that may have been previously undiagnosed. However, that distinction may not be as important to ascertain as is a nuanced understanding of the specific neuropsychological dysfunction causing the patient's symptoms and/or functional deficits, the latter of which is essential to provide appropriately targeted treatment.

For this reason, the inclusion of a neuropsychologist in concussion management is invaluable. As one example, neuropsychological evaluation can help determine whether declining academic performance is a result of a lack of motivation in the setting of depression, impairments in attention or concentration, difficulty with memory or processing, or some combination thereof. This becomes particularly important in targeting treatment for patients with prolonged symptoms and those with cognitive and/or psychological sequelae that persist and/or emerge after apparent recovery.

Psychologists, Psychiatrists, and Other Licensed Mental Health Providers

Even in the absence of any underlying mental health problems, several patients experience psychological symptoms after concussion, but not all will require referrals to mental health professionals. Addressing these concerns early in treatment, educating patients and families on common post-concussive symptoms, offering reassurance around the expected trajectory of recovery, and providing resources and tools to aid in symptom management can be beneficial [26]. Recognizing that not all centers will have access to a psychologist with particular expertise in concussion, most providers will refer to child and adolescent psychologists or sport psychologists.

Indications for referral to a mental health professional include but are not limited to (1) pre-existing mental health conditions exacerbated by concussion in patients who are not currently in treatment, (2) worsening of psychological symptoms over time, (3) depression, anxiety, or post-traumatic symptoms affecting social and/or academic functioning distinct from or disproportionate to the degree of post-concussive symptoms as a whole, and (4) concerns that psychological symptoms are a driving force in prolonging recovery in the form of persistent headaches, sleep-related difficulties, cognitive impairments, or otherwise.

Patients endorsing psychological symptoms, and particularly depression, should routinely be screened for safety. This includes not only asking about thoughts of dying or harming oneself or others, but also inquiring about access to lethal means such as firearms or medications in the home, and discussing specific safety plans including ways in which patients are realistically willing to reach out for help should the need arise. Those endorsing current suicidal ideation with intent and/or a plan should be referred to an emergency department for urgent evaluation.

Relative Energy Deficiency in Sport

Relative energy deficiency in sport (RED-S) refers to the impairment of physiologic function due to insufficient caloric intake to meet the metabolic demands of one's energy expenditure [27]. Insufficient caloric intake and resultant energy deficiency can occur in the setting of a clinical eating disorder, but in many cases the failure to maintain an appropriate balance between intake and energy expenditure is unintentional. It is also important to note that athletes with various types of eating disorders may not develop the caloric deficits associated with RED-S. In other words, not every athlete with RED-S has an eating disorder, and not every athlete with an eating disorder will meet the criteria for RED-S. Still, each of these entities can lead to physical and psychological consequences, and many of the same principles of multidisciplinary care apply.

Chronic reduction in energy availability can lead to metabolic dysfunction and suppression of menstrual hormones. This results in varying degrees of degradation of bone health, which can render athletes susceptible to stress fractures due to low bone density. Male athletes often have decreased testosterone, while female athletes experience menstrual irregularities including cessation of the menstrual cycle [27, 28].

The relationship between low energy availability and psychological problems is bidirectional. Maladaptive perfectionism, obsessive tendencies, low self-esteem, and striving for thinness can perpetuate a spectrum of restrictive eating and/or excessive training behaviors. Low energy availability can in turn adversely impact mood and performance, thereby exacerbating many of the psychological problems that are likely to fuel further imbalance. RED-S is similar to concussion in as much as it affects multiple organ systems and the fact that addressing the psychological needs of the athlete is critical. It is perhaps distinct in that beyond treatment and rehabilitation of the individual athlete, there are tremendous opportunities for the multidisciplinary team model to be used to prioritize screening and prevention efforts as well.

Primary Care, Adolescent Medicine, and Sports Medicine Physicians

One of the keys to developing a successful multidisciplinary model is to clearly define and agree upon the role of each team member. The role of the physician in caring for patients with RED-S is generally to monitor biophysiological metrics including weight, body mass index, vital signs, and laboratory measures of metabolic and hormonal function as indicated. This role can be filled by a single physician or shared among two or more providers, with appropriate consideration to ensuring adequate monitoring without overburdening the patient and family with excessive appointments.

The frequency of visits can vary based on acuity and severity, but weight should generally be followed by a provider who is seeing the patient regularly to ensure continued progress. It may also be preferable for weight checks to be carried out in an office that is accustomed to caring for patients with weight-related concerns. In this type of setting, it is often more feasible to have standardized protocols in place to minimize patient distress (e.g., patients agree to be weighed in a manner in which they are not made aware of the number on the scale), and to avoid tactics used to falsely increase one's measured weight such as carrying coins or other weighted objects in pockets. Similarly, in addition to standard vital signs, many patients require monitoring of orthostatic vital signs, and staff members should be adequately trained and equipped for this as well.

In practice, when specialists such as adolescent medicine or sports medicine physicians are available, they will take on the role of seeing the patient regularly and closely monitoring these parameters, whereas the pediatrician may see the patient at their standard frequency (generally annual well visits and sick visits as needed). Regardless, all providers involved in the patient's care should be kept informed of their progress through regular communication.

Beyond primary care, adolescent medicine, and sports medicine physicians, consultation with additional specialists is sometimes warranted. The complex nature of hormonal dysfunction and associated physiological changes may warrant consultation with an endocrinologist or other specialist with expertise in that area. For example, while in the past secondary amenorrhea may have been treated with oral contraceptives to generate a regular menstrual cycle, we now know that this simply masks the underlying hormonal suppression, eliminating what could be a valuable biological marker of recovery, and is now not generally recommended in this population. Given the complex nature of RED-S and its effects on multiple organ systems, it may be wise to have a low threshold for consulting appropriate specialists in these cases.

Lastly, patients with eating disorders or significant malnourishment may require treatment in emergency rooms, pediatric hospitals, or even psychiatric facilities that may or may not specialize in eating disorders. To whatever extent possible, having clear contingency plans, criteria for referrals to higher levels of care, and avenues of communication with providers at hospitals and other facilities can be invaluable. Ideally, when a patient requires a higher level of care, the outpatient treatment team should collaborate with the admitting facility to best support the patient and family, with the goal of transitioning back to outpatient management with close follow-up whenever it is safe to do so.

Psychologists, Psychiatrists, and Other Licensed Mental Health Providers

The role for psychologists, psychiatrists, and other licensed mental health providers should be catered to the needs of the individual patient. The standard of care for children and adolescents with clinical eating disorders is a family-centered approach. The Maudsley Model is a standardized family-based therapy that starts by empowering parents to take on the early stages of weight restoration and recovery, and gradually shifts toward allowing the adolescent greater responsibility for maintaining their progress [29]. When family dynamics prohibit effective implementation of this approach, referral to an individual therapist with expertise in eating disorders may be more appropriate. In other cases, particularly for athletes with concomitant depression, anxiety, trauma, and/or psychosomatic symptoms, it may be most appropriate to refer *both* to family-based treatment and individual therapy.

Of course, many patients with RED-S do not have clinical eating disorders, but all patients should routinely be screened for mental health concerns nonetheless.

While low energy availability may not be the result of an underlying psychological disorder, the associated physiological changes can adversely impact mood, sleep, and performance. Further, for those requiring treatment for medical sequelae of RED-S such as stress fractures, referral to a mental health specialist can help to mitigate depression, anxiety, and difficulties around self-esteem or identity that often accompany time away from sports due to injury [9]. Some athletes may be more receptive to mental health referrals presented as a means of supporting them through recovery and return to sports, whereas existing stigma around mental health may still elicit resistance to mental health treatment due to fears of being perceived as flawed or mentally or emotionally weak.

Provided there is no concern for a clinical eating disorder, these athletes do not necessarily need family-based treatment or therapists with expertise in eating disorders. For athletes with depression, anxiety, or other psychosocial stressors, referral to a therapist specializing in the care of children and adolescents may be optimal, allowing the therapist to evaluate the patient and determine the most appropriate therapeutic approach. Lastly, for athletes for whom there is low suspicion for clinical eating disorder or other psychological problems contributing to RED-S, sports psychologists can still be incredibly valuable resources. In addition to supporting the athlete with any challenges they encounter throughout the treatment process, a sports psychologist can foster healthy coping mechanisms, address maladaptive or negative thoughts, and in some cases may help to advocate for the patient by helping them to express concerns they may not be comfortable sharing with other medical providers.

While many psychiatrists practice psychotherapy, due in part to limited mental health resources, referrals to psychiatrists are often reserved for patients for whom existing providers feel psychopharmacological management may be helpful. A sports psychiatrist is ideal but not entirely necessary, provided there is open communication between providers regarding the introduction of any psychotropic medications. There are important considerations not only for athletes in general but particularly for athletes with RED-S, many of whom may have orthostasis or other cardiovascular sequelae that could be exacerbated by certain medications. Further, patients and families should be informed of potential weight-related side effects regardless of whether the pharmacological agent is intentionally selected in part to promote weight gain.

Nutritionists

Although medical providers have access to nutrient recommendations and guidelines for athletes and are well-equipped to identify deficiencies and provide general nutritional counseling, RED-S requires a thorough evaluation and nuanced approach. Registered dieticians and other nutritionists may be better suited to complete the detailed assessment of dietary practices and nutritional needs required in these cases, and to develop and implement a comprehensive plan to correct existing deficits.

For athletes with clinical eating disorders, collaboration between physicians, therapists, and nutritionists is essential when making recommendations pertaining to dietary practices. There should be clear communication and consensus on the role of each provider, not only to avoid conveying mixed messages, but also to provide the structure and boundaries necessitated by the complexities of this patient population. For example, nutritionists and family therapists may need to specifically address mealtime behaviors, whereas individual therapists might allow the patient to share their experiences around mealtimes but not necessarily give explicit instructions. Physicians may not need to address the details of these elements at all. Physicians and nutritionists might agree to both regularly monitor the patient's weight, or they might instead agree that one provider is better suited for this task, depending on frequency of visits and office capabilities.

Importantly, nutritional counseling for children and adolescents is inextricably linked to addressing family dynamics and the psychological factors that influence eating behaviors. As such, the treating nutritionist almost inevitably functions as an additional source of psychological and emotional support. Further, the pervasive stigma of mental illness and the meaning that patients and families might attribute to the need for mental health treatment can lead to resistance not only to seeking help, but also to fully engaging with mental health providers. Nutritionists, however, are generally not perceived as mental health providers. Consequently, patients and families may initially be more comfortable sharing the emotional challenges around mealtimes and other aspects of implementing treatment recommendations in the home with this type of provider. This underscores the importance of ensuring that families understand the framework of the multidisciplinary team and consent to sharing of information between providers at the start of treatment. This also highlights the multifaceted role of the nutritionist, which often includes supporting patients and families, acknowledging the psychological aspects of treatment, and encouraging utilization of mental health resources to optimize recovery.

Surgical Patients

The psychological impacts of injury in sport have tremendous implications for athletes at every level, and this may be particularly true for those requiring surgical intervention. In addition to what might be considered within the realm of a normal emotional reaction to a stressful life event, injuries have been associated with symptoms of depression, anxiety, post-traumatic stress, and maladaptive responses manifesting as eating disorders or substance misuse [9–11]. A prospective cohort study of division I collegiate athletes found that 51% of injured athletes met the criteria for at least mild depression, while 12% met the criteria for moderate depression [30]. Consistent with findings in the adult literature, a small case series of athletes aged 21 years and younger found that in the aftermath of anterior cruciate ligament (ACL) injury, the majority experienced symptoms of post-traumatic stress disorder, including avoidance, hyperarousal, and intrusive symptoms [13].

Although athletes with pre-existing mental health issues may be at greater risk for experiencing psychological difficulty after an injury, those without any such history are susceptible as well [9, 30, 31]. One important consideration is athletic identity, which is a cognitive and social construct generally defined as the degree to which one identifies as an athlete. Higher levels of athletic identity can result in a greater sense of loss and heightened emotional response to injury, and have been associated with difficulty seeking help [9, 32, 33]. Additional factors that can influence the psychological impact of injury include support from family and peers, ability to implement healthy coping skills, and potential implications for the team or individual, including scholarship opportunities and missing high stakes competitions.

Orthopedic Surgeons

One of the most important means of supporting an athlete after injury is setting realistic expectations for recovery. Orthopedic surgeons are uniquely positioned to have detailed conversations based on the severity of the injury, the specific surgical procedure, and level of play of each individual. In doing so they can help to minimize uncertainty and can partner with the athlete in setting reasonable goals for recovery and return to sports. By acknowledging the emotional and psychological impact of the injury during routine conversations with patients and families, providers can mitigate the stigma of mental health, encourage open communication, and provide appropriate referrals when indicated.

As the mind-body relationship is bidirectional, it follows that psychological factors can impact physical health, and recovery from injury is no exception. A multicenter prospective cohort study of patients undergoing primary ACL reconstruction found that the degree of depressive symptoms was inversely related to patient-reported outcomes, including decreased perceived knee function and higher likelihood of post-operative complications [34]. Most patients have at least one office visit with the orthopedic surgeon prior to the procedure, followed by multiple post-operative visits to monitor their progress with healing and rehabilitation. This presents an opportunity to screen for mental health symptoms not only before surgery, but throughout the recovery process, and can be implemented via routine administration of validated screening tools at each visit [19], or simply asking patients how they are recovering mentally in addition to their physical recovery.

Physical Therapists and Athletic Trainers

While the specific approach to rehabilitation can vary across settings, physical therapists and/or athletic trainers are invariably highly involved in the process, working directly with the athlete throughout the duration of their recovery. The frequency and duration of these interactions provides an opportunity to build relationships with athletes, offer support and motivation, and potentially identify mental health issues and coordinate appropriate referrals when indicated. In addition to setting short- and long-term goals and partnering with the athlete to achieve them, physical therapists and athletic trainers can play an important role in empowering athletes to actively participate in their own recovery, which can mitigate the sense of loss of control so often associated with injury. An important concept that has emerged in the literature is the internal health locus of control (HLOC), defined as the degree to which an individual perceives their ability to control life events [35]. Multiple studies have demonstrated that higher HLOC in patients undergoing ACL reconstruction is associated with improvements in physical and social function, bodily pain, mental health, and both subjective and objective measures of knee function [35, 36].

Two of the most widely recognized constructs influencing successful return to sport include kinesiophobia and psychological readiness to return to sport, both of which have primarily been studied in patients undergoing ACL reconstruction. Although perhaps most accurately defined as a fear of movement, *kinesiophobia* is a term widely used to refer to a fear of re-injury, and is associated with inferior postoperative outcomes including objective measures of function, as well as decreased likelihood of returning to sports and an increased risk for sustaining a recurrent ACL tear within the first 24 months of returning to sport [19, 37]. Psychological readiness to return to sport has similarly been identified as an independent predictor for successful return to pre-injury level of play and decreased risk of re-injury [38–40]. Physical therapists and athletic trainers can theoretically play an important role in mitigating kinesiophobia and enhancing psychological readiness by acknowledging the natural apprehension that follows a significant injury, creating an environment in which athletes can express their fears or concerns, and by incorporating high-level sports-specific drills and exercises to build confidence.

Psychologists, Psychiatrists, and Other Licensed Mental Health Providers

Though psychological consequences of sport-related injury are well-documented, access to mental health resources varies across settings, and in many cases the demand far exceeds availability. Unfortunately, the perceived or actual lack of mental health resources may be a deterrent for medical providers to implement regular screening, citing an inability to provide effective referrals. As a result, utilization of these resources may require a creative approach.

A comprehensive multidisciplinary team may be an effective means of optimizing available resources, and athletes with sport-related injury represent a population in which various models might be implemented. For example, a single psychiatrist may not be able to see every injured athlete but can share their expertise in the form of psychoeducation and/or case consultation with other providers on the team. For athletes who require individual therapy, a model that provides short-term treatment in the aftermath of injury might be an effective means of increasing availability by limiting the duration of treatment. This approach can also be used as a "bridge" for patients who will likely require long-term management and are working on establishing care in the community, as mental health providers often have very long wait lists. Lastly, in a pediatric healthcare setting, the majority of injured athletes tend to be adolescents, many of whom struggle with feeling isolated from friends and teammates after the injury. This provides an opportunity for a group therapy approach (injury support group), which would allow a greater number of athletes to access a licensed mental health professional. Perhaps even more importantly, the benefits of social connection and shared experiences are inherently therapeutic, and can alleviate feelings of isolation, loneliness, and hopelessness.

Conclusion

Caring for young athletes is a privilege that comes with unique challenges and responsibilities. It requires a thoughtful and comprehensive approach to treatment, with considerations specific to each patient and family. As is true for any medical specialty, we earn the confidence of our patients by accurately diagnosing and successfully treating illness and injury. But in many ways, we earn their trust by demonstrating familiarity with the culture of their sports, respect for their athletic goals and endeavors, and a genuine desire and effort to learn about aspects in which we are not as well-versed. This includes but is not limited to understanding the specific demands of their sport and/or position on the team and having an appreciation for their perspective on the potential consequences of our recommendations, particularly regarding time away from sports. Our ability to provide personalized comprehensive care in this manner is significantly enhanced by utilizing a multidisciplinary team model, which not only benefits the patients and families, but provides an opportunity for medical providers across specialties to continually learn from one another and from so many remarkable young athletes.

References

1. Carter S, Garside P, Black A. Multidisciplinary team working, clinical networks, and chambers; opportunities to work differently in the NHS. Qual Saf Heal Care. 2003;12(SUPPL. 1):25–8.
2. Laffel LMB, Vangsness L, Connell A, Goebel-Fabbri A, Butler D, Anderson BJ. Impact of ambulatory, family-focused teamwork intervention on glycemic control in youth with type 1 diabetes. J Pediatr. 2003;142(4):409–16.
3. Sporer BC, Windt J. Integrated performance support: facilitating effective and collaborative performance teams. Br J Sports Med. 2018;52(16):1014–5.
4. Roncaglia I. A practitioner's perspective of multidisciplinary teams: analysis of potential barriers and key factors for success. Psychol Thought. 2016;9(1):15–23.
5. Eime RM, Young JA, Harvey JT, Charity MJ, Payne WR. A systematic review of the psychological and social benefits of participation in sport for children and adolescents: informing development of a conceptual model of health through sport. Int J Behav Nutr Phys Act. 2013;10:98.
6. Wolanin A, Gross M, Hong E. Depression in athletes: prevalence and risk factors. Curr Sports Med Rep. 2015;14(1):56–60.

7. Yang J, Peek-Asa C, Corlette JD, Cheng G, Foster DT, Albright J. Prevalence of and risk factors associated with symptoms of depression in competitive collegiate student athletes. Clin J Sport Med. 2007;17:481.
8. Proctor SL, Boan-Lenzo C. Prevalence of depressive symptoms in male intercollegiate student-athletes and nonathletes. J Clin Sport Psychol. 2010;4:204.
9. Daley MM, Griffith K, Milewski MD, Christino MA. The mental side of the injured athlete. J Am Acad Orthop Surg. 2021;29(12):499–506.
10. Putukian M. The psychological response to injury in student athletes: a narrative review with a focus on mental health. Br J Sports Med. 2016;50(3):145–8.
11. Herring SA, Boyajian-O'Neill LA, Coppel DB, Daniels JM, Gould D, Grana W, et al. Psychological issues related to injury in athletes and the team physician: a consensus statement. Med Sci Sports Exerc. 2006;38(11):2030–4.
12. Aron CM, Harvey S, Hainline B, Hitchcock ME, Reardon CL. Post-traumatic stress disorder (PTSD) and other trauma-related mental disorders in elite athletes: a narrative review. Br J Sports Med. 2019;53(12):779–84.
13. Padaki AS, Noticewala MS, Levine WN, Ahmad CS, Popkin MK, Popkin CA. Prevalence of posttraumatic stress disorder symptoms among Young athletes after anterior cruciate ligament rupture. Orthop J Sport Med. 2018;6(7):1–5.
14. Arthur-cameselle J, Sossin K, Quatromoni P. A qualitative analysis of factors related to eating disorder onset in female collegiate athletes and non-athletes. Eat Disord. 2017;25(3):199–215. https://doi.org/10.1080/10640266.2016.1258940.
15. Van Slingerland KJ, Durand-Bush N, Bradley L, Goldfield G, Archambault R, Smith D, et al. Canadian Centre for Mental Health and Sport (CCMHS) position statement: principles of mental health in competitive and high-performance sport. Clin J Sport Med. 2019;29(3):173–80.
16. International Society for Sports Psychiatry. 2022. https://www.sportspsychiatry.org/.
17. International Olympic Committee. 2022.
18. Lopez-Leon S, Lopez-Gomez MI, Warner B, Ruiter-Lopez L. Psychotropic medication in children and adolescents in the United States in the year 2004 vs 2014. DARU. 2018;26(1):5–10.
19. Burland JP, Toonstra JL, Howard JS. Psychosocial barriers after anterior cruciate ligament reconstruction: a clinical review of factors influencing postoperative success. Sports Health. 2019;11:528. https://doi.org/10.1177/1941738119869333.
20. Hunt DL, Oldham J, Aaron SE, Tan CO, Iii WPM, Howell DR. Dizziness, psychological function, and postural stability following sport-related concussion. Clin J Sport Med. 2021;00:1–7.
21. Leddy J, Master C, Mannix R, Wiebe D, Grady M, Meehan WP, et al. Early targeted heart rate aerobic exercise versus placebo stretching for sport-related concussion in adolescents: a randomised controlled trial. Lancet Child Adolesc Health. 2021;5(11):792–9.
22. Howell DR, Taylor JA, Tan CO, Orr R, Meehan WP. The role of aerobic exercise in reducing persistent sport-related concussion symptoms. Med Sci Sports Exerc. 2019;51(4):647–52.
23. Howell DR, Hunt DL, Oldham JR, Aaron SE, Meehan WP, Tan CO. Postconcussion exercise volume associations with depression, anxiety, and dizziness symptoms, and postural stability: preliminary findings. J Head Trauma Rehabil. 2021;37:249.
24. Master CL, Master SR, Wiebe DJ, Storey EP, Lockyer JE, Podolak OE, et al. Vision and vestibular system dysfunction predicts prolonged concussion recovery in children. Clin J Sport Med. 2018;28(2):139–45.
25. Shah AS, Raghuram A, Kaur K, Lipson S, Shoshany T, Stevens R, et al. Specialty-specific diagnoses in pediatric patients with postconcussion syndrome. Clin J Sport Med. 2021;32:114.
26. Bailey C, Meyer J, Briskin S, Tangen C, Hoffer SA, Dundr J, et al. Multidisciplinary concussion management: a model for outpatient concussion management in the acute and post-acute settings. J Head Trauma Rehabil. 2019;34(6):375–84.
27. Mountjoy M, Sundgot-Borgen J, Burke L, Carter S, Constantini N, Lebrun C, et al. The IOC consensus statement: beyond the female athlete triad-relative energy deficiency in sport (RED-S). Br J Sports Med. 2014;48(7):491–7.

28. Mountjoy M, Sundgot-Borgen JK, Burke LM, Ackerman KE, Blauwet C, Constantini N, et al. IOC consensus statement on relative energy deficiency in sport (RED-S): 2018 update. Br J Sports Med. 2018;52(11):687–97.
29. Mairs R, Nicholls D. Assessment and treatment of eating disorders in children and adolescents. Arch Dis Child. 2016;101(12):1168–75.
30. Leddy MH, Lambert MJ, Ogles BM. Psychological consequences of athletic injury among high-level competitors. Res Q Exerc Sport. 1994;65(4):347–54.
31. Appaneal RN, Levine BR, Perna FM, Roh JL. Measuring postinjury depression among male and female competitive athletes. J Sport Exerc Psychol. 2009;31:60–76.
32. Christino MA, Fantry AJ, Vopat BG. Psychological aspects of recovery following anterior cruciate ligament reconstruction. J Am Acad Orthop Surg. 2015;23(8):501–9.
33. Edison BR, Christino MA, Rizzone KH. Athletic identity in youth athletes: a systematic review of the literature. Int J Environ Res Public Health. 2021;18(14):7331.
34. Garcia GH, Wu HH, Park MJ, Tjoumakaris FP, Tucker BS, Kelly JD, et al. Depression symptomatology and anterior cruciate ligament injury. Am J Sports Med. 2016;44(3):572–9.
35. Nyland J, Cottrell B, Harreld K, Caborn DNM. Self-reported outcomes after anterior cruciate ligament reconstruction: an internal health locus of control score comparison. Arthroscopy. 2006;22(11):1225–32.
36. Christino MA, Fleming BC, Machan JT, Shalvoy RM. Psychological factors associated with anterior cruciate ligament reconstruction recovery. Orthop J Sport Med. 2016;4(3):1–9.
37. Paterno MV, Flynn K, Thomas S, Schmitt LC. Self-reported fear predicts functional performance and second ACL injury after ACL reconstruction and return to sport: a pilot study. Sports Health. 2018;10(3):228–33.
38. Ardern CL, Taylor NF, Feller JA, Whitehead TS, Webster KE. Psychological responses matter in returning to preinjury level of sport after anterior Cruciate ligament reconstruction surgery. http://ajsm.sagepub.com/supplemental. Accessed 24 Sep 2019.
39. Ardern CL, Taylor NF, Feller JA, Whitehead TS, Webster KE. Sports participation 2 years after anterior cruciate ligament reconstruction in athletes who had not returned to sport at 1 year a prospective follow-up of physical function and psychological factors in 122 athletes. http://ajsm.sagepub.com/supplemental. Accessed 24 Sep 2019.
40. McPherson AL, Feller JA, Hewett TE, Webster KE. Psychological readiness to return to sport is associated with second anterior cruciate ligament injuries. Am J Sports Med. 2019;47(4):857–62. https://doi.org/10.1177/0363546518825258.

Index

A

Abstract thinking, 197
Acceptance and commitment therapy (ACT), 71, 109, 111, 126
ACL-Return to Sport after Injury (ACL-RSI) scale, 144
ACT-based strategies, 171
Actigraphic assessment, 90, 93
Activity pacing, 171
Adolescents, 100, 103
Adversity, 22
Age-appropriate training, 195
Alcohol use, 43
American Academy of Pediatrics (AAP), 93, 204
American Academy of Sleep Medicine, 82, 93
American College of Sports Medicine (ACSM), 60
American Development Model (ADM), 184
Anabolic androgenic agents (AAS), 45
Anderson's Athletic Identity Questionnaire (AIQ), 9
Anorexia nervosa (AN), 38
ANOVA, 105
Anterior cruciate ligament (ACL) injuries, 34, 120, 136
Antidepressants, 25
Anxiety, 26, 119, 122
Athlete identity measurement scale (AIMS), 9
Athletes' self-efficacy, 142
Athletic community, 73
Athletic Coping Skills Inventory-28 (ACSI-28), 145

Athletic identity, 8–12, 100, 186
Athletic pursuits, 22
Athletic trainers (AT), 109, 256, 257
Attention deficit hyperactivity disorder (ADHD), 39
Autism spectrum disorder (ASD), 40
Autonomous self-identity, 100
Avoidant/restrictive food intake disorder (ARFID), 37

B

Beck Depression Inventory, 112
Binge-eating disorder (BED)'s core criteria, 38
Bipolar disorders, 24, 25
Bipolar presentations, 24–25
Bulimia nervosa (BN), 38

C

Cannabis, 43
Causal attribution, 197
CBT for insomnia (CBT-I), 124
Cell phone applications, 91
Centers for Disease Control and Prevention guidelines, 104
Certificate of Additional Training, 246
Children's Report of Sleep Patterns (CRSP), 90
Chronic pain, 157
Chronic postsurgical pain (CPSP), 157
Chronic traumatic encephalopathy (CTE), 130
Clinical eating disorders, 255

Printed by Printforce, the Netherlands